D0857070

Statistical Issues in Drug Research and Development

STATISTICS: Textbooks and Monographs

A Series Edited by

Vol. 1: The Generalized Jackknife Statistic, *H. L. Gray and W. R. Schucany*
Vol. 2: Multivariate Analysis, *Anant M. Kshirsagar*
Vol. 3: Statistics and Society, *Walter T. Federer*
Vol. 4: Multivariate Analysis: A Selected and Abstracted Bibliography, 1957-1972, *Kocherlakota Subrahmaniam and Kathleen Subrahmaniam* (out of print)
Vol. 5: Design of Experiments: A Realistic Approach, *Virgil L. Anderson and Robert A. McLean*
Vol. 6: Statistical and Mathematical Aspects of Pollution Problems, *John W. Pratt*
Vol. 7: Introduction to Probability and Statistics (in two parts), Part I: Probability; Part II: Statistics, *Narayan C. Giri*
Vol. 8: Statistical Theory of the Analysis of Experimental Designs, *J. Ogawa*
Vol. 9: Statistical Techniques in Simulation (in two parts), *Jack P. C. Kleijnen*
Vol. 10: Data Quality Control and Editing, *Joseph I. Naus* (out of print)
Vol. 11: Cost of Living Index Numbers: Practice, Precision, and Theory, *Kali S. Banerjee*
Vol. 12: Weighing Designs: For Chemistry, Medicine, Economics, Operations Research, Statistics, *Kali S. Banerjee*
Vol. 13: The Search for Oil: Some Statistical Methods and Techniques, *edited by D. B. Owen*
Vol. 14: Sample Size Choice: Charts for Experiments with Linear Models, *Robert E. Odeh and Martin Fox*
Vol. 15: Statistical Methods for Engineers and Scientists, *Robert M. Bethea, Benjamin S. Duran, and Thomas L. Boullion*
Vol. 16: Statistical Quality Control Methods, *Irving W. Burr*
Vol. 17: On the History of Statistics and Probability, *edited by D. B. Owen*
Vol. 18: Econometrics, *Peter Schmidt*
Vol. 19: Sufficient Statistics: Selected Contributions, *Vasant S. Huzurbazar (edited by Anant M. Kshirsagar)*
Vol. 20: Handbook of Statistical Distributions, *Jagdish K. Patel, C. H. Kapadia, and D. B. Owen*
Vol. 21: Case Studies in Sample Design, *A. C. Rosander*
Vol. 22: Pocket Book of Statistical Tables, *compiled by R. E. Odeh, D. B. Owen, Z. W. Birnbaum, and L. Fisher*

Vol. 23: The Information in Contingency Tables, *D. V. Gokhale and Solomon Kullback*
Vol. 24: Statistical Analysis of Reliability and Life-Testing Models: Theory and Methods, *Lee J. Bain*
Vol. 25: Elementary Statistical Quality Control, *Irving W. Burr*
Vol. 26: An Introduction to Probability and Statistics Using BASIC, *Richard A. Groeneveld*
Vol. 27: Basic Applied Statistics, *B. L. Raktoe and J. J. Hubert*
Vol. 28: A Primer in Probability, *Kathleen Subrahmaniam*
Vol. 29: Random Processes: A First Look, *R. Syski*
Vol. 30: Regression Methods: A Tool for Data Analysis, *Rudolf J. Freund and Paul D. Minton*
Vol. 31: Randomization Tests, *Eugene S. Edgington*
Vol. 32: Tables for Normal Tolerance Limits, Sampling Plans, and Screening, *Robert E. Odeh and D. B. Owen*
Vol. 33: Statistical Computing, *William J. Kennedy, Jr. and James E. Gentle*
Vol. 34: Regression Analysis and Its Application: A Data-Oriented Approach, *Richard F. Gunst and Robert L. Mason*
Vol. 35: Scientific Strategies to Save Your Life, *I. D. J. Bross*
Vol. 36: Statistics in the Pharmaceutical Industry, *edited by C. Ralph Buncher and Jia-Yeong Tsay*
Vol. 37: Sampling from a Finite Population, *J. Hajek*
Vol. 38: Statistical Modeling Techniques, *S. S. Shapiro*
Vol. 39: Statistical Theory and Inference in Research, *T. A. Bancroft and C.-P. Han*
Vol. 40: Handbook of the Normal Distribution, *Jagdish K. Patel and Campbell B. Read*
Vol. 41: Recent Advances in Regression Methods, *Hrishikesh D. Vinod and Aman Ullah*
Vol. 42: Acceptance Sampling in Quality Control, *Edward G. Schilling*
Vol. 43: The Randomized Clinical Trial and Therapeutic Decisions, *edited by Niels Tygstrup, John M. Lachin, and Erik Juhl*
Vol. 44: Regression Analysis of Survival Data in Cancer Chemotherapy, *Walter H. Carter, Jr., Galen L. Wampler, and Donald M. Stablein*
Vol. 45: A Course in Linear Models, *Anant M. Kshirsagar*
Vol. 46: Clinical Trials: Issues and Approaches, *edited by Stanley H. Shapiro and Thomas H. Louis*
Vol. 47: Statistical Analysis of DNA Sequence Data, *edited by B. S. Weir*
Vol. 48: Nonlinear Regression Modeling: A Unified Practical Approach, *David A. Ratkowsky*
Vol. 49: Attribute Sampling Plans, Tables of Tests and Confidence Limits for Proportions, *Robert E. Odeh and D. B. Owen*
Vol. 50: Experimental Design, Statistical Models, and Genetic Statistics, *edited by Klaus Hinkelmann*
Vol. 51: Statistical Methods for Cancer Studies, *edited by Richard G. Cornell*
Vol. 52: Practical Statistical Sampling for Auditors, *Arthur J. Wilburn*
Vol. 53: Statistical Signal Processing, *edited by Edward J. Wegman and James G. Smith*
Vol. 54: Self-Organizing Methods in Modeling: GMDH Type Algorithms, *edited by Stanley J. Farlow*
Vol. 55: Applied Factorial and Fractional Designs, *Robert A. McLean and Virgil L. Anderson*
Vol. 56: Design of Experiments: Ranking and Selection, *edited by Thomas J. Santner and Ajit C. Tamhane*
Vol. 57: Statistical Methods for Engineers and Scientists. Second Edition, Revised and Expanded, *Robert M. Bethea, Benjamin S. Duran, and Thomas L. Boullion*
Vol. 58: Ensemble Modeling: Inference from Small-Scale Properties to Large-Scale Systems, *Alan E. Gelfand and Crayton C. Walker*

Vol. 59: Computer Modeling for Business and Industry, *Bruce L. Bowerman and Richard T. O'Connell*
Vol. 60: Bayesian Analysis of Linear Models, *Lyle D. Broemeling*
Vol. 61: Methodological Issues for Health Care Surveys, *Brenda Cox and Steven Cohen*
Vol. 62: Applied Regression Analysis and Experimental Design, *Richard J. Brook and Gregory C. Arnold*
Vol. 63: Statpal: A Statistical Package for Microcomputers – PC-DOS Version for the IBM PC and Compatibles, *Bruce J. Chalmer and David G. Whitmore*
Vol. 64: Statpal: A Statistical Package for Microcomputers – Apple Version for the II, II+, and IIe, *David G. Whitmore and Bruce J. Chalmer*
Vol. 65: Nonparametric Statistical Inference, Second Edition, Revised and Expanded, *Jean Dickinson Gibbons*
Vol. 66: Design and Analysis of Experiments, *Roger G. Petersen*
Vol. 67: Statistical Methods for Pharmaceutical Research Planning, *Sten W. Bergman and John C. Gittins*
Vol. 68: Goodness-of-Fit Techniques, *edited by Ralph B. D'Agostino and Michael A. Stephens*
Vol. 69: Statistical Methods in Discrimination Litigation, *edited by D. H. Kaye and Mikel Aickin*
Vol. 70: Truncated and Censored Samples from Normal Populations, *Helmut Schneider*
Vol. 71: Robust Inference, *M. L. Tiku, W. Y. Tan, and N. Balakrishnan*
Vol. 72: Statistical Image Processing and Graphics, *edited by Edward J. Wegman and Douglas J. DePriest*
Vol. 73: Assignment Methods in Combinatorial Data Analysis, *Lawrence J. Hubert*
Vol. 74: Econometrics and Structural Change, *Lyle D. Broemeling and Hiroki Tsurumi*
Vol. 75: Multivariate Interpretation of Clinical Laboratory Data, *Adelin Albert and Eugene K. Harris*
Vol. 76: Statistical Tools for Simulation Practitioners, *Jack P. C. Kleijnen*
Vol. 77: Randomization Tests, Second Edition, *Eugene S. Edgington*
Vol. 78: A Folio of Distributions: A Collection of Theoretical Quantile-Quantile Plots, *Edward B. Fowlkes*
Vol. 79: Applied Categorical Data Analysis, *Daniel H. Freeman, Jr.*
Vol. 80: Seemingly Unrelated Regression Equations Models : Estimation and Inference, *Virendra K. Srivastava and David E. A. Giles*
Vol. 81: Response Surfaces: Designs and Analyses, *Andre I. Khuri and John A. Cornell*
Vol. 82: Nonlinear Parameter Estimation: An Integrated System in BASIC, *John C. Nash and Mary Walker-Smith*
Vol. 83: Cancer Modeling, *edited by James R. Thompson and Barry W. Brown*
Vol. 84: Mixture Models: Inference and Applications to Clustering, *Geoffrey J. McLachlan and Kaye E. Basford*
Vol. 85: Randomized Response: Theory and Techniques, *Arijit Chaudhuri and Rahul Mukerjee*
Vol. 86: Biopharmaceutical Statistics for Drug Development, *edited by Karl E. Peace*
Vol. 87: Parts per Million Values for Estimating Quality Levels, *Robert E. Odeh and D. B. Owen*
Vol. 88: Lognormal Distributions: Theory and Applications, *edited by Edwin L. Crow and Kunio Shimizu*
Vol. 89: Properties of Estimators for the Gamma Distribution, *K. O. Bowman and L. R. Shenton*
Vol. 90: Spline Smoothing and Nonparametric Regression, *Randall L. Eubank*
Vol. 91: Linear Least Squares Computations, *R. W. Farebrother*
Vol. 92: Exploring Statistics, *Damaraju Raghavarao*

Vol. 93: Applied Time Series Analysis for Business and Economic Forecasting, *Sufi M. Nazem*
Vol. 94: Bayesian Analysis of Time Series and Dynamic Models, *edited by James C. Spall*
Vol. 95: The Inverse Gaussian Distribution: Theory, Methodology, and Applications, *Raj S. Chhikara and J. Leroy Folks*
Vol. 96: Parameter Estimation in Reliability and Life Span Models, *A. Clifford Cohen and Betty Jones Whitten*
Vol. 97: Pooled Cross-Sectional and Time Series Data Analysis, *Terry E. Dielman*
Vol. 98: Random Processes: A First Look, Second Edition, Revised and Expanded, *R. Syski*
Vol. 99: Generalized Poisson Distributions: Properties and Applications, *P.C. Consul*
Vol. 100: Nonlinear L_p-Norm Estimation, *René Gonin and Arthur H. Money*
Vol. 101: Model Discrimination for Nonlinear Regression Models, *Dale S. Borowiak*
Vol. 102: Applied Regression Analysis in Econometrics, *Howard E. Doran*
Vol. 103: Continued Fractions in Statistical Applications, *K.O. Bowman and L.R. Shenton*
Vol. 104: Statistical Methodology in the Pharmaceutical Sciences, *Donald A. Berry*
Vol. 105: Experimental Design in Biotechnology, *Perry D. Haaland*
Vol. 106: Statistical Issues in Drug Research and Development, *edited by Karl E. Peace*
Vol. 107: Handbook of Nonlinear Regression Models, *David A. Ratkowsky*
Vol. 108: Robust Regression: Analysis and Applications, *edited by Kenneth D. Lawrence and Jeffrey L. Arthur*

ADDITIONAL VOLUMES IN PREPARATION

Statistical Issues in Drug Research and Development

edited by

Karl E. Peace

Biopharmaceutical Research Consultants, Inc.
Ann Arbor, Michigan

MARCEL DEKKER, INC. New York and Basel

Library of Congress Cataloging-in-Publication Data

Statistical issues in drug research and development / edited by Karl E. Peace
p. cm -- (Statistics, textbooks and monographs ; vol. 106)
ISBN 0-8247-8290-9 (alk. paper)
1. Drugs--Testing--Statistical methods. 2. Drugs--Research.
I. Peace, Karl E., II. Series: Statistics, textbooks and monographs ; v. 106.
RM301.27.S727 1990
615.1'072--dc20 89-23727
CIP

This book is printed on acid-free paper.

MARCEL DEKKER, INC.
270 Madison Avenue, New York, New York 10016

Current printing (last digit):
10 9 8 7 6 5 4 3 2 1
PRINTED IN THE UNITED STATES OF AMERICA

Preface

In 1983, the concept of establishing work groups within the Biopharmaceutical Section of the American Statistical Association (ASA) was formally established. The concept had been proposed by the future goals committee and was endorsed by the Executive Committee of the Section. The idea was that work groups addressing statistical issues of widespread interest, particularly to pharmaceutical industry statisticians, would contribute to the vitality of the section.

I underscore the *formal establishment* of the concept of work groups in 1983, since the Executive Committee in 1971 identified two topics of general interest to be studied by interested volunteers. The topics were titled "Bioavailability" and "Enhancing the Process of Statistical Evaluation and Review in NDA Submissions." These topics and attendant activity contributed to the identity and growth of the Section.

Current work group activity essentially began in August, 1984, with peak activity during 1986 being highest. Work groups were formulated to address 12 topics: "Summarization, Analysis and Monitoring of Adverse Experiences," "The Two-by-Two Crossover and Other Multi-Period Designs in Drug Efficacy Studies," "Positive Control or Active Control Equivalence Studies," "Combination Drug Development," "Dose Response/Dosing in the Elderly," "Intention to Treat/Who to Include in Analysis," "Dual Control Groups in Rodent Carcinogenicity Studies," "Pooling of Data," "Assessment of Statistical Methodology in Analgesic Studies," "Recent Advances in Bioassay," "Analysis of Trials with Incomplete Data," and "Issues in Epidemiology." Through the annual joint statistical meetings in August, 1988, these groups have been responsible for 10 sessions (the majority of which were invited), 29 roundtable discussions, and at least 47 individual presentations, at the spring and summer annual statistical meetings.

Most of these contributions to the programs for these meetings came from the first seven groups; particularly, the groups addressing "Crossover Designs," "Active Control Equivalence Studies," and "Combination Drug Development." These groups were ably led by Sylvan Wallenstein and Harji Patel, Bob Makuch, and Gene Laska and Hans Carter, respectively. This book reflects some of the accomplishments of the first seven work groups (Chapters 2–8). It is being published as part of the contribution of the Biopharmaceutical Section to the ASA sesquicentennial celebration, which was held in Washington, D.C., August 6–10, 1989, with the annual joint summer meetings of the ASA, the Biometric Society and the Institute of Mathematical Statistics.

The chapters of this book reflect topics addressed by the ASA Biopharmaceutical Section work groups that have been most active and productive. Specifically, the work of seven groups is reflected in Chapters 2–8.

The first chapter presents in detail the etiology and evolution of the work groups. Background, work group guidelines, work group leaders and members, and issues and problems to be addressed are presented. The topics of Chapters 2, 4, 6, and 7 pertain exclusively to statistical issues associated with clinical trials in clinical drug development programs. The topics of Chapters 3 and 5 are most relevant to clinical trials, except that some concepts also apply to other biological experimentation. The topic of Chapter 8 pertains only to a particular safety screen of a new drug tested in rodents.

The chapters are self-contained. Even though some sections reflect the efforts of individual members of the work groups, all sections of each chapter have a common reference.

I wish to express deep and sincere thanks to the work group members who have made contributions to this book, particularly to the leaders of the work groups. Their collective efforts should be illuminating to professional statisticians, especially those engaged in pharmaceutical drug development. Special thanks go to the publisher for interest in this project as well as to my previous secretary, Nora Coury, whose help proved invaluable.

Karl E. Peace

Contents

Contributors

Kenneth S. Crump Executive vice-president, K. S. Crump Division, Clement Associates, Inc., Ruston, Louisianna

Dennis O. Dixon Associate Professor, Department of Biomathematics, University of Texas, M.D. Anderson Cancer Center, Houston, Texas

Satya D. Dubey Chief, Statistical Evaluation and Research Division, Department of Biometrics, Center for Drug Evaluation and Research, Food and Drug Administration, Rockville, Maryland

Suzanne Edwards Senior Statistician, Department of Clinical Statistics, Burroughs Wellcome Corporation, Research Triangle Park, North Carolina

Gerald M. Fava Director of Statistics, Research Data Services, Knoll Pharmaceuticals, a unit of BASF K & F Corporation, Whippany, New Jersey

Lloyd D. Fisher Professor, Department of Biostatistics, University of Washington, and Director, Department of Clinical Statistics, Fred Hutchinson Cancer Research Center, Seattle, Washington

Ralph F. Frankowski Professor, Department of Biometry, School of Public Health, University of Texas, Houston, Texas

Gerald Hajian Head, Preclinical Statistics, Department of Statistical Services, Burroughs Wellcome Corporation, Research Triangle Park, North Carolina

David B. Hall Chief, Biometrics, Division of Viral Diseases, Center for Infectious Diseases, Centers for Disease Control, Atlanta, Georgia

Joseph K. Haseman Research Mathematical Statistician, Division of Biometry and Risk Assessment, National Institute of Environmental Health Sciences, Research Triangle Park, North Carolina

Martha S. Hearron Senior Medical Biostatistician, Department of Medical Biostatistics III, The Upjohn Company, Kalamazoo, Michigan

Jay Herson President, Applied Logic Associates, Inc., Houston, Texas

Jiann-Ping Hsu* Mathematical Statistician, Division of Biometrics, Center for Drugs and Biologics, Food and Drug Administration, Rockville, Maryland

Arthur F. Johnson† Director of Clinical Statistics, Department of Statistical Science, Smith, Kline and French Laboratories, Philadelphia, Pennsylvania

Mary F. Johnson Executive Director, Department of Biostatistics, G. H. Besselaar Associates, Princeton, New Jersey

Ronald P. Kershner Director, Department of Biometrics, Sterling-Winthrop Research Institute, Rensselaer, New York

Gary G. Koch Professor, Department of Biostatistics, School of Public Health, University of North Carolina, Chapel Hill, North Carolina

Matthew Koch University of North Carolina, Chapel Hill, North Carolina

Eugene M. Laska Director, Statistical Sciences and Epidemiology and World Health Organization Collaborating Center for Training and Research in Mental Health Program Management, Nathan S. Kline Institute for Psychiatric Research, Orangeburg, New York and Research Professor of Psychiatry, New York University Medical Center, New York, New York

George Lynch Ancaster, Ontario, Canada

Robert W. Makuch Associate Professor, Laboratory of Epidemiology and Public Health, Yale University, New Haven, Connecticut

Morris J. Meisner Head, Statistical Sciences Laboratory, Statistical Sciences and Epidemiology Division, Nathan S. Kline Institute for Psychiatric Research, Orangeburg, and Research Associate Professor, Department of Psychiatry, New York University Medical Center, New York, New York

Joel W. Novak President, The EMMES Corporation, Potomac, Maryland

Harji I. Patel Assistant Director, Department of Biostatistics, Hoechst-Roussel Pharmaceuticals, Inc., Somerville, New Jersey

---

Present affiliations:

*Manager, Department of Biometrics, Parke-Davis Pharmaceutical Research Division, Warner-Lambert Company, Ann Arbor, Michigan.

†Adjunct Full Professor, Department of Biometrics and Computing, Hahnemann University, Philadelphia, Pennsylvania.

Karl E. Peace* President, Biopharmaceutical Research Consultants, Inc., Ann Arbor, Michigan

Gordon Pledger Chief, Technical Information Section, Epilepsy Branch, National Institute of Neurological Disorders and Stroke, National Institutes of Health, Bethesda, Maryland

Marcia Polansky Associate Professor, Department of Biometrics and Computing, School of Allied Health, Hahnemann University, Philadelphia, Pennsylvania

Rukmini Rajagopalan Statistician, Department of Medical Data, Boehringer Ingelheim Pharmaceuticals, Inc., Ridgefield, Connecticut

David S. Salsburg Senior Research Fellow, Department of Clinical Research, Pfizer Central Research, Pfizer Laboratories, Inc., Groton, Connecticut

Murray R. Selwyn President, Statistics Unlimited, Inc., Auburndale, Massachusetts

William A. Sollecito Vice President of Operations, Quintiles, Inc., Chapel Hill, North Carolina

Donald M. Stablein Vice-president, The EMMES Corporation, Potomac, Maryland

Sylvan Wallenstein† Associate Professor, School of Public Health, Columbia University, New York, New York

---

**Previous affiliation:* Vice-president of Technical Operations, Parke-Davis Pharmaceutical Research Division, Warner-Lambert Company, Ann Arbor, Michigan.

†*Present affiliation:* Associate Professor, Department of Biomathematical Sciences, Mount Sinai Medical Center, New York, New York.

1
ASA Biopharmaceutical Section Work Groups

Karl E. Peace* *Biopharmaceutical Research Consultants, Inc., Ann Arbor, Michigan*

I. INTRODUCTION

The Executive Committee of the Biopharmaceutical Section of the American Statistical Association (ASA), at its August 1983 meeting in Toronto, decided to develop work groups to address topics of widespread interest to the statistical profession. It was thought that work groups would provide a vehicle for greater and wider participation in section activities, particularly among younger members. Some topics had already been suggested at that time. Kathleen Lamborn, 1984 program chair, asked me at the March 1984 meeting of the Executive Committee in Orlando, FL, to coordinate efforts of the work groups.

By April 1984, ten topics for possible work-group activity had been selected. These were Intention to Treat, Combination Drug Trials, Dose Response, Dosing in the Elderly, Positive Control Trials, Who Should Be Included in Analyses, The Composite Randomization Trial as a Quicker Route to Establishing Efficacy, The Two-by-Two Crossover and Other Multiperiod Designs in Efficacy Trials, An Assessment of the Statistical Methodology in Analgesic Trials: Recommendations for Change, and Dual Control Groups in Drug Safety Studies. These topics were

* *Previous affiliation:* Warner-Lambert Company, Ann Arbor, Michigan.

announced in the April 1984 issue of *Amstat News*, along with an invitation to interested readers to contact the work groups coordinator.

By May 1984, draft guidelines for work-group activity were developed by the work-groups coordinator. These were circulated to members of the Executive Committee and to the ASA office for review and comment.

By June 1984, approximately 70 people had responded to the April 1984 announcement in *Amstat News*. All were initially added as members to potential work groups in which they expressed interest. Each received a letter of acknowledgment and thanks from the work-groups coordinator.

In addition, as the initial effort to get certain work groups started, six of the topics were selected for discussion at four round-table luncheons (four of the six topics were combined and reduced to two) at the 1984 Joint Statistical meetings in Philadelphia. Discussion leaders were also selected. The topics were Dose Response/Dosing in the Elderly, discussion to be led by Art Johnson; Intent to Treat/Who to Include in Analyses, discussion to be led by Lloyd Fisher; Dual Control Groups in Drug Safety Studies, discussion to be led by Gerry Hajian; and The Composite Randomization Trial as a Quicker Route to Efficacy, discussion to be led by Richard Simon. Round-table luncheon topics and discussion leaders were announced in the June 1984 issue of *Amstat News*.

By July 1984, comments received from reviewers of the work-group draft guidelines were incorporated and the guidelines were finalized. Copies of these were made available to any interested individuals. The round-table luncheons were also filled (quickly). Materials for the discussion leaders were sent. This included a list of the attendees via the June 1984 *Amstat News* notice, a list of names of all individuals who had expressed interest to the work-groups coordinator in any of the topics, a draft problem statement for the particular topic(s), and a copy of the guidelines. The charge from the work-groups coodinator to the discussion leaders was to assess whether the topic(s) was sufficiently viable to warrant work-group formulation. In addition, the discussion leaders were asked to lead the efforts of the respective work groups or to assist in the identification of a work-group leader.

There was lively discussion at all four round table luncheons at the summer meetings, August 15, 1984, in Philadelphia. The assessment as to work-group viability of the topic(s) was positive from three of the discussion leaders. Those in attendance at the luncheon discussion of The Composite Randomization Trial as a Quicker Route to Efficacy thought the topic insufficient to warrant work-group formulation. They selected the topic Poolability of Data as a replacement. In addition, several attendees at the summer meetings indicated the desire to have Summarization and Analysis of Adverse Experience Data as a potential work-group topic.

By November 1984, work groups were partially or completely formulated to address nine topics. Work-group leaders had also been identified for five. This represented interest from approximately 100 people. A report from the work-groups coordinator listing topics and leaders appeared in the November 1984 issue of *Amstat News*. The report also solicited additional interest either as members or as leaders.

By March 1985, an additional work-group leader was identified. In addition, the Executive Committee of the Biopharmaceutical Section of the ASA at its meeting in Raleigh, NC, expressed interest in setting up work groups to address additional topics furnished from members of the statistical profession through the ASA questionnaire developed by Barbara Tilley and mailed after the 1984 annual statistical meetings.

As of the August 1985 annual statistical meetings, nine viable topics for work-group activity and leaders and membership of groups addressing six of the topics had been identified. In addition, draft problem statements for all nine groups had been developed by the work-group coordinator.

The draft problem statements were formulated to facilitate initial discussion. They could be changed as deemed appropriate by the leaders and members of the work groups. Although everyone who expressed interest in a particular work group was added to the membership of that work group by the work-groups coordinator, the work-group leader could modify the membership as deemed appropriate.

The six groups with leaders were rather active prior to and including the 1985 Las Vegas meetings. Many met on several occasions—locally and in concert with professional meetings. Dave Salsburg's group was the most active. Two papers emanating from Dave's group, one by Art Johnson and the other by Dave, were presented in Las Vegas at a contributed paper session on work-group activity organized and chaired by the work-group coordinator. One paper emanating from Lloyd Fisher's group was also presented at the session. It was jointly presented by Lloyd and Martha Hearron. Two other papers, authored or co-authored by members of Sylvan Wallenstein's group, were also presented at the session. One was presented by Joe Fleiss. The other was presented by Andrew Willan. In addition, Joe Haseman presented an invited paper at the Las Vegas meetings on the topic of Dual Control Groups in Drug Safety Studies. Also, Dave's group, Lloyd's group, and Joe's and Gerry's group met at round-table luncheons at these meetings. An open round-table luncheon for discussion of the topic Summarization and Analysis of Adverse Experience Data was also held.

Three open round table discussions were also held. These reflected feedback from the ASA membership solicited via the Barbara Tilley questionnaire. The topics discussed and discussion leaders were: Continuing Education in the Biopharmaceutical Section with Nina Mocniak, Recent Advances in Bioassay with Neeti R. Bohidar, and Statistical Assessment of Bias in Unblinded Reading of Pathology Slides with Jay Chmiel. Nina, Neeti, and Jay attempted to assess whether the viability of these topics or related topics was sufficient to warrant additional work-group formulation.

Finally, the work-groups coordinator made a presentation to the ASA Publications Committee at its 1985 meeting in Las Vegas. The purpose of the presentation was to provide background to the committee on the work-groups program and to request guidance and sanction for publication of work-group efforts. The committee acknowledged and lauded the Biopharmaceutical Section through the efforts of the work groups and was supportive of publication efforts.

Work-group activity was perhaps highest in 1986, culminating with several sessions, presentations, and round-table luncheons at 1986 statistical meetings. There were two invited paper sessions at the spring meetings of the Eastern North American Region (ENAR) of the Biometric Society in Atlanta. One reflected efforts of the Combination Drug Development Work Group and other efforts of the Crossover Designs Work Group. Nine members of these work groups presented papers or were discussants at these sessions. They were Hans Carter, Gordon Pledger, Gene Laska, Karl Peace, Walt Federer, Sylvan Wallenstein, Ron Kerchner, Harji Patel, and Byron Jones. At the 1986 summer meetings in Chicago, there were two invited paper sessions, one organized contributed paper session, and six round-table luncheons. The invited paper sessions reflected efforts of the Active Control Equivalence Studies (originally named Positive Control Trials) and the Combination Drug Development work groups. Participants were Bob Makuch, Bob Davis, Jay Herson, Gordon Pledger, Stu Bessler, Gene Laska, Hans Carter, Bill Beaver, Bill Vodra, and Hoi Leung. The organized Contributed paper session reflected efforts of the Crossover Design work group. Participants were Hareji Patel, Matthew Koch, Ed Stanek, David Rosa, Doug Gause, Karl Peace, Mohammed Alhobali, and Marcia Polansky. The six round-table luncheons addressed the topics Multiperiod Designs in Drug Efficacy Trials, Pooling Data, Combination Drug Development, Summarization and Analysis of Adverse Experience Data, Active Control Equivalence Studies, and Analysis of Trials with Incomplete Data. Discussion was led by Sylvan Wallenstein, Judy Goldberg, Hans Carter, Janet Elashof, Bob Makuch, and Ron Helms, respectively.

Work-group activity continued during 1987, 1988, and 1989. Some members of the work groups who were more active earlier elected to publish their (largely individual efforts) research in peer journals. In addition, several groups felt that they had adequately addressed the issues. There were also several presentations at the spring and summer meetings during the period by individuals from various work groups but only two (organized/contributed) sessions at the spring and summer meetings. One session reflected efforts of the work group addressing Recent Advances in Bioassay and was a part of the 1987 program in San Francisco. The other reflected efforts of the work group addressing Summarization and Analysis of Adverse Experiences and was a part of the 1988 program in New Orleans. Participants at these sessions were Neeti Bohidar, Gary O. Zerbe, E. M. Carter, J. J. Hubert, Tom Copenhaver, Tsai-Lein Lin, Ken Goldberg, Patrick D. O'Meara, Clement Maurath, Sharon Anderson, Walter W. Offen, Paul Leber, and Donald A. Berry. In addition, several groups met at these annual meetings via round-table luncheons. They were Dual Control Groups in Animal Carcinogenicity Studies, Crossover Designs, Summarization and Analysis of Trials with Incomplete Data, Combination Drug Trials, Positive Control Trials, and Bioassay Issues'. Discussions were led by Joe Haseman and Gerry Hajian; Harji Patel and Gerry Fava; Clement Maurath, Patrick O'Meara, and Sharon Anderson; Ron Helms, Gene Laska, Hans Carter, and Karl Peace; Bob Makuch and Jay Herson; and Charlie Goldsmith, respectively. Obviously, much activity occurred between August 1988 and January 1989, culminating with the publication of this volume during the ASA sesquicentennial year.

Currently, there are 12 work groups in various stages of development and work. Seven of these contributed work to this volume. These contributions appear as Chapters 2–8. Work-group guidelines are presented in this chapter as Section II, work-group problems and issues statements are presented as Section III, and work-group participants are identified as Section IV. Finally, some concluding remarks are offered in Section V.

II. ASA BIOPHARMACEUTICAL SECTION WORK-GROUP GUIDELINES

A. Background

From time to time the statistical profession derives benefit from the collective efforts of statisticians focusing on technical topics of widespread interest relevant to statistical practice. An example is the work of the FDA Biometric and Epidemiological Methodology Advisory Committee (BEMAC) in 1976 and 1977. One of the goals of the Biopharmaceutical Section of the ASA is to generate topics of widespread interest and to establish work groups to address such topics.

B. Statement of Purpose

It is not necessarily intended that the work groups undertake original research on the topics. The thrust is to put the topic (problem) in perspective and to present an integrated discussion of information relevant to the topic.

The purpose of the work groups is:

- To study topics of widespread interest to the Biopharmaceutical Section.
- To develop a report that would:
    - Contain a detailed description of the problem and its history.
    - Contain an assessment of the impact of the problem on the applied area of research, for example, on Drug Development.
    - Contain a (re)solution of the problem, if possible.
    - Contain conclusions and recommendations from the (re)solution of the problem.
    - Contain a bibliography.

N.B. If a (re)solution of the problem is not possible, then the third and fourth development goals should be replaced by:

- Contain an adequate characterization of the pros and cons of possible (re)solutions (e.g., segments of the work group may have different views as to *the* solution).

C. Administrative Procedures

Administration of the program is through the Executive Committee of the Biopharmaceutical Section of the ASA by the work-group coordinator. The responsibilities of the coordinator are:

- To develop a list of work-group topics.
- To develop a list of potential work-group members.
- To formulate work-group constituency including work-group leaders.
- To provide problem statements to the work-group leaders.
- To coordinate and review work-group activities.

- To disseminate efforts of the work groups to the executive committee of the Biopharmaceutical Section of the ASA and to other relevant audiences as necessary.
- To organize sessions at the spring and annual joint statistical meetings reflecting the efforts of the work groups.

D. Work-Group Constituency

Work-group membership is the responsibility of the work-group coordinator. Potential members should contact the work-group coordinator directly, by phone or in writing. It is appropriate for potential members to submit to the coordinator information about relevant topics of interest and familiarity/competence with the topic. This is particularly important for the selection of group leaders. Potential members should clear with their management their participation in work-group efforts. Work groups shall consist of:

- A group leader.
- Work-groups coordinator.
- At least three but no more than ten other members.
- Members so as to minimize travel for group meetings insofar as possible.

E. Work-Group Leader Responsibilities

The work-group leader is responsible for:

- Directing the activities of the group toward topic (re)solution.
- Administrative clerical support for the groups' activities and reports.
- Submitting to the work-groups coordinator draft and final reports of work-group efforts on the topics.
- Chairing session(s) at the spring and annual joint meetings on results of group efforts.

F. Work-Group Responsibilities/Guidelines

The work group through the work-group leader will provide the work-group coordinator:

- A detailed description of the problem, an assessment of the impact of the problem on the applied area of research, and recommendation as to whether study is warranted further. This would occur within 3 ± 1 months of group formulation.
- A draft (preliminary) report to include:
  - Problem statement

- Background/history
- Findings/solution/resolution
- Discussion of findings
- Conclusions
- Recommendations

This should occur within 15 ± 3 months of group formulation.

- A final report. This should occur with 2.5 ± 0.5 years of group formulation.

In addition the work group shall:

- Participate in work-group sessions at statistical meetings.

III. WORK-GROUP TOPICS AND PROBLEMS/ISSUES STATEMENTS

A. Summarization, Analysis, and Monitoring of Adverse Experiences

Adverse experience (AE) data are most often summarized by the crude rate, that is, the ratio of the number of persons experiencing the event to the number of persons exposed to the drug. A criticism of the crude rate as a summary measure is that it ignores differential exposure to the drug. Recently, life-table methods for cumulative rates or time specific rates have been applied, which theoretically overcome this objection. It may be possible to incorporate explanatory variables or risk factors into either methodology. There are issues surrounding use of either methodology. Some are design/analysis/interpretation oriented. Others are definitional. For example, since AE data prior to market approval usually comes from trials designed to assess efficacy (and not designed to answer a specific safety question), should inferential analysis be made on AE data? Since many data post market approval may not be viewed as experimental, what special problems does this pose in applying the methodology? How (or) should data from different protocols be summarized? The efforts of the work group on this topic should be directed toward developing a report that could be used as a guide for summarizing/analyzing AE data. The report should pay due attention to all relevant issues. It should follow to the extent possible the format suggested in the statement of purpose section of the guidelines for the work groups.

B. The Two-byTwo Crossover and Other Multiperiod Designs in Efficacy Trials

The decade following Grizzles' paper on two-by-two crossover designs heard much discussion concerning its use in drug efficacy studies. Much of the discussion was triggered by analysis/conclusion considerations in the presence of unequal residual drug effects and the inclusion of baseline measurements to validate the lack of such effects. The discussion perhaps was culminated by the report issued in 1976 by the FDA-assembled BEMAC. The conclusion of that report was essentially that the two-by-two crossover should be avoided in trials aimed at establishing unequivocal efficacy. Should this recommendation be taken carte blanche? Are there some efficacy trials where the two-by-two crossover may be the design of choice, either on purely statistical grounds or in concert with what is known about the disease process or on ethical grounds? Should or does the BEMAC recommendation apply to other more complex crossover designs? For example, the addition of two sequences in which patients are not crossed over to the alternative treatment to the two-by-two crossover design permits a valid comparison of direct effects of the drugs based on all the data regardless of the conclusion about residual effects. The same may be said for the three-period crossover of three drugs where patients are randomized to the six possible sequences of drug administration. In addition, some drugs, antianginal, for example, have been approved when much of the efficacy data came from crossover trials with more than two periods. The efforts of the work group on this topic should be directed toward developing a report that would address the pros and cons of the above issues as well as any other pertinent ones. The pros and cons should be based to the extent possible on statistical methodological grounds. Attention should also be given to the substantive application areas. The report should follow the format suggested in the statement of purpose section of the guidelines for the work groups.

C. Active Control Equivalence Studies

Essentially there are two types of clinical trials that may be pursued in establishing efficacy of a new drug at a given dose. One, almost definitionally, is to use a placebo control. The other is to use a dose of a drug that has already been established as efficacious. The latter trial is known as the positive control or the active control equivalence study (ACES). Ostensibly, the objective of the placebo controlled trial is to show superior efficacy. Consequently, a one-sided alternative may be argued. The positive controlled trial is thought of as an "equivalence" trial. Equivalence is most often interpreted in terms of a two-sided alternative. This may be interpreted as "The new drug is not worse than the positive control (by $-w$) but neither is it better (by w)." Is this really the research objective? Or is it just "The new drug is not worse than the positive control"? Sidedness is one issue in designing positive controlled trials. Other design and analysis issues are the magnitude of the difference (w), the choice of endpoint(s) particularly for chronic diseases, multiple comparisons, sample size, power, minimizing variability, assessment of benefit to risk, and method of analysis/summary (e.g., confidence intervals or hypothesis testing?). The efforts of the work group on this topic should be directed to developing a report that would provide a review of the design and analysis issues in positive controlled trials. The review should include statistical methodology as warranted. Attention should also be given to the substantive application areas. The report should also contain recommendations regarding design and analyses. Perhaps this would be dependent on the type of disease and drug class. The report should follow the format suggested in the statement of purpose section of the guidelines for the work groups.

D. Optimization in Clinical Trials and Combination Drug Development

"Minimally effective dose" or "dose comparison" issues aside, approval to market a single-entity drug requires adequate demonstration of effectiveness of a single dose. This is usually provided from clinical trials comparing the drug at the dose to a placebo. Fixed-combination drugs require adequate demonstration that each component (of the combination) contributes to the claimed effects of the combination for approval. Interpreted literally, this requires comparing the combination to each of its components. Should combination trials be placebo-controlled? In either case, what are the hypotheses to be tested? What is the most efficient design? What is the most appropriate analysis? To what extent are the answers to these questions influenced by the "claimed effects"? For example, is the development approach the same when both components are geared toward the same effect or for different effects? To what extent is the approach dependent on the number of components? For example, for a two-component (A or B) drug (AB), one might argue that AB should be compared to A and to B. But what about a three-component drug? Is it merely sufficient to compare ABC to A, to B, and to C, individually? Or would ABC be compared to AB, to AC, and to BC, as well? The efforts of the work group on this topic should be directed to developing a report that would offer guidance concerning these issues regarding combination drug development. The report should be based on valid statistical methodological grounds. However, attention should be paid to issues from the substantive application areas—for example, analgesics versus antiinflammatory or cough/cold.

The report should follow the format suggested in the statement of purpose section of the guidelines for the work groups.

E. Dose Response/Dosing in the Elderly

Much attention has been focused recently on the topics of dose response in the clinical setting and dosing in the elderly. The attention to dose response in the clinical setting has been kindled in large part by the inclusion of the dose comparison trial in the recent rewrite of the FDA IND/NDA guidelines. Attention to dosing in the elderly has also been kindled by position pieces by members of the regulatory agency and coverage in the Pink Sheet. These two topics are interrelated and potentially impact heavily on drug development programs. The efforts of the work group on these topics should be directed to developing a report following the format suggested in the statement of purpose section of the work group guidelines. The background, introductory, or description section of the report should address sufficiently the topic of dose response, primarily in a nonclinical setting (e.g., What is the aim? How is the information obtained?) and also should integrate the current topics. This could then lead logically into an impact assessment of the current topics on drug development. The main body (solution) of the report could (1) address a scientifically defensible plan for developing dose-response information (which would include experiments or trials and the attendant designs and analysis methodologies) and (2) address a scientifically defensible plan for developing information for dosing in the elderly.

F. Intention to Treat

There appear to be two schools of thought within the statisical community regarding the handling in data analyses of patients who were randomized to treatment in a clinical trial yet were never treated. One position is that all patients, whether treated or not, should be accounted for in analyses. The other is that only patients who received treatment should be accounted for in analysis. The efforts of the work group on this topic should be directed to developing a report that would reflect the pros and cons of each position and provide direction to choosing between the two. The pros and cons should be based to the extent possible on statistical methodological grounds. The report should follow the format suggested in the statement of purpose section of the guidelines for the work groups.

G. Dual Control Groups in Rodent Carcinogenicity Studies

Much attention is currently being focused on the design, analysis, and interpretation of drug safety studies, particularly long-term chronic toxicity studies. An aspect of the design of such studies at some research facilities, and therefore impacting on their analysis and interpretation, is to use two identical control groups rather than one. The efforts of the work group on this topic should be directed to developing a report that would reflect the pros and cons of one versus two control groups. The pros and cons should be based to the extent possible on statistical methodological grounds. The report should follow the format suggested in the statement of purpose section of the guidelines for the work groups.

H. Pooling of Data

Rarely is it possible to conduct a clinical trial whose objective is to furnish both clinical and statistical evidence of efficacy at a single site. Rather, it is most often necessary to use several sites. The usual statistical design for such a trial is a completely randomized block design (with replication) with sites (or investigator or clinics) as blocks. Almost invariably, even though the greatest precautions are taken with protocol development, recruitment of investigators and patients, monitoring, and data collection, there are questions raised relative to the "poolability" of the data. Contributing to this are those occasions where the directions and magnitudes of treatment group differences across all sites are inconsistent with "expectations." The efforts of the work group on this topic should be directed to developing a report that would provide a review of the issues in pooling data. The review should include statistical methodology. Attention should also be given to issues from the substantive application areas. Criteria as to when data may be pooled without question, when data should not be pooled without question, and when data fall intermediately may be possible. The report should follow the format statement of purpose section of the guidelines for the work groups.

I. An Assessment of Statistical Methodology in Analgesic Trials

Many measures and statistical analysis methodologies for the measures have been proposed for assessing effectiveness of analgesic drugs. Some measures are sum of pain intensity differences (SPID), sum of pain analog intensity differences (SPAID), total pain relief (TOTPR), and onset and duration of relief. Are all three measures SPID, SPAID, and TOTPR necessary? For example, aren't SPID and TOTPR complementary?

Don't SPID and SPAID attempt to measure the same parameter? In addition, the measures are difficult to apply to the data on patients who drop out. Perhaps time-to-event methods should be incorporated into the analgesic methodology armentaria. Events of interest may be pain relief, partial or complete, drop out, etc. The efforts of the work group on this topic should be directed toward developing a report that would address the pros and cons of the current (non time-to-event methods) measures and methodologies for analgesic drug assessment and make a case for incorporating time-to-event methods. This should be based to the extent possible on statistical methodological grounds. Attention should also be given to the substantive application areas. The report should follow the format suggested in the statement of purpose section of the guidelines for the work groups.

J. Recent Advances in Bioassay

Bioassay statistical methods are applied to three distinct areas in the pharmaceutical industry, viz. Pharmacology, Pathology/Toxicology and Risk Assessment. Initial efforts will be primarily confined to the area of Pharmacology. The following topics are proposed for specific study:

1. Multivariate Bioassay
   (Time dependent, Multi-response)
2. Joint Drug Action I
   (Quantitative Response)
3. Joint Drug Action II
   (Qualitative Response)
4. Drug Receptor Interaction
5. Bioassay Software Review

The efforts of the Work Group on this topic should be directed toward developing a report which would address the applicability, methodology, computer algorithm, and numerical example and interpretation of each topic. This should be based to the extent possible on statistical methodological grounds. Attention would also be given to the substantive application areas. The report should follow the format suggested in the statement of purpose section of the guidelines for the work groups.

K. Analysis of Trials with Incomplete Data

Longitudinal clinical trials are often afflicted with incomplete data, a problem which can have a substantial impact on the statistical analysis. Missing data are often classified in two different ways: (a) the mechanism leading to missing values, and (b) the statistical method used to handle the incomplete data. D. B. Rubin (1976, *Biometrika*, **63**, 581–592) classified mechanisms into three categories:

1. The missing data are said to be *missing at random* and the observed data are said to be *observed at random* when the process leading to missing values of a dependent variable, Y, does not depend upon the values of Y or upon the values of concomitant variables X.

2. The missing data are *missing at random* but the observed data are *not observed at random* when the missing-data process depends upon the observed values of Y and X, but not upon the missing values of Y.

3. The missing data are *not missing at random* if the missing-data process depends on the missing values of Y.

"Missing by design" would be considered as a fourth category by some investigators; as a practical matter this category can be included in the "missing at random" category. Some investigators classify missing data as *ignorably missing* or *non-ignorably missing*. In some cases the *pattern* of missing data is important, as for example, a hierarchical pattern (e.g., when a subject drops out of a longitudinal study and does not return).

Although incomplete data are the rule, rather than the exception, incompleteness almost always has serious implications for the statistical analysis. In the least serious case (a small proportion of data missing at random) missing data lead to loss of power (both by smaller sample size and loss of orthogonality) and to more complicated analyses. In the most serious cases (substantial proportions of data missing for reasons related to the processes under study) there may be no legitimate statistical analysis of the data and, therefore, no reasonable scientific inferences from the trial.

This Work Group will address issues related to determining whether data are observed/missing at random, specification of appropriate statistical methods for various types of incomplete clinical trials data, and determination of possible adverse side effects of the statistical analysis (e.g., undesirable effects of adjusting for non-comparable distributions of baseline values resulting from randomly missing data).

L. Recent Advances in Epidemiology

Applied statisticians take a scientific question (often with already collected data) as the raw material and attempt to build a study design or a data analysis to answer the question. Often, a major accomplishment is redefining the question so that it can be answered. Although we can collect data when the facts are known or knowable, in epidemiological studies we cannot control who is exposed, nor can we adjust for unknown and unsuspected factors, which may exist and which may affect the outcome. Thus, there are a number of substantive issues involved in judging an epidemiological study.

There are a number of questions to be addressed:

1. What are reasonable expectations of an epidemiological study? What makes a study acceptable? or even exceptional?

2. Can standards for judging epidemiological studies be developed? How do we assess the potential for bias in a study?

3. We have reasonably well defined designs when needed to assess the outcome of a well defined exposure (cohort studies) or potential exposure leading to a specific disease (using case-control studies). In some problems in environmental epidemiology it is not clear what the exposure is, who is at risk of being exposed, whether they were actually exposed, if so, how much, and what the actual adverse event is. How does one approach these environmental epidemiological studies?

4. Can a book of "case studies" be developed to show how specific problems are approached? This would include a protocol and an explanation of why the decisions in the protocol were made. We could have one section devoted to each major design.

The efforts of the Work Group on this topic should be directed toward developing a report which would address these issues and questions. This should be based to the extent possible on statistical methodological grounds. Attention would also be given to the substantive application areas. The report should follow the format suggested in the statement of purpose section of the guidelines for the work groups.

IV. WORK-GROUP PARTICIPANTS

A. Summarization, Analysis, and Monitoring of Adverse Experiences Work Group

Leaders: Suzanne Edwards, Janet Elashof, Clement Maurath, Sharon Anderson, Patrick O'Meara.

Participants: Gary Koch, Arthur Itkin, David Carlin, John Ondrasik, Gladys Reynolds, Walter W. Offen, Robert Small, Ling-Ling Tsao, Phillip Lavin, Donald A. Berry, Amy Kunes, Denise Kinch, Robert O. Chen, Rukmini Rajagopalan, Paul Leber, Marjorie Keshmeri, Bill Sollecito, Karl Peace.

B. Crossover Designs Workgroup

Leaders: Sylvan Wallenstein, Harji I. Patel.

Participants: Phillip Banks, George Lynch, Curtis Wiltse, Andrew

Wilan, Marcia Polansky, Gerald Fava, Jack Green, Ronald Kershner, Matthew Koch, Karl Peace.

C. Active Control Equivalence Studies

Leader: Robert Makuch.
Participants: Stuart Bessler, Robert Davis, David Hall, Jay Herson, Mary Johnson, Gordon Pledger, J. P. Hsu, Lloyd Fisher, Karl Peace.

D. Optimization in Clinical Trials and Combination Drug Development Work Group

Leaders: Eugene Laska, Hans Carter.
Participants: Lee Huang, Donald Stablein, David Salsburg, Morris Meisner, David Carlin, Vernon Chinchilli, Jay Herson, Gordon Pledger, Polly Feigl, Hoi Leung, Jeff Meeker, Karl Peace.

E. Dose Response/Dosing in the Elderly Work Group

Leader: David Salsburg.
Participants: Arthur Johnson, Rukmini Rajagopalan, Jeff Meeker, David Carlin, Sandy Heft, Christopher Cox, Tony L. Ona, George Lynch, Annette Moore, Andrew Willan.

F. Intention to Treat Work Group

Leader: Lloyd Fisher.
Participants: Martha S. Hearron, Robert Davis, Jay Herson, Dennis Dixon, Ralph Frankowski, Thomas Spradlin, Katherine Freeman, Albert Getson, Phillip Banks, Karl Peace.

G. Dual Control Groups in Rodent Carcinogenicity Studies Work Group

Leaders: Joe Haseman, Gerald Hajian.
Participants: Bob Condon, J. P. Hsu, Kenny Crump, Murray Selwyn, Paul Sanders, Karl E. Peace.

H. Pooling of Data Work Group

Leaders: Judy Goldberg, Joe Fleiss, Richard Simon.
Participants: Arlene Ash, Robert Scheer, Donald Boxer, John Taulbee, David Thomas, Ray Bain, Karl E. Peace.

I. An Assessment of the Statistical Methodology in Analgesic Trials Work Group

Leaders: Alan Izu, Larry Gould.

Participants: Timothy Bain, Christopher Cox, Jim Crowe, Jack Green, Charles Locke, Curtis Wiltse, Gene Laska, Kathleen Lamborn.

J. Recent Advances in Bioassay Work Group

Leader: Neeti Bohidar.

Participants: Gene Laska, Hans Carter, Arthur Itkin, Alan Izu, John J. Hubert, Charlie Goldsmith, Ed M. Carter, Tom Copenhaver, Gary O. Zerbe, Tsai-Lein Lin, Ken Goldberg.

K. Analysis of Clinical Trials with Incomplete Data

Leader: Ron Helms.

Participants: Timothy Bain, Christopher Cox, Jim Crowe, Jack Green, Charles Locke, Curtis Wiltse, Gene Laska, Kathleen Lamborn.

L. Issues in Epidemiology

Leaders: Gladys Reynolds, Bob Parker, Bill Jenkins.

Participants: Being identified.

V. CONCLUDING REMARKS

The decision by the Executive Committee of the Biopharmaceutical Section of the ASA in August 1983, in the interest of viability of the section, to formulate work groups to address topics of widespread interest to statisticians appears to have been a good one. There certainly has been a great deal of interest expressed in the work groups. In addition, many of the work groups have been very active and accomplished quite a lot. Interest and input have come from younger members of the profession, from less known though not necessarily younger members, and from well-known members held in highest esteem. Academia has been represented by students and faculty. Private consultants have been represented. The pharmaceutical industry has been represented. Governmental agencies have been represented and I'm sure other segments as well. I would anticipate work-group activity for many more years. As some groups finish, others will no doubt start.

I have enjoyed my involvement in all aspects of this project. I would not kid anyone if I said that it has not been time-consuming. It has. In fact, it has on many occasions been labor intensive, particularly, the last two months prior to getting this volume off to the publisher. However, the rewards have been ample.

Intellectual conversations have been stimulating. I've gotten to know old friends better and made many new ones. All interactions have been exemplary. This may represent the largest and most concentrated effort yet exhibited by the section. Thanks are in order to work-group leaders, to all participants identified in Section IV, and especially to all contributors to Chapters 2–8 of this volume. It is my hope that the five groups not contributing to this volume will continue their work and that there will be a follow-up volume that will house their efforts.

BIBLIOGRAPHY

Peace, K. E. (1984). Attn: Members of the Biopharmaceutical Section. *Amstat News*, *104*, 4, April.

Program and Abstracts 1984 Joint Statistical Meetings. 144th Meeting of the American Statistical Association. Philadelphia, August 13–16.

Proceedings of the Biopharmaceutical Section. American Statistical Association, Washington, DC, 1984.

Peace, K. E. (1984). Report from Work Groups Coordinator. *Amstat News*, *100*, 14, December.

Programme and Abstracts 1985 Joint Statistical Meetings. 145th Meeting of the American Statistical Association, Las Vegas, August 5–8.

Proceedings of the Biopharmaceutical Section. American Statistical Association, Washington, DC, 1985.

Peace, K. E. (1985). *Summary of ASA Biopharmaceutical Section Work Groups*. Proceedings of the Biopharmaceutical Section. ASA, 806 15th Street, N.W., Washington, DC 20005, pp. 77–82.

Program and Abstracts 1986 Joint Statistical Meetings. 146th Meeting of the American Statistical Association, Chicago, August 18–21.

Proceedings of the Biopharmaceutical Section. American Statistical Association, Washington, DC, 1986.

Program and Abstracts 1987 Joint Statistical Meetings. 147th Meeting of the American Statistical Association, San Franscisco, August 17–20.

Proceedings of the Biopharmaceutical Section. American Statistical Association, Washington, DC, 1987.

Program and Abstracts 1988 Joint Statistical Meetings. 148th Meeting of the American Statistical Association, New Orleans, August 22–25.

Proceedings of the Biopharmaceutical Section. American Statistical Association, Alexandria, VA, 1988.

2
Summarization, Analysis, and Monitoring of Adverse Experiences

Suzanne Edwards *Burroughs Wellcome Corporation, Research Triangle Park, North Carolina*

Gary G. Koch *University of North Carolina, Chapel Hill, North Carolina*

William A. Sollecito *Quintiles, Inc., Chapel Hill, North Carolina*

Karl E. Peace* *Biopharmaceutical Research Consultants, Inc., Ann Arbor, Michigan*

I. INTRODUCTION TO ADVERSE EXPERIENCE DATA IN CLINICAL TRIALS

Suzanne Edwards, Gary G. Koch, and William Sollecito

A. Introduction

In clinical trials of new drugs, the analysis of safety data, particularly the analysis of adverse experiences, is often not as extensive as the analysis of efficacy data. There are many reasons for this. Adverse experience data are difficult to quantify and standardize, since many of the commonly occurring reactions are subjective, such as headache or nausea. Furthermore, the determination of a causal link between an adverse

**Previous affiliation:* Warner-Lambert Company, Ann Arbor, Michigan.

experience and a particular drug can be exceedingly difficult. During the course of a clinical trial, the adverse experiences occurring in the group treated with the experimental drug are not necessarily due to the pharmacological action of the drug. They may be due to the illness being treated or an unrelated illness, due to some aspect of the drug-taking experience (for instance, the placebo effect), or due to the action of or interaction with other medications.

From a statistical point of view, the analysis of safety data is often awkward because one wants to confirm, rather than disprove, a null hypothesis, that is, that the drug is safe. Failure to show the drug is unsafe does not imply, of course, that the hypothesis of safety is true. Furthermore, clinical trials are generally not designed to provide statistically powerful tests of safety. The early phase clinical trials enroll very few subjects, and the later trials are designed primarily to address questions of efficacy rather than safety.

The types of adverse reactions most amenable to statistical analysis are those that occur with some frequency. The investigators may be able to anticipate some of these reactions based on their knowledge of the pharmacological activity of the drug and the results of animal experiments. Unexpected and unusual drug reactions may also occur, especially if a sufficiently large population is studied for a sufficiently long period of time. However, in the entire series of premarketing clinical trials, the new drug is tested in at most a few thousand subjects, most of whom are treated for less than a year. Therefore it is not possible before marketing to discover adverse drug reactions that have either a low incidence rate or a long latency period. Although postmarketing surveillance is undeniably important in the detection of adverse reactions, careful collection and analysis of the data from premarketing trials are important for several reasons (Skegg and Doll, 1977): (1) the commonest reactions are often the most important, (2) common minor reactions may be clues to rarer, more serious ones, and (3) suspicions raised in premarketing trials may lead to more effective postmarketing monitoring.

The drug sponsor needs to determine the extent and intensity of the adverse reactions the drug may be expected to produce in the potential user population in order to decide whether use of the drug poses an unacceptable level of discomfort or risk. If the drug is marketed, this information is also necessary for labeling, so that the drug can be appropriately prescribed.

Currently, adverse experience data are presented to the Food and Drug Administration (FDA) in the form of listings and tabulations, often without any accompanying statistical analysis; for trials where few adverse experiences are reported this may be sufficient. The purpose of this chapter is to explore alternative strategies for analysis of this type of data in premarketing clinical trials. The analyses will be illustrated using data from several clinical trials. Two of these are randomized parallel-designed placebo-controlled clinical trials, a short-term trial of a combination antihistamine/decongestant (see Section IV), and a medium-length trial of an antidepressant (see Section V). A third example involves the analysis of a series of active-controlled trials for a new analgesic (see Section VI), and a fourth is based on a crossover trial concerning an aspect of cardiovascular function (see Section VII). The data are used only to illustrate the methodology, and the statistical results presented are not intended to have specific implications for the four general classes of drugs under consideration.

B. Terminology

In the literature, several terms are commonly used to denote a non-beneficial effect from a drug: adverse drug reaction (ADR), side effect, and drug toxicity, among others. The term "adverse drug reaction" is frequently used in the context of postmarketing surveillance. The World Health Organization has defined an ADR as "any response to a drug which is noxious and unintended, and which occurs at doses used in man for prophylaxis, diagnosis, or therapy." This definition requires a judgement as to noxiousness of the response as well as to the intentions of an unspecified party. Kramer (1981) argues that whether an event is adverse (noxious) depends on the clinical setting and the intentions of the treating physician, and that this judgement should be made separately for each case.

The term "side effect" does not imply that the response is adverse. In its broadest usage, side effect includes any response other than the main therapeutic effect of the drug. Side effects can range from harmless epiphenomena (e.g., transient liver enzyme changes) to innocuous nuisances to harmful and possibly irreversible injuries to death. The term "side effect" and "ADR" both imply that the observed effect is caused by a particular drug.

Leaving aside the question of adverseness, Kramer (1981) uses the term "clinical manifestation" to refer to "an abnormal sign, symptom, or laboratory test, or a cluster of abnormal signs, symptoms, and tests" that is not necessarily caused by the administration of a particular drug. Signs and symptoms differ in that signs are observable by the examining physician, whereas symptoms are sensations perceived only by the patient. For the purposes of this chapter, a symptom or sign that is not measurable on an interval or ratio scale will be referred to as an "adverse experience." Thus, fever would be considered an adverse experience, but, according to this restricted definition, body temperature would not. The analysis of adverse experiences is only one part of the safety evaluation of a new drug. Other indicators of adverse drug reactions include abnormalities in laboratory examinations, changes in vital signs, findings from physical examinations, and the results of special tests (e.g., electrocardiograms).

C. Overview of Adverse Experience Evaluations in Clinical Trials

The series of clinical trials that are conducted in support of an application to the FDA for the marketing of a new drug (a New Drug Application, NDA) is customarily divided into Phase I, Phase II, and Phase III. As the trials progress, an increasing number of subjects are enrolled in studies of greater length. Phase IV refers to the monitoring done after the drug is marketed.

The experimental drug is first introduced to man in Phase I trials that involve a small number (typically between 10 and 20) of very closely monitored subjects. The trials are designed to assess dose tolerance and to determine the fate of the drug in the human body. They may also provide early efficacy testing, if the study subjects are patients with the disorder to be treated. In most Phase I trials, the subjects are healthy adult male volunteers. Some reactions may occur in Phase I trials with volunteers that might not occur in later trials with patients. These include the following types (Idanpaan–Heikkela, 1983):

1. Reactions occurring in normal volunteers that would be masked or modified in patients, due to their underlying disease(s) or concomitant medication(s).
2. Reactions induced by higher doses of the drug.
3. Reactions that are extensions of the pharmacological actions of the drug.
4. Reactions related to interactions between the drug and common events in the daily life to which hospitalized patients might not be exposed. Idanpaan-Heikkila cites the example of a drug that caused adverse reactions following a few drinks of alcohol in healthy subjects up to 60 h after the last drug dose.

Phase II trials are used to demonstrate the effectiveness and relative safety of the new drug with respect to a control (other treatment or no treatment), and to determine the optimum dose range for particular indications. These trials may detect the most common reactions in the patient population expected to benefit from the drug. They may also be used to predict the target organ system(s) for reactions found in the Phase III trials. Trials using intensively monitored inpatients may uncover some reactions that would not be found with outpatients.

Phase III trials are conducted after the drug's efficacy has been demonstrated to some extent. They are intended to further establish the efficacy and safety profiles in populations resembling the population expected to use the drug. These trials usually involve a larger number of subjects under a larger number of investigators in studies of longer duration than Phase II trials. The length of the trials depends on the intended use of the drug. For example, psychoactive drugs, which are intended for chronic or long-term intermittent use, must be tested in longer trials than antimicrobial drugs, which are intended to be used for only a few days or weeks. Large short-term Phase III trials may uncover acute ADRs and ADRs that occur only in certain subgroups (e.g., patients with hepatic or renal disease). Longer-term trials may uncover ADRs that appear only after a certain length of time or cumulative dose.

Knowledge of the drug's effects is still incomplete at the time of an NDA approval. Phase IV studies are conducted to monitor for ADRs that may have been missed in the premarketing phases due to the size and length of the trials. In Phase IV, knowledge is accumulated by means of two primary methods (Jones, 1982a):

1. Experimental studies (i.e., clinical trials) requested to clarify specific issues, such as the effect of the drug in children.
2. Nonexperimental methods, including evaluation of spontaneous reports, and epidemiologic case-control studies.

Late-developing or rare ADRs may be discovered in Phase IV, as well as ADRs occurring in subgroups of the population in which the drug was not tested prior to marketing. Also, increases in the incidence of common disease, or reactions that are not usually looked for unless signaled (e.g., low sperm count) may be discovered.

D. Adverse Drug Reaction Mechanisms and Predisposing Factors

Adverse drug reactions may be classified according to their proposed mechanisms (Eadie et al., 1981):

1. Pharmacologic
2. Allergic
3. Idiosyncratic
4. Others, including those leading to
   a. Dysmorphogenesis (e.g., thalidomide-induced fetal anomalies)

b. Carcinogenesis (e.g., diethylstilbesterol-induced vaginal cancer in offspring)

Most ADRs occur on the first day of treatment, and two-thirds develop within 4 days (Prescott, 1979). The early reactions are often pharmacologic ADRs; allergic ADRs tend to occur later. Dysmorphogenesis and carcinogenesis may appear months or years, respectively, after drug administration, and since most premarketing clinical trials exclude women of child-bearing potential, both of these types of reactions may be detected only after marketing.

Pharmacological ADRs, which are direct extensions of the drug's pharmacological effects, are the most commonly occurring type. The severity is usually dose and plasma drug concentration dependent, and, if the drug's pharmacological effects in humans are known, the qualitative nature of such ADRs is predictable.

Allergic ADRs result from a previous sensitization to the drug or to a closely related one. A period of time (usually 7–14 days) is necessary for the synthesis of drug-specific antibodies before the allergic reaction can appear. In contrast to the pharmacological ADR, this type of reaction often bears no resemblance to the drug's usual effects, and its severity is dose and plasma drug concentration independent.

An idiosyncratic ADR is a genetically determined abnormal reactivity to a drug, which is characterized by a discontinuity from the ordinary distribution of dose sensitivities (Eadie et al., 1981). This is the least common type of ADR. An example is the aplastic anemia that occurs in one person in approximately every 20,000 treated with choramphenicol.

Some ADRs result from the indirect effects of the drug, which makes the detection of their drug relationship more difficult. Corticosteroids, for example, may interfere with the body's defense mechanisms, causing latent pulmonary tuberculosis to become active (Wade, 1970). An example of a more tenuous relationship is injury from an accident caused by drug-induced drowsiness.

Certain groups of individuals are at higher risk than others of developing ADRs. Davies (1981) lists the following as predisposing factors: age, sex, race, genetic differences, allergic disorders, previous ADRs, renal and hepatic disease, and decreased plasma protein binding. Fitness, body weight, and diet may also modify the drug's effects. Psychiatric variables, such as attitude toward medication, may be important also, especially in studies of psychoactive drugs.

Age is a predisposing factor not only because of changes due to the aging process, but also because of differences in life-style. The old and the very young are especially prone to ADRs. Some investigators have found that ADRs of all types are more common in white than in dark races, and more common in women than in men, but others have found no such differences. Patients with a history of allergic disorders are more likely than others to develop ADRs, including those that are not allergic in character (Davies, 1981).

Many drugs are transported through the body by plasma proteins, are metabolized by the liver, and then eliminated by the kidneys. Pathological problems with any of these tissues or organs may increase the likelihood of an adverse reaction. Abnormally slow or fast metabolism may predispose to adverse reactions, depending on whether the parent drug or its metabolites are responsible (Prescott, 1979).

Interacting with the human factors are factors relating to the administration of the drug, such as dose, drug formulation (e.g., tablet versus capsule), route of administration, and duration of treatment. Even with the same daily dose, a decreased frequency of administration, which necessarily increases the peak–trough difference in plasma concentration, may lead to more dose-related side effects (Temple, 1982). The frequency of side effects may also depend on how fast the body develops a tolerance to the drug. If the drug is given in gradually increasing doses, there may be fewer side effects than if a maintenance-level dose is given on the first day of treatment.

Dose may be specified in absolute units (e.g., milligrams), or, if the drug has a narrow therapeutic range, in units relative to the patient's weight (e.g., milligrams per kilogram). If an absolute amount of the drug is given, the plasma concentration of the drug depends on the patient's size. Thus, sex differences in the incidence of adverse experiences may sometimes be due to weight differences between males and females.

Of all the factors that may influence the occurrence of adverse reactions, the main ones that are likely to be collected routinely in a clinical trial are age, race, sex, height, weight, and information pertaining to the dosing regimen.

E. Adverse Experiences Not Due to Drugs

In a survey of the epidemiologic literature of adverse drug reactions, Kramer (1981) found that the most common symptoms attributed to ADRs were as follows: nausea/vomiting, diarrhea, abdominal pain, rash, pruritus, drowsiness, insomnia, weakness, headache, dizziness, tremulousness, muscle twitching, and fever. This list accounts for about two-thirds of the ADRs reported in most studies. Kramer comments on the nonspecificity of these symptoms and cites a study by Reidenberg and

Lowenthal (1968) in which healthy people not on medication reported a similar list of symptoms. Hospitalized patients would be expected to have a higher background incidence of symptoms, and, since they generally have disorders that cause them some worry, they may also have a higher incidence of psychosomatic complaints.

In addition to the background occurrence of symptoms are the symptoms produced by the act of taking a drug, whether or not the drug is pharmacologically active. Buncher (1972) notes that the side effects from placebo therapy are even more extensive than the list of conditions that have been helped by placebo. Although the side effects attributed to placebo are mostly changes in mood and emotion (Salzman et al. 1972), they may involve almost every organ and system in the body (Trouton, 1957). Pogge and Coats (1962) found that the most common side effects of placebo are those associated with central nervous system depression, such as fatigue, drowsiness, and dizziness. They further observed, as did Green (1962), that the incidence of side effects attributed to placebo increases with dosage (i.e., number of tablets).

Many researchers have tried to ascertain the characteristics that would differentiate potential placebo responders from nonresponders. Salzman et al. note that, in the literature, little difference has been demonstrated between the two as regards age, sex, race, or education. Theories advanced to explain the placebo response phenomenon include suggestibility and increased awareness of somatic experience. Salzman et al. report that therapeutic response to placebo is usually highest during the earliest stages of treatment, gradually disappearing after a few weeks. If the mechanisms of placebo-induced symptoms and placebo-induced improvement are similar, placebo side effects may also disappear with time.

In the studies of placebo toxicity cited above, the subjects were not told that they might receive placebos. In clinical trials of new drugs, however, subjects must give an informed consent in order to participate. The conclusions and theories given above may not apply if the study subjects are informed about the possibility of receiving placebo. During the consent process, subjects are also told of the potential toxicities of the experimental drug. Hassar and Weintraub (1976) tested subjects about the information presented during the consent process and found that they retained very little of the toxicity information. They note, however, that the subjects who listened closely to the negative aspects of the trial may have refused to participate.

F. Collection of Adverse Experience Data in Clinical Trials

The frequency with which adverse experience assessments are performed depends on the type of trial. With Phase I trials, the assessment is nearly continuous for a certain length of time after administration of the drug. In Phase II and Phase III trials, adverse experiences are usually assessed at discrete predetermined times, unless a subject has a serious adverse experience, in which case closer monitoring may occur.

Assessments may be scheduled for one or more times during the period between admission and the start of treatment (baseline assessments), several times during the treatment phase, and one or more times post-treatment. At the assessments, subjects are asked about all adverse experiences that have occurred in the interval since the last assessment. A higher frequency of assessments will result in a greater number of adverse experiences being reported, since the subjects must recall the experiences over shorter periods of time. There is some question as to what interval should be used for the baseline assessments. Often, just the adverse experiences happening at the time of the baseline assessment are recorded.

An adverse experience may have happened once, several times, or continuously in the interval between assessments. If the adverse experience is a sign, rather than a symptom, and is continuing at the time of assessment, the investigator may be able to observe it. Otherwise, the investigator must rely on the subject's account, which may be sketchy if the adverse experience was not a serious one.

FDA regulations require the collection of all adverse experiences whether or not they are considered to be drug-related. Causality is regarded as a separate entity. Skeggs and Doll (1977) present a strong case for the collection of all adverse events in clinical trials. They argue that if this method had been used in studies of practolol, the ocular toxicity of this drug might have been discovered before it was marketed.

1. Methods of Obtaining Adverse Experience Data

Adverse experience data may be collected either by an interviewer or through a self-administered questionnaire. Interviewer-administered questionnaires are used more often; however, self-administered questionnaires are commonly used in studies where the subjects are being treated for chronic pain (e.g., ulcers, angina). Each method has its advantages and disadvantages (see Bulpitt, 1983). With the self-administered questionnaire, the conditions under which the subject answers the questions are standardized; thus, interviewer bias is eliminated. However, the subject must be able to read and understand the questions. With interviewer-administered questions, the interviewer can sometimes tell when a question is not understood, and supply more information. Also, the completion rate for individual questions is likely to be higher with interviewer-administered questionnaires.

Two types of questioning may be used to elicit adverse experiences: an open-ended procedure or a check list. An advantage of the open-ended procedure is that it does not suggest side effects to the subject. However, as Grady (1976) pointed out, open-ended questions such as "How are you feeling today?" or "How you noticed any ill effects from the treatment?" do not indicate to the patients that they should mention all types of adverse experiences, such as vivid dreams, constipation, or loss of libido. Furthermore, subjects' responses, such as "I feel yukky," may be difficult to interpret clinically. The check list has the potential to elicit adverse experiences the subject had forgotten or considered unimportant.

Downing, Rickels, and Meyers (1970) and Huskisson and Wojtulewski (1974) analyzed the differences between the two methods. Both studies confirmed the findings of Greenblatt (1964) that more adverse experiences will be reported if a check list is used. Downing et al. concluded that the check list will elicit a greater number of drug-related adverse experiences than the open-ended procedure. However, Huskisson et al. found that the use of a check list interferes with the collection of adverse experiences by increasing the incidence of irrelevant complaints in both the treated and control groups. They further conclude that subjects are more likely to report adverse experiences not included in the check list if a check list is not used. Wallin and Sjovall (1981) recommend that the two methods be used in conjunction.

Responses to an open-ended adverse experience assessment procedure will need to be coded before they can be analysed. At present, various dictionaries (e.g., COSTART, DART, WHO, or hybrids of these) are used for this purpose by different pharmaceutical companies, although the need for consensus terminology is recognized (see Westland, 1982; Streichenwein and Blomer, 1982).

2. Length of Observation Period

Treatment-related adverse experiences may occur after the patient has stopped taking the study medication if the sequence of medical events leading to the adverse experience started during the treatment period. There are four choices for the length of time allowed for observation of adverse experiences (Shultz and Assenzo, 1982):

a. Include only adverse experiences that occur while the patient is taking the study drug. Since the drug may produce a delayed reaction, this is not an optimal choice. It is, however, frequently used in premarketing studies.
b. Include adverse experiences that occur while the patient is on the study drug and for a short prespecified interval afterward

(e.g., 10 blood-level half-lives). This includes all adverse experiences that occur while the drug is pharmacologically active, although some drug-related adverse experiences may not become observable until after this period. If the drug is withdrawn abruptly, adverse experiences observed after discontinuation of treatment may be due to withdrawal, rather than to delayed reactions. They may also be due to the recrudescence of the symptoms of the disorder the drug was intended to treat (Routledge, 1977).

c. Include all adverse experiences that occur during the protocol-specified study duration. For example, if the study is to last for 1 year, all adverse experiences that occur during the year are included regardless of how long the patients remain on treatment. This method is also frequently used in premarketing studies.

d. Include all adverse experiences, no matter how long they occur after the end of treatment. This method is likely to be used only for epidemiologic Phase IV studies.

Adverse experiences may also occur too early in the treatment phase to be treatment-related, for example, those that occur between randomization and the start of treatment, or shortly after treatment but before the drug has a chance to become pharmacologically active. There is no universally accepted procedure for handling such events; the method to be used must be specified before looking at the data, however. If the early adverse experiences are due to chance, their inclusion should not greatly affect the results of the study.

3. Collection of Concomitant Information

The investigator may collect data pertaining to any of the following aspects of a subject's adverse experiences: date and time of onset, pattern (i.e., isolated, intermittent, or continuous), duration, who reported it (i.e., subject and/or observer), severity, action taken, relationship to drug, or other relevant information. The interpretation to be used for each of these variables under a variety of possible circumstances must be specified before the study begins. It must be decided, for example, what duration to use for intermittent adverse experiences, or what date of onset to use if the onset was before the beginning of the assessment interval.

The severity of an adverse experience is often classified according to a three-point scale: mild, moderate, or severe. The term "severity" can be interpreted in at least two ways, however: (1) the degree of interference with the subject's ability to function normally, or (2) the intensity of the adverse experience relative to all other cases of the same experience the physician has seen. Thus it would be possible to rate a heart attack as "mild" according to the second interpretation, but not according to the first.

A judgment of the extent to which an adverse experience is drug-related usually depends on the temporal relationship between the administration of the drug and the appearance and disappearance of the experience, knowledge of the underlying disease, and knowledge of the pharmacological properties of the drug. There is some debate as to who should make this judgement: the physician, because of closeness to the patient, or the medical monitor, because of perspective for a wide range of adverse experiences across many studies of the drug. The degree of drug relationship, or causality, is often defined in terms of a five-point scale: not related, unlikely, possible, probable, and definite. Many investigators are hesitant to use either of the extreme classifications (Jones, 1982b). An adverse experience is likely to be considered "not related" only if its occurrence preceded the administration of the drug. Several authors have proposed algorithms for assigning causality in postmarketing monitoring so as to minimize the subjective aspects (e.g., Kramer et al., 1979; Karch and Lasagna, 1977). In these, the determination of "definite" drug relationship is linked to procedures such as dechallenge (withdrawal of the drug) and rechallenge (reintroduction of the drug). These procedures may not be feasible or ethical in a premarketing clinical trial.

G. Potential Sources of Bias

In this section, the difficulties of obtaining unbiased adverse experience information are discussed in general. Since one of the examples involves a clinical trial of an antidepressent (see Section V), the additional data-collection problems in trials of psychoactive drugs will also be discussed. Sources of bias in the collection of specific variables are discussed in Section II.

In any multicenter clinical trial, the centers will differ with respect to the populations from which they draw patients, diagnostic methods employed, and aspects of subject selection and study management not controlled by the protocol. In clinical trials using psychiatric patients, the investigator or center effect may be especially pronounced (Metzler and Schooley, 1981). Diagnosis of psychiatric disease is less straightforward than diagnosis of many other diseases (see Lal, Fielding, and Karkalas, 1975, for discussion of the problems of diagnosis and classification of clinical depression). Also, the response of psychiatric patients to medicine may depend heavily on environmental factors, as well as the therapeutic style of the investigator.

Two common sources of bias in clinical trials involve compliance in taking medicine and dropouts from study. Compliance is more of a problem with outpatients than inpatients (Calimlim and Weintraub, 1981), and both compliance and dropout problems may be more severe in subjects with psychiatric disorders, since they have more than the usual amount of difficulty in making decisions and following through with prescribed courses of action (Metzler and Schooley, 1981).

Dropouts may be due to efficacy (subject believes he is cured and so needs no more medication), lack of efficacy (why take a drug that is not doing any good?), spontaneous remission of disease, or adverse experiences. Dropouts due to lack of efficacy are a particular problem with the placebo group in longer studies. In fact, placebo recipients who fail to drop out (i.e., placebo responders) may create a problem with selection bias. Dropouts due to adverse experiences may cause important adverse experiences to be missed if the subjects drop out before the adverse experiences have been assessed.

The assessment of adverse experiences may be complicated by the similarity of the adverse experience to the symptoms of the disease and vice versa (see Vere, 1976). Infection, for example, may cause non-specific symptoms that mimic the side effects of the antimicrobial drug (Idanpaan-Heikkila, 1983). Busfield et al. (1962) noted that apparent side effects in depressed patients are often identical to the complaints they present prior to treatment, thus emphasizing the importance of baseline assessments (see also Beaumont, 1976). Behavioral toxicity in psychologically disturbed patients is particularly difficult to assess and to classify as desirable or adverse. A drug effect (e.g., mood suppression) may be be considered adverse for one patient and desirable for another, or valuable for treatment of a patient at one stage and harmful at another (Shader and DiMascio, 1970). Withdrawal symptoms may be extremely difficult to differentiate from the symptoms of underlying disease. Idanpaan-Heikkila mentions two studies in which the symptoms in healthy volunteers after the abrupt withdrawal of medication were similar to those observed in patients with psychoneurotic disorders.

The severity of a patient's disease may affect the ability to perceive or communicate an adverse experience. The relationship between the patient and the physician may also influence whether or not the patient reports a symptom, and how it is recorded (Bulpitt, 1983). Communication between the patients in a clinical trial may produce a "halo" effect, resulting in an epidemic-like spread of the reporting of an adverse experience (Lasagna, 1981).

Another potential source of bias is the unintentional "unblinding" of treatment in one or more patients due to the occurrence of adverse experiences that are characteristic of one of the treatments, or the necessity to decode due to an emergency situation. The recording of subsequent adverse experiences in these patients may be influenced by the knowledge or suspicion of their treatment. The patients, themselves, may care less about whether the study is blinded than about what treatment they are receiving. In some cases, outpatient subjects have had their medication analyzed to find out whether they were taking an active drug or a placebo.

II. STATISTICAL CONSIDERATIONS

Suzanne Edwards, Gary G. Koch, and William Sollecito

The choice of statistical methodology depends on the research question of interest, the sampling and measurement processes used to obtain the data, the target population to which conclusions are to be generalized, and the assumptions the analyst is willing to make in order to facilitate generalization from the study to the target population (see Koch, Gillings, and Stokes, 1980; Koch and Sollecito, 1984; Koch and Edwards, 1988). In this section, the data structure of adverse experience information, the types of research questions that can be addressed statistically, and the underlying assumptions and rationale for several alternative analysis strategies will be discussed.

A. Sampling Process Issues

In most clinical trials, neither the investigators nor the study subjects are chosen by random sampling methods. The investigators are usually specialists in the area being studied, and are chosen for their potential to provide good study management. The subjects are a convenience sample, chosen for their ability to satisfy the admission (inclusion/exclusion) criteria.

In Phase II and III studies, the drug is tested in subjects with the indication the drug is intended to treat. The following types of subjects are usually excluded:

1. Subjects unsuitable for ethical reasons (e.g., women of child-bearing potential).
2. Subjects at increased risk of adverse reactions (e.g., very old or young subjects, subjects with kidney or liver damage).
3. Subjects with characteristics (e.g., concomitant pathology) that could compromise determination of efficacy parameters.

4. Subjects having taken medication prior to the study that could affect the efficacy of the test drug or interact with it to produce adverse reactions.

In general, subjects who, for medical or social reasons, seem likely to provoke protocol deviations should also be excluded (Armitage, 1983), so that the number of protocol deviations can be kept to a minimum. The study may be further restricted to those with a particular set of medical characteristics (e.g., diagnosis, stage of disease), the only limitation on the restrictions being the availability of a large enough pool of subjects. In order for the drug's efficacy to be demonstrated, the subjects selected should be ill enough that substantial improvement is possible, but not so ill as to make response to any kind of medication unlikely.

The restrictiveness of the admission criteria affects the potential to detect treatment differences, the generalizability of the conclusions, and also the choice of analysis strategies (Koch and Gillings, 1982). The more exclusive the admission criteria, the more homogeneous the study population, and thus the greater the likelihood of detecting treatment-group differences if they exist. However, the conclusions obtained from a narrowly defined study population are applicable to only a small segment of the population of potential users of the drug. With less restrictive admission criteria (i.e., a more heterogeneous group of subjects), the increased variability of response variables may decrease the likelihood of detecting treatment differences, unless the sample size is increased. Also, more sophisticated methods of analysis (e.g., covariance adjustment or stratified analysis) may be necessary to ensure that the differences detected between treatment groups are due to the drug. However, the conclusions drawn from a study with broad coverage of the target population have a stronger basis for generalization.

Whereas the demonstration of efficacy may be made more efficient by narrowing the definition of the study population, for the demonstration of safety, generalizability is the overriding consideration. For the drug's safety profile to be established, the drug must be given to a broad spectrum (and large number) of patients. As discussed above, premarketing clinical trials exclude many types of subjects who may be potential users of the marketed drug.

Furthermore, the subjects in a clinical trial are selectively different in many respects from the population of patients who satisfy the admission criteria (see Friedman, Furberg, and DeMets, 1981, Chapter 3). One difference is socioeconomic status: clinical trial participants are usually not wealthy. As Chalmers (1982) pointed out, a physician who has received payment from a private patient for decisions regarding health care may feel uncomfortable about randomizing that patient to treatment. Another difference is severity of illness. Most trials are based in hospitals, often hospitals that are referral centers, so the patients who come to the attention of a study investigator may tend to be sicker than other patients with the same disorder. Many of the available patients may have already failed on existing therapies. Trials with an active control treatment tend to attract (via physician selection and patient self-selection) patients who are more severely ill then do placebo-controlled trials (Hadler and Gillings, 1983).

B. Measurement Process Issues

The measurement process includes consideration of the choice of variables to be measured, methods of obtaining the data, the form of data expression and structure, and the quality of the data. Ideally, data from which inferences are to be drawn should be relevant from a medical viewpoint, reliable (measurements of the same variable for an individual yield consistent values), and valid (measurements approximate the true value of the variable for the individual). A discussion of the adverse experience variables and concomitant data that may be collected and the possible methods of data collection is given in Section I. This section concerns the form of adverse experience data expression and structure, in particular, the construction of variables reflecting whether or not particular adverse experiences occurred, and, if so, their severity (in the sense of either seriousness or intensity), frequency, duration, and timing. Possible sources of ambiguity and measurement error are also discussed.

1. Occurrence/Nonoccurrence and Severity

At each assessment, the occurrence of adverse experiences during the previous interval is collected via a checklist, an open-ended procedure, or a combination of both. Dichotomous summary measures are often constructed by combining related adverse experiences (e.g., all neurological adverse experiences) or by combining over time. A commonly used statistical approach is to compare treatment groups with respect to the proportion of subjects who had a particular adverse experience, or any of a group of related ones, at least once during the treatment period.

As discussed in Section I, the set of adverse experiences reported in any clinical trial may fail to include all of those that are due to the pharmacological action of the drug (i.e., true ADRs), and may include some that are due to other factors but that have a physiological basis, as well as some that are due only to the power of suggestion. If a particular adverse experience was assessed via a checklist and was not reported, its nonoccurrence is more of a certainty than if it was not reported in response to an open-ended procedure. Regardless of the assessment procedure, some adverse experiences will fail to be reported due to reasons such as the state of the subject's health, memory, or rapport with the investigator.

Since many of the adverse experiences commonly reported are symptoms, rather than signs, and are thus observable only by the individuals in whom they occur, adverse experience data is inherently low in reliability and validity. A variety of terms may be used to denote the same experience, and any one term may denote different experiences to different individuals. The investigator must understand and record what the patient means and not just what he says. For example, when a patient reports that he is "tired," does he mean that he is fatigued, sleepy, weak, or lethargic?

After the adverse experience is reported by the patient, it is recorded, edited for data entry, possibly coded, and entered into a data base. Bias, as well as transcription errors, may be introduced at each step in this process. In extreme cases, the final version is qualitatively different from the original event. An example of this is as follows: a patient sees spots before eyes because of standing up too quickly; the investigator records "saw spots," and the event is coded "hallucination."

Determination of the severity of an adverse experience is made by the investigator on the basis of the patient's account of the experience, and by direct observations if the adverse experience is a sign. This judgment is necessarily subjective, and opinions may vary between investigators and within the same investigator over time.

Information pertaining to serious (i.e., potentially life-threatening or irreversible) adverse experiences is collected as soon as possible after they occur, rather than at at the next scheduled assessment. Adverse experiences that are not life-threatening or irreversible may also be considered serious, depending on the seriousness of the condition being treated. Patients having serious and unexpected adverse experiences are often removed from the study, and if the experiences are considered to be drug-related and are serious enough to outweigh the benefits from the drug, the study itself may be terminated.

Severity is often presented together with occurrence/nonoccurrence as one ordinal variable with categories such as none, mild, moderate, severe. If the subject had an adverse experience several times during the assessment interval, the severity of the most severe episode is usually recorded. A summary measure for the severity of a particular adverse experience during a trial is the severity of the most severe episode that occurred.

Ambiguity in the interpretation of both occurrence/nonoccurrence and severity arises when an adverse experience is reported by a patient during the treatment period but also at baseline. Although it is possible for a baseline adverse experience to disappear spontaneously and then to reappear due to the action of the drug, it is more likely that the baseline adverse experience continued into the treatment period, especially if it occurred shortly after the start of treatment. The drug may also cause a baseline adverse experience to become more (or less) severe during the treatment period, but a change in severity can also occur spontaneously.

A response variable that incorporates the baseline data can be constructed as follows. Using a scale of 0 = none, 1 = mild, 2 = moderate, and 3 = severe, subtract the baseline score from the treatment-period score. Values of −3 to 0, inclusive, indicate that either the adverse experience never occurred, or that it was equally or less severe at the treatment period assessment than at baseline. Values of +1 to +3 indicate that the adverse experience occurred for the first time during the treatment period, or that it was more severe during treatment than at baseline. Metzler and Schooley (1981) propose the use of this difference score in studies of psychoactive drugs as a way to separate the symptoms of the disease under study from potential side effects of the drug. Symptoms can be artificially defined as those adverse experiences that remained stable or improved from baseline (scores of −3 to 0), and side effects as those that showed a decrement (scores of +1 to +3). Other methods of incorporating baseline data are discussed in Sections IV and V.

2. Frequency, Duration, and Timing

Unless additional information about the overall frequency, duration, and timing of the adverse experiences of interest is collected at the time of the patient's termination from the trial, this information must be determined from the pattern of occurrence/nonoccurrence reported at the assessments. These determinations are complicated by the fact that an adverse experience may have occurred once, several times, or continuously in the interval preceding each of the assessments. So the number of times any one adverse experience is reported is not necessarily indicative of the number of times it occurred. For example, if a subject reports a particular adverse experience at each of four weekly assessments, he may have had four separate episodes, many episodes occurring intermittently throughout the trial, or only one episode, which continued into all four assessment intervals. Furthermore, the assessment intervals are usually not all the same length; assessments are often performed more frequently toward the beginning of the treatment period than toward the end.

One variable that can be used as a crude surrogate for both frequency and duration is the ratio of the number of assessments at which a subject reports a particular adverse experience to the number of assessments made for that subject. This measure is appropriate only if the assessments are equally spaced throughout the trial. An alternative measure is the ratio of the sum of the lengths of the assessment intervals for which a subject reported a particular adverse experience to that subject's length of time on trial. Neither of these variables truly reflects either frequency or duration, but they may be the most useful measures available.

Timing refers to when the adverse experience occurs relative to the start of treatment. Some adverse experiences may occur early in the study and then disappear as the patient's tolerance to the drug increases. Adverse experiences may also not appear until after a certain cumulative dose or length of time. One variable that reflects the timing is the time until the first occurrence of the adverse experience. Often, only the interval containing the first occurrence is known. Also, patients who leave the study early, for whatever reason, may not be at risk for developing delayed adverse reactions or available for the reporting of any that might occur.

Whether frequency/duration or timing is of more interest depends on what Riis (1982) calls the "signal-to-noise ratio" of the adverse experience under consideration. With adverse experiences such as headaches or drowsiness, which commonly occur spontaneously (i.e., low signal-to-noise ratio), it is of interest to determine whether the group treated with the test drug has increased frequency/duration relative to the background frequency/duration, which can be provided by a placebo control group. For adverse experiences with high signal-to-noise ratios (e.g., rash, convulsions) what is of primary interest is whether they occurred at all, and if so, how long after initiation of treatment. Serious adverse experiences, such as convulsions, are likely to occur only once before the patient is removed from the study.

C. Effect of Noncompliance to Protocol

For the purpose of comparison of treatments, the selection process must be the same for all subjects (for example, randomization to treatment), and patients must be managed uniformly and measured uniformly (for example, double-blindedness). However, substantial bias may still be introduced by failure of subjects or investigators to comply with the study protocol. The types of noncompliance can be classified (Koch and

Sollecito, 1984) as major protocol violations, minor protocol deviations, and incomplete data. Major protocol violations, which may have profound influence on patient response, include the following: inclusion of subjects not satisfying the admission criteria, subject noncompliance to the dosage regimen, subject usage of excluded concomitant medications, and investigator or subject awareness of the assigned treatment in double-blind studies. Minor protocol deviations, which can be regarded as random effects of the clinical testing environment, include variations in the timing of assessments or in the prescribed schedule of daily activities, when these variations do not affect the relevance of the data obtained. Incomplete data may be due to early withdrawal, missing assessments, or missing data values from an assessment.

A patient's willingness to comply with the protocol may be closely associated with other characteristics (Blum, 1982). For example, a tendency to drink alcohol excessively may affect a patient's compliance with the protocol, as well as prognosis, the benefit received from treatment, and/or the predisposition to adverse reactions. Conversely, prognosis and beneficial or adverse reactions to treatment also affect compliance. An example of the possible association between compliance and response was shown in the analysis of the Coronary Drug Project (Canner, 1979). Patients in both the active and placebo groups who faithfully followed the treatment regimen had significantly longer survival times than those who did not.

Since compliance influences response and vice versa, and patient characteristics influence both compliance and response, bias is introduced if the types of subjects not complying to the protocol or the reasons for noncompliance differ between the treatment groups. Special analysis may be warranted to assess the nature of the noncompliance and its impact on treatment-group comparability (see Koch and Sollecito, 1984).

There is no way to know the direction or extent of bias in response variables from noncompliance (or to know the true values in the case of missing data). However, exclusion of noncompliant subjects from the analyses also introduces bias. DeMets, Friedman, and Furberg (1980) and Armitage (1983) recommend that all randomized subjects be included in all primary analyses, unless it is clear that no bias is introduced by their exclusion (see Sackett and Gent, 1979, for a more lenient viewpoint). The exclusion of patients may be admissible in supplementary safety analyses if the direction of the resulting bias is such as to put the test drug at a disadvantage. For example, patients who never received any of their assigned treatment are often excluded from analyses.

D. Statistical Analysis Issues

In most Phase II and III clinical trials, the evaluation of efficacy is the primary research objective, and thus the study design, length and size of study, and admission criteria are geared to assessing whether or not the drug works. However, a research design that provides an appropriate framework for efficacy testing is likely to be inadequate for the evaluation of safety in several respects. Two shortcomings are lack of generalizability due to protocol-specified exclusions (see Section II.A) and insufficient sample size; the implications of both of these on the statistical analysis of adverse experiences are discussed in subsequent sections.

In general, statistical significance testing for safety data is far less straightforward than for efficacy data. As pointed out by Friedman, Furberg, and DeMets (1981, Chapter 2), it is not always possible to specify the research questions in advance of seeing the data, because which adverse experiences occur, and their severity, may be unpredictable. Furthermore, when many adverse experiences are monitored in a single study, the problem of multiple inference becomes an issue. In order to have enough events to make statistical analysis worthwhile, adverse experiences must often be grouped in some way (e.g., by body system). Although this may lessen the multiple inference problem and improve statistical power, it also results in a loss of information. Rigorous, convincing statistical analysis of serious adverse experiences is rarely possible because once a test drug is suspected of having an unfavorable risk-benefit ratio, it is generally considered unethical to continue to expose trial subjects to it.

1. Implications of Sample Size and Study Length

Ethical as well as economic considerations dictate that as few subjects be exposed to the test drug as are necessary to answer the primary research question (efficacy). For a drug to be considered efficacious, a relatively large difference between treatment groups is usually required. For safety analyses, however, if suspected side effects are serious, then small differences between treatment groups are clinically relevant, and a much larger sample is required to detect such differences (Lachin, 1982a). Also, large sample sizes are necessary to detect treatment-group differences with respect to the incidence of rare adverse experiences.

Since the study sample size is likely to be smaller than desired from a safety analysis perspective, statistical analysis methods should be chosen partly for their ability to optimize power. Some discussion of the power of the statistical tests used to detect treatment group differences should be presented when the results are negative (i.e., no treatment-group difference). Hadler and Gillings (1983) suggest that the minimum incidence level of adverse reactions that can be identified by a study, given the size of the drug group, should also be specified.

Methods for calculating sample sizes for clinical trials are given by Halperin et al. (1968), Lachin (1981), and Donner (1984), among others. Lachin (1979) provides a discussion of sample size considerations with reference to Phase II–III clinical trials of potentially hepatotoxic drugs. A discussion of the sample sizes needed for postmarketing surveillance is given by Lewis (1981), who provides tables of the necessary size for the treated group under various conditions. His calculations are based on the expected incidence of the adverse reaction, the desired significance level, and the background incidence. When the adverse reaction is quite unusual (i.e., no background incidence), only a few cases are necessary to provide sufficient proof of potential danger. With increasing levels of background incidence, there is a corresponding increase in the sample sizes required. Sample size calculations, allowing for background incidence, also depend on the size of the control group relative to the treated group and the additional incidence of the adverse reaction due to treatment. Even larger sample sizes are needed for studies in which many adverse reactions are monitored simultaneously.

Given the near impossibility of detecting rare adverse reactions in premarketing trials, Hadler and Gillings (1983) recommend (in the context of rheumatoid arthritis trials) restricting consideration of safety factors in Phase III trials to those having a given expected incidence, and deferring investigation of rarer adverse reactions to formalized Phase IV studies. They also propose curtailing the length of Phase III studies (recommendation: 6 months for rheumatoid arthritis trials) and relying more heavily on Phase IV for detection of delayed adverse reactions.

Idanpaan-Heikkila (1983) conducted a study for the FDA to explore the role of Phase III studies in providing relevant safety information. Specific objectives included (1) study of what adverse effects were uncovered in long-term drug exposure (greater than 6 months) that were not observed during short-term or medium-term exposure, (2) study of what adverse experiences were uncovered in the second 500 or so patients receiving short-term therapy that were not uncovered in the first 500 patients, and (3) investigation of the timing of Phases I–II and III. The recommendations from this study included the extension of appropriate Phase II trials for collection of medium-term and long-term safety data while conducting Phase III, and the extension of the short-term Phase III trials rather than expansion of the short-term subject population.

Idanpaan-Heikkila also recommended the use of survival data

analysis methods, such as life tables, for the presentation of safety results. The importance of such analyses has been discussed further by O'Neill (1988). A commonly used method for summarizing adverse experience data has been the ratio of the number of subjects having a particular adverse experience to the total number treated with the test drug. This crude proportion is determined from subjects who are treated for varying lengths of time, including some subjects who might have had adverse reactions but were not in the study long enough for their development or observation. Thus, the crude proportion is likely to be much lower than a life-table estimated probability of adverse experience, and, based on the crude proportion, the drug may appear to be safer than it actually is.

Provided that the assumptions for its use are met, a life-table approach can account for changes in the rate of adverse experiences over time, and can appropriately handle the problem of incomplete data from subjects who drop out or are withdrawn. As previously discussed, the time to first occurrence of a particular adverse experience may be of more interest for some adverse experiences than others. Survival data analysis methods are used in the analysis of the example in Section VI.

2. Implications of Choice of Control Group

By law, the sponsor of a new drug does not have to show the drug to be better in any way than the existing forms of treatment. Therefore, in the United States, placebo-controlled trials, where ethical, are used most often to provide the primary evidence of efficacy. There are also compelling reasons to use active-controlled trials (Hsu, 1983). Both clinicians and patients may be more easily recruited for studies in which the patient is to receive either an approved drug or one with the potential to be approved. Also, blinding is more effectively maintained in active-controlled studies, and fewer patients are likely to withdraw due to lack of efficacy. However, there are substantial difficulties in the evaluation of efficacy in active-controlled trials (see Temple, 1983), some of which may be avoided by the use of both an active and a placebo control group.

With respect to the evaluation of adverse experiences, it is more straightforward to compare the test drug to placebo, rather than to another active treatment, which may have its own associated side effects, unless the absence of a particular side effect is one of the main selling points of the new drug. Another complication in the comparison of two active drugs is that the relative incidence of true adverse reactions depends on the relative doses. This is, of course, not the case with placebo control.

One way in which the choice of control group can affect the statistical analysis is by influencing the degree to which necessary assumptions seem reasonable. For example, in survival data analysis, one must sometimes assume that withdrawal is unrelated to treatment. If one of the groups is receiving an effective treatment and the other is receiving placebo, this assumption may not be valid.

3. Generalizability Considerations

Given that neither clinics nor subjects within clinics are selected by probability sampling, and that study subjects are not representative of the population of potential users of the marketed drug, or even of the population of individuals satisfying the admission criteria for the geographic region(s) covered by the clinic(s), the subjects in a clinical trial may not be representative of any well-defined target population. If assumptions that would extend inference to a general target population are controversial, then design-based inference (using, e.g., nonparametric randomization-based methods) may be more effective than model-based inference (see Koch and Gillings, 1983).

Nonparametric randomization-based methods (e.g., Fisher's exact test, the Mantel–Haenszel test) require no assumptions other than the randomization of subjects to treatment groups and the integrity of the measurement process. However, the conclusions drawn apply only to those subjects who were actually randomized. Furthermore, randomization-based methods are primarily used for hypothesis testing. Other methods must be used for confidence-interval construction and estimation of relationships.

Model-based methods may be used if the study subjects are considered to be conceptually equivalent to a (possibly stratified) simple random sample of some larger population. Assumed probability models can be used to describe the relationship of the response variable to explanatory variables such as treatment, investigator, and pretreatment subjects' characteristics. The choice of models depends on the measurement scale of the response variable. An example of a well-known model-based method for the analysis of continuous response variables is multiple linear regression. For adverse experience data, the response variables to be considered here are either dichotomous (e.g., occurrence/nonoccurrence), discrete ordinal (e.g., severity), counts or rates (e.g., the number of assessments at which an adverse experience is reported, the number of adverse experiences per unit of exposure), or the time to the first occurrence of an adverse experience.

The advantages of model-based methods over design-based methods include (Koch and Sollecito, 1984) more powerful analysis through reduced variance, the capacity to assess the homogeneity of effects for responses across strata, and the capacity to adjust for explanatory variables that are not equivalently distributed for the treatment groups. Although randomization-based methods may also be used to adjust for possible nonequivalence of the treatment groups via stratification on the variables for which the treatment groups are not comparable, model-based methods may incorporate a larger number of (possibly continuous) such variables. The disadvantages of model-based methods are that they may be more difficult to implement, interpret, and explain to non-statisticians than are design-based methods. Also, since the assumptions necessary for model-based methods cannot be proven, the results of such analyses are more likely to be subject to debate. A reasonable strategy is thus to use both design-based and model-based methods in combination.

III. STATISTICAL METHODOLOGY

Suzanne Edwards, Gary G. Koch, and William Sollecito

In this section the statistical theory is presented for the primary design and model-based methods used in the examples of Sections IV–VII. Methods of analysis for summary variables relating to adverse experience occurrence, severity, and frequency/duration are presented, as well as survival data analysis methods for the analysis of time to first adverse experience. Software used for the implementation of the methods in this chapter is also referenced.

A. The Mantel–Haenszel Method and Extensions

The method of Mantel and Haenszel (1959) is one of the most well-known design-based methods of analysis in clinical trials. It can be used to provide a test of treatment differences with respect to a dichotomous response variable (e.g., occurrence/nonoccurrence of adverse experiences), combined over strata (e.g., centers in a multicenter trial), and adjusted for the effect of the stratification variables. When the response variable has consistently higher values for one treatment than another across strata, the Mantel–Haenszel procedure has a greater power than an unstratified chi-square statistic. Some caution in the use of this statistic is necessary, however, when the pattern of treatment differences varies across strata.

Mantel (1963) proposed an extension of the Mantel–Haenszel procedure to the analysis of a set of $(2 \times r)$ tables; further discussion of such extensions for $(s \times r)$ tables is given by Landis et al. (1978) and Kuritz, Landis, and Koch (1988). When the r response categories are ordinarily scaled (as for severity), various scores can be assigned to the responses, and the test statistics can thus be based on the resulting mean score.

When the s subpopulations (treatment groups) are ordinally scaled as well (say, for treatment groups of placebo, low dose, and high dose), a correlation-type statistic can be used. A discussion of alternative scoring techniques is given in Landis et al. (1979) and Koch and Edwards (1988).

A further generalization of the Mantel–Haenszel strategy allows the analysis of case-record data, using univariate or multivariate response variables, and allowing explanatory variables to be used as either stratification variables or covariables. The methodology for these randomization statistics is presented in some detail in the next three subsections. Univariate and multivariate randomization statistics methodology is presented in Section III.A.1, covariate adjustment is presented in Section III.A.2, and stratification adjustment is presented in Section III.A.3.

Both stratification and covariate adjustment may be used to clarify the degree to which differences between treatment groups are due to treatment. Variables for which the treatment groups are comparable may be used as covariables. These variables may be either categorical or continuous, and no assumptions need be made regarding the relationship of the covariables to the response variable. Variables that are not randomized when patients are randomized to treatment groups (e.g., center, season of enrollment) and variables for which the treatment groups are not comparable may be used as stratification variables. If these variables are continuous, they must first be categorized. Disadvantages of analyses with stratification and covariate adjustment (Koch and Sollecito, 1984) include their increased complexity in terms of implementation and interpretation, and their greater susceptibility to controversy, arising from the choice of stratification variables and covariables.

The methodology presented in the next three subsections is a synthesis of the material presented in Koch and Bhapkar (1982), Koch, Amara, Davis, and Gillings (1982), and Amara (1983). The principal software used in this chapter for the implementation of this methodology is the FREQ Procedure of SAS Institute, Inc. (1985) and a related macro documented in Amara and Koch (1980).

1. Unadjusted Randomization Statistics for Case Record Data

Let y_{ik} denote the observed value of the response variable of interest for the k-th subject ($k = 1, 2, \ldots, n_i$) in the i-th subpopulation ($i = 1, 2, \ldots, s$). In the applications covered herein, i typically corresponds to treatment group, of which there are two, the experimental group and the control group, so $s = 2$. Each of the s subpopulations is of size n_i so that

$\sum_{i=1}^{s} n_i = n$, the total sample size. The question of investigation is the extent to which there is an association between the response variable and the subpopulations. If subjects are randomly assigned to subpopulations, between which there is no difference in effect, then the subset of observed response values for any subpopulation should be equivalent to a simple random sample from the set of n response values. This argument gives rise to the randomization hypothesis of no assocation:

> H_0: There is no association between the response variable and the subpopulations in the sense that the observed partition of the response values, y_{ik}, into s subpopulations can be regarded as equivalent to a successive set of simple random samples of sizes $n_1, n_2, \ldots, n_s$.

The hypothesis H_0 can be tested by assessing the compatibility of the data for the subpopulations with their expected values under a randomization sampling process. Let

$$\bar{y}_i = (1/n_i) \sum_{k=1}^{n_i} y_{i1}/n_i$$

denote the mean response value for the i-th subpopulation. Then, under H_0, the expected value for $\bar{y}_i$ is

$$E\{\bar{y}_i \mid H_0\} = \bar{y} = \sum_{i=1}^{s} \sum_{k=1}^{n_i} y_{ik}/n$$

that is, the pooled subpopulation mean, and the covariance structure is

$$\text{Cov}\{\bar{y}_i, \bar{y}_{i'} \mid H_0\} = \{v/(n-1)\}\{(n\delta_{ii'}/n_i) - 1\} \tag{2.1}$$

where $\delta_{ii'} = 1$ if $i = i'$ and $\delta_{ii'} = 0$ otherwise, and

$$v = \left\{\sum_{i=1}^{s} \sum_{k=1}^{n_i} (y_{ik} - \bar{y})^2\right\} \Big/ n$$

denotes the finite population variance.

If the subpopulation sample sizes $n_1, n_2, \ldots, n_s$ are sufficiently large, then randomization central limit theory (see Puri and Sen, 1971) can be used to construct a chi-square test statistic:

$$\begin{aligned} Q &= \bar{\mathbf{y}}'\mathbf{C}'[\mathbf{C}\,\mathbf{Cov}\,\mathbf{C}']^{-1}\mathbf{C}\bar{\mathbf{y}} \\ &= \{(n-1)/nv\}\bar{\mathbf{y}}'\mathbf{C}'[\mathbf{C}\mathbf{D}_n^{-1}\mathbf{C}']^{-1}\mathbf{C}\bar{\mathbf{y}} \end{aligned} \tag{2.2}$$

where $\bar{\mathbf{y}} = (\bar{y}_1, \bar{y}_2, \ldots, \bar{y}_s)'$ is the vector of subpopulation means, **Cov** has the structure given in (2.1), $\mathbf{D_n}$ is a diagonal matrix with $n_1, n_2, \ldots, n_s$ on the diagonal, and $\mathbf{C} = [\mathbf{I}_{(s-1)}, -\mathbf{1}_{(s-1)}]$ is a contrast matrix, where $\mathbf{I}_{(s-1)}$ is the $(s-1)$-th order identity matrix, and $\mathbf{1}_{(s-1)}$ is an $(s-1) \times 1$ vector of ones. Q has, asymptotically, a chi-square distribution with $(s-1)$ degrees of freedom.

Expression (2.2) can be shown to be equal to

$$Q = \{(n-1)/nv\} \sum_{i=1}^{s} n_i(\bar{y}_i - \bar{y})^2 \tag{2.3}$$

by use of the matrix lemma given in Koch and Bhapkar (1982). Since expression (2.3) involves the ratio of between subpopulations sum of squares to total sum of squares, Q can be interpreted as a one-way analysis of variance statistic. When the $\{y_{ik}\}$ are dichotomous, $nQ/(n-1)$ is the Pearson chi-square statistic for the $(s \times 2)$ contingency table from the subpopulation versus response classification, and when the $\{y_{ik}\}$ are ranks, Q is the Kruskal–Wallis statistic.

An analogous chi-square statistic can be formulated to test the association between the subpopulations and a multivariate set of d response variables. Let $\mathbf{y}_{ik} = \{y_{ijk}\} = \{y_{i1k}, y_{i2k}, \ldots, y_{idk})'$ denote the $(d \times 1)$ response vectors, and let

$$\bar{\mathbf{y}}_i = \{\bar{y}_{ij}\} = (\bar{y}_{i1}, \bar{y}_{i2}, \ldots, \bar{y}_{id})' \tag{2.4}$$

denote the observed mean vector for the i-th subpopulation. Then, under the multivariate version of H_0, the expected value vector for $\bar{\mathbf{y}}_i$ is

$$E\{\bar{\mathbf{y}}_i \mid H_0\} = \bar{\mathbf{y}}_* = \{\bar{y}_j\} = (\bar{y}_{*1}, \bar{y}_{*2}, \ldots, \bar{y}_{*d})' \tag{2.5}$$

which is the pooled sample mean vector, and the covariance structure can be expressed as

$$\mathbf{Cov}\{\bar{\mathbf{y}}_i, \bar{\mathbf{y}}_{i'} \mid H_0\} = \{\mathbf{V}/(n-1)\}\{(n\delta_{ii'}/n_i) - 1\}$$

where

$$\mathbf{V} = (1/n) \sum_{i=1}^{s} \sum_{k=1}^{n_i} [(\mathbf{y}_{ik} - \bar{\mathbf{y}}_*)(\mathbf{y}_{ik} - \bar{\mathbf{y}}_*)'] \tag{2.6}$$

The chi-square test statistic is

$$Q = \{(n-1)/n\} \left\{ \sum_{i=1}^{s} n_i(\bar{\mathbf{y}}_i - \bar{\mathbf{y}}_*)'\mathbf{V}^{-1}(\bar{\mathbf{y}}_i - \bar{\mathbf{y}}_*)\right\} \tag{2.7}$$

where **V** is given in expression (2.6). If the subpopulation sizes are sufficiently large (e.g., at least 20), Q has a chi-square distribution with $d(s-1)$ degrees of freedom. In this regard, when the $\{y_{ijk}\}$ are d dichotomous indicators for any d of the outcomes of a categorical variable with $(d+1)$ possible outcomes, $nQ/(n-1)$ is the Pearson chi-square for the $s \times (d+1)$ contingency table from the subpopulation versus response classification.

2. Covariate-Adjusted Randomization Statistics

As an extension of the notation in the previous section, let $\mathbf{x}_{ik}$ denote the $(t \times 1)$ vector of covariables associated with the k-th subject in the i-th subpopulation. Let $\bar{\mathbf{x}}_i = (\bar{x}_{i1}, \bar{x}_{i2}, \ldots, \bar{x}_{it})'$ denote the mean covariable vector for the i-th subpopulation and let $\bar{\mathbf{x}}_* = (\bar{x}_{*1}, \bar{x}_{*2}, \ldots, \bar{x}_{*t})'$ be the pooled subpopulation mean covariable vector. Then the multivariate randomization test statistic given in (2.7) can be rewritten so as to differentiate the response variables from covariables as follows:

$$Q(\mathbf{y}, \mathbf{x}) = \{(n-1)/n\} \sum_{i=1}^{s} n_i[(\bar{\mathbf{y}}_i - \bar{\mathbf{y}}_*)', (\bar{\mathbf{x}}_i - \bar{\mathbf{x}}_*)'] \begin{bmatrix} \mathbf{V}_y & \mathbf{V}'_{xy} \\ \mathbf{V}_{xy} & \mathbf{V}_x \end{bmatrix}^{-1} \begin{bmatrix} \bar{\mathbf{y}}_i - \bar{\mathbf{y}}_* \\ \bar{\mathbf{x}}_i - \bar{\mathbf{x}}_* \end{bmatrix}$$

where

$$\begin{bmatrix} \mathbf{V}_y & \mathbf{V}'_{xy} \\ \mathbf{V}_{xy} & \mathbf{V}_x \end{bmatrix} = (1/n) \left\{ \sum_{k=1}^{n} \begin{bmatrix} (\mathbf{y}_{ik} - \bar{\mathbf{y}}_*) \\ (\mathbf{x}_{ik} - \bar{\mathbf{x}}_*) \end{bmatrix} [(\bar{\mathbf{y}}_{ik} - \bar{\mathbf{y}}_*)', (\mathbf{x}_{ik} - \bar{\mathbf{x}}_*)'] \right\}$$

$Q(\mathbf{y}, \mathbf{x})$ has asymptotically a chi-square distribution with $(d+t)(s-1)$ degrees of freedom.

Under the (joint) multivariate randomization hypothesis of no association, $Q(\mathbf{y}, \mathbf{x})$ can be partitioned into two independent components,

$$\begin{aligned} Q(\mathbf{y}, \mathbf{x}) &= Q(\mathbf{x}) + \{Q(\mathbf{y}, \mathbf{x}) - Q(\mathbf{x})\} \\ &= Q(\mathbf{x}) + Q(\mathbf{y} \mid \mathbf{x}) \end{aligned}$$

where $Q(\mathbf{x})$ [which has the form of (2.7) with $\mathbf{x}$ and $\mathbf{V}_x$ substituted for $\mathbf{y}$ and $\mathbf{V}$] is the multivariate statistic for testing the randomization hypothesis for the covariables.

If the randomization hypothesis for the covariables is true, $Q(\mathbf{y} \mid \mathbf{x})$ can be interpreted as a covariate-adjusted test statistic that has approximately a chi-square distribution with $d(s-1)$ degrees of freedom. $Q(\mathbf{y} \mid \mathbf{x})$ can be shown [by the matrix lemma given in Koch and Bhapkar (1982)] to have the form

$$Q(\mathbf{y}\,|\,\mathbf{x}) = \{(n-1)/n\}\left\{\sum_{i=1}^{s} n_i \bar{\mathbf{g}}_i' \mathbf{V}_g^{-1} \bar{\mathbf{g}}_i\right\}$$

where

$$\bar{\mathbf{g}}_i = (\bar{\mathbf{y}}_i - \bar{\mathbf{y}}_*) - \mathbf{V}_{xy}' \mathbf{V}_x^{-1}(\bar{\mathbf{x}}_i - \bar{\mathbf{x}}_*)$$

and

$$\mathbf{V}_g = \mathbf{V}_y - \mathbf{V}_{xy}' \mathbf{V}_x^{-1} \mathbf{V}_{xy} \tag{2.8}$$

This form of the statistic shows $Q(\mathbf{y}\,|\,\mathbf{x})$ to be a multivariate randomization statistic like (2.7) with respect to the residuals

$$\mathbf{g}_{ik} = (\mathbf{y}_{ik} - \bar{\mathbf{y}}_*) - \mathbf{V}_{xy}' \mathbf{V}_x^{-1}(\mathbf{x}_{ik} - \bar{\mathbf{x}}_*)$$

of a pooled sample set of multiple regressions of the $\mathbf{y}_{ik}$ on the $\mathbf{x}_{ik}$. $Q(\mathbf{y}\,|\,\mathbf{x})$ is thus analogous to the rank analysis of covariance methods of Quade (1967).

The randomization hypothesis for the covariables should be verified via the statistic $Q(\mathbf{x})$. If the hypothesis is rejected, it may indicate an imbalance in the allocation of subjects to subpopulations, thus implying that the randomization model framework is possibly not appropriate for the analysis of the response variables. In this case, poststratification on the covariable(s) may be used to reduce the imbalance. If, however, $Q(\mathbf{x})$ is significant with respect to covariables whose values were known prior to randomization, and the randomization is assumed to have been properly conducted, then the randomization model framework may still be considered appropriate.

The primary rationale for the covariate-adjusted statistic $Q(\mathbf{y}\,|\,\mathbf{x})$ is that it can be viewed as providing adjustments that induce equivalence of the subpopulations with respect to the covariables, and thus subpopulation differences with respect to the response variables can be attributed more definitely to subpopulation effects rather than partially to random imbalances in the covariables. The covariate-adjusted statistic $Q(\mathbf{y}\,|\,\mathbf{x})$ may also be more significant than its unadjusted counterpart $Q(\mathbf{y})$ due to a more precise covariance structure. However, the tendency for $Q(\mathbf{y}\,|\,\mathbf{x})$ to be larger than $Q(\mathbf{y})$ is partly a random event depending on the tendency for subjects with "less favorable" covariable status (i.e., likely to have less favorable response) to be assigned to the "more favorable" subpopulation.

3. Stratification-Adjusted Randomization Statistics

Let $h = 1, 2, \ldots, q$ index a set of strata for some partition of the n subjects. The hypothesis of no association between the responses and the subpopulations that takes stratification into account (i.e., the randomization hypothesis of no partial association, H_{0P}) is the same as the randomization hypothesis H_0, or its multivariate counterpart, expressed for each of the q strata simultaneously.

One method for testing H_{0P} involves average partial association statistics, which are extensions of those of Mantel and Haenszel (1959) and Mantel (1963). Let the sample size of the i-th subpopulation in the h-th stratum be denoted by n_{hi} so that $\sum_{i=1}^{s} n_{hi} = n_h$. Let $\bar{\mathbf{y}}_{hi}$, $\bar{\mathbf{y}}_{h*}$, and $\mathbf{V}_h$ denote the h-th stratum counterparts of $\bar{\mathbf{y}}_i$, $\bar{\mathbf{y}}_*$, and $\mathbf{V}$ in (2.4), (2.5), and (2.6), respectively. Let

$$\mathbf{F}_i = \sum_{h=1}^{q} n_{hi}\bar{\mathbf{y}}_{hi}$$

denote the vector of across strata sums of the response vectors for the i-th subpopulation. The expected value and variance structure for $\mathbf{F} = (\mathbf{F}_1', \mathbf{F}_2', \ldots, \mathbf{F}_s')'$ can be expressed as

$$\mathbf{E}\{\mathbf{F} \mid H_{0P}\} = \sum_{h=1}^{q} \mathbf{I}_d \otimes \mathbf{D}_{\mathbf{n}_h}\bar{\mathbf{y}}_{h*}$$

and

$$\mathbf{Var}\{\mathbf{F} \mid H_{0P}\} = \sum_{h=1}^{q} [n_h^2/(n_h - 1)]\{\mathbf{V}_h \otimes [\mathbf{D}_{\mathbf{P}_h} - \mathbf{P}_h\mathbf{P}_h']\}$$

where $\mathbf{n}_h = (n_{h1}, n_{h2}, \ldots, n_{hs})$, $\otimes$ denotes left Kronecker product multiplication, and

$$\mathbf{P}_h = (P_{h1}, P_{h2}, \ldots, P_{hs})' = (1/n_h)(n_{h1}, n_{h2}, \ldots, n_{hs})'$$

The average partial association chi-square test statistic has the form

$$Q_G = \mathbf{G}'\mathbf{V}_\mathbf{G}^{-1}\mathbf{G}$$

where

$$\mathbf{G} = (\mathbf{I}_d \otimes \mathbf{C})(\mathbf{F} - \mathbf{E}\{\mathbf{F} \mid H_{0P}\})$$
$$\mathbf{V}_\mathbf{G} = (\mathbf{I}_d \otimes \mathbf{C})(\mathbf{Var}\{\mathbf{F} \mid H_{0P}\})(\mathbf{I}_d \otimes \mathbf{C})'$$

such that $\mathbf{I}_d$ denotes a $(d \times d)$ identity matrix, and $\mathbf{C} = [\mathbf{I}_{(s-1)}, -\mathbf{I}_{(s-1)}]$. Under H_{0P}, Q_G has an approximate chi-square distribution with $d(s-1)$ degrees of freedom, provided that the across-strata subpopulation sample sizes, $n_{+i} = \sum_{h=1}^{q} n_{hi}$, are sufficiently large. When $d = 1$ and the $\{y_{ik}\}$ are dichotomous, Q_G is the Mantel–Haenszel statistic; in other cases, it is an extended Mantel–Haenszel statistic.

The covariate-adjustment methods of the preceding section can be used to formulate covariate-adjusted stratification statistics. Let

$$\mathbf{g}_{hik} = (\mathbf{y}_{hik} - \bar{\mathbf{y}}_{h*}) - \mathbf{V}_{h,xy}\mathbf{V}_{h,x}^{-1}(\mathbf{x}_{hik} - \bar{\mathbf{x}}_{h*})$$

denote the within stratum residual vectors. Let

$$\bar{\mathbf{g}}_h = (\bar{g}_{h11}, \ldots, \bar{g}_{h1d}, \ldots, \bar{g}_{hs1}, \ldots, \bar{g}_{hsd})'$$

denote the vector of mean residuals for responses within subpopulations for stratum h. The vector

$$\mathbf{g} = \sum_{h=1}^{q} [n_h \mathbf{I}_d \otimes \mathbf{D}_{\mathbf{P}_h}] \bar{\mathbf{g}}_h$$

(where $\mathbf{P}_h = \{n_{hi}/n_h\}$, for $i = 1, 2, \ldots, s$) is a vector of across-strata sums of the residuals for each of the response measures within subpopulations. Under H_{0P}, this vector has expected value $\mathbf{0}_{(s\times d)}$ and variance

$$\mathbf{Var}(\mathbf{g} \mid H_{0P}) = \sum_{h=1}^{q} [n_h^2/(n_h - 1)]\{\mathbf{V}_{h,g} \otimes [\mathbf{D}_{\mathbf{P}_h} - \mathbf{P}_h \mathbf{P}'_h]\}$$

where $\mathbf{V}_{h,g}$ is the h-th stratum counterpart to (2.8).

A $d(s-1)$-th order vector of contrasts can be formulated as $\mathbf{f} = [\mathbf{I}_d \otimes \mathbf{C}]\mathbf{g}$. The covariate-adjusted stratification statistic is then

$$Q_G(\mathbf{y} \mid \mathbf{x}) = \mathbf{f}'\{[\mathbf{I}_d \otimes \mathbf{C}][\mathbf{Var}(\mathbf{g} \mid H_{0P})][\mathbf{I}_d \otimes \mathbf{C}]'\}^{-1}\mathbf{f}$$

which is asymptotically distributed as a chi-square with $d(s-1)$ degrees of freedom when the overall sample sizes n_{+i} are sufficiently large.

An alternative covariance-adjusted stratification statistic, formulated from the difference of two average partial association statistics, is

$$Q_G^*(\mathbf{y} \mid \mathbf{x}) = Q_G(\mathbf{y}, \mathbf{x}) - Q_G(\mathbf{x})$$

$Q_G(\mathbf{y}, \mathbf{x})$ the joint multivariate chi-square statistic for the responses and covariances, has $(d+t)(s-1)$ degrees of freedom, and $Q_G(\mathbf{x})$, the chi-square statistic for the covariates, has $t(s-1)$ degrees of freedom, so $Q_G^*(\mathbf{y}\,|\,\mathbf{x})$ has $(d+t)(s-1)-t(s-1)=d(s-1)$ degrees of freedom. This alternative statistic is not an extension of the Mantel–Haenszel strategy, and its properties are not well known. However, it usage may be preferable to $Q_G(\mathbf{y}\,|\,\mathbf{x})$ when some of the $\mathbf{V}_{h,x}$ are singular, or when there is a large number of strata each with small sample sizes. Additional discussion of covariance-adjusted stratification statistics like $Q_G(\mathbf{y}\,|\,\mathbf{x})$ and an illustrative example are given in Koch, Carr et al. (1989).

B. Exact Tests

Often the most salient feature of adverse experience data is that each of the adverse experiences reported occurs in a small number of patients. The sample sizes for the treatment groups may also be relatively small. A commonly used rule for the suitability of the Pearson chi-square test to a fourfold table such as the following

	Adverse experience		
Treatment	Yes	No	
Experimental	n_{11}	n_{12}	n_{1+}
Control	n_{21}	n_{22}	n_{2+}
	n_{+1}	n_{+2}	n

is that the expected value, $m_{ij}=n_{i+}n_{+j}/n$, for all cells should exceed 5.0. An alternative to the chi-square test when cell counts are small is Fisher's exact test. Given that the marginals for the observed table are fixed, then if there is no difference between the treatments with respect to adverse experience incidence, the probability of a given cell is given by the hypergeometric distribution, that is,

$$\Pr\{n_{ij}\,|\,H_0\}=\frac{n_{1+}!\,n_{2+}!\,n_{+1}!\,n_{+2}!}{n!\,n_{11}!\,n_{12}!\,n_{21}!\,n_{22}!}$$

The p value for Fisher's (two-sided) exact test can be found by enumerating all tables with the same marginals as the observed table, calculating the probability of each, and then summing the probabilities of those tables that are equally or less likely than the observed table.

For $r\times c$ tables, the principle is the same, but the probabilities are calculated using the multiple hypergeometric distribution. Pagano and

Halvorsen (1981) and Mehta and Patel (1983) have developed algorithms for calculating the exact significance levels of $r \times c$ tables that are computationally faster than previously proposed algorithms because they do not require total enumeration of the tables.

For a set of fourfold tables, such as

	Adverse experience		
Treatment	Yes	No	
Experimental	n_{h11}	n_{h12}	n_{h1+}
Control	n_{h21}	n_{h22}	n_{h2+}
	n_{h+1}	n_{h+2}	n_h

for $h = 1, 2, \ldots, q$, the Mantel–Haenszel statistic may be appropriate even if the within-stratum sample sizes are small, as long as the combined stratum sample sizes

$$n_{+1+} = \sum_{h=1}^{q} n_{h1+} \quad \text{and} \quad n_{+2+} = \sum_{h=1}^{q} n_{h2+}$$

are sufficiently large. Mantel and Fleiss (1980) proposed the following criterion for the suitability of the Mantel–Haenszel procedure for a set of fourfold tables:

$$\min\left\{\left[\sum_{h=1}^{q} m_{h11} - \sum_{h=1}^{q} (n_{h11})_{\mathrm{L}}\right], \left[\sum_{h=1}^{q} (n_{h11})_{\mathrm{U}} - \sum_{h=1}^{q} m_{h11}\right]\right\} \geq 5$$

where $m_{h11} = n_{h1+}n_{h+1}/n_h$ is the expected value for n_{h11}, and $(n_{h11})_{\mathrm{L}}$ and $(n_{h11})_{\mathrm{U}}$ are respectively the lowest and the highest possible values for that cell, given that the marginals are fixed. Thus, the criterion requires that the potential variation in the across-strata sum of expected values for a particular cell should be at least 5.0. The criterion, of course, does not depend on which of the four cells is chosen. If the Mantel–Fleiss criterion is not met for a set of fourfold tables, an exact test may be carried out using algorithms like those of Thomas (1975) or Mehta, Patel, and Gray (1985).

C. Nonparametric Tests for Censored Survival Data

A variety of nonparametric tests for censored survival data can be used for treatment (or other group) comparisons of time to first adverse experience. The most commonly used tests are based on generalizations of either the Savage (1956) or Wilcoxon (1945) statistics. Gehan (1965) proposed a generalization of the Wilcoxon statistic with a permutation-based variance, calculated under the assumption of equal censoring patterns for the groups. Breslow (1970) proposed an asymptotic variance for the Gehan statistic, which does not require the assumption of equal censoring. Alternative generalizations of the Wilcoxon statistic, using scores based on estimates of the survival function, have been proposed by Peto and Peto (1972) and Prentice (1978). The generalized Savage test, often referred to as the log rank test, was first proposed by Mantel (1966) and later derived by Cox (1972) from likelihood theory under the Cox regression model (see Section III.F). The Mantel–Cox version of the test uses the Mantel–Haenszel variance. An alternative permutation-based variance, which requires the assumption of equal censoring, was proposed by Peto and Peto (1972). Similarities in the construction of the log rank and generalized Wilcoxon tests are discussed in Tarone and Ware (1977) and elsewhere, and are summarized below.

For simplicity, let us assume that only two treatment groups are to be compared. A parallel presentation using matrices for multiple group comparisons is given in Schemper (1984). Let z_h $(h = 1, 2, \ldots, q)$ be the distinct ordered times to first adverse experience (failure) in the pooled sample. A fourfold table can be formed at each of the q failure times. Let n_{h11} and n_{h21} be the number of failures at time z_h for the experimental and control groups, respectively. The respective numbers at risk just prior to z_h are n_{h1+} and n_{h2+}, and the total number at risk is n_h. A statistic for group comparisons is

$$G = \sum_{h=1}^{q} w_h[n_{h11} - (n_{h1+}n_{h+1}/n_h)]$$

which is a weighted sum of the differences between the observed and expected number of failures. A variance for G based on the hypergeometric distribution is given by

$$V = \sum_{h=1}^{q} w_h^2 n_{h1+}n_{h2+}n_{h+1}n_{h+2}/[n_h^2(n_h - 1)]$$

where the last term in the sum is defined to be zero if $n_h = 1$. A test for group comparison is then given by G^2/V, which is asymptotically distributed as chi-square with one degree of freedom. The choice of $w_h = 1$ corresponds to the Mantel–Cox test, and $w_h = n_h$ leads to the Breslow (1970) test. The difference in weighting schemes for the two tests explains the difference in their sensitivities. The Breslow test, which is weighted by the number at risk, is sensitive to early-occurring differences, whereas the Mantel–Cox test, in which all intervals are weighted equally, is more sensitive to late-occurring differences. The use of both tests together may thus provide insight into the nature of the group differences.

When the number of failures is small, the validity of asymptotic tests is questionable. The Mantel–Cox test is sometimes adjusted by a continuity correction (i.e., $(G-\frac{1}{2})^2/V$) in order to address this problem. Simulation studies have shown that the continuity-corrected Mantel–Cox test tends to be overly conservative (Lininger et al., 1979). It may also be nonconservative in the case of unequal sample sizes where the larger event rate occurs in the smaller sample (Kellerer and Chmelevsky, 1983). The uncorrected Mantel–Cox test and the Breslow test may be seriously nonconservative, especially in this situation (Kellerer and Chmelevsky, 1983; Latta, 1981).

Exact log rank or generalized Wilcoxon tests may be conducted, based on the permutation distribution of the score statistics, G, associated with the corresponding asymptotic tests. These tests assume equal censoring patterns for the groups to be compared, however, and this is often not the case. Jennrich (1984) proposed the use of conditional tests after artificial censoring as a method of producing analogies to standard tests (e.g., log rank, generalized Wilcoxon) that are exact even in the presence of unequal censoring. However, artificial censoring involves randomly censoring one observation in the other group after each failure, and thus the test result depends not only on the data, but also on the randomization used for the artificial censoring.

In this chapter, the Mantel–Cox and Breslow tests are used for group comparisons provided that the Mantel–Fleiss (1980) criterion is met for the set of fourfold tables produced by stratifying on time of failure t_h. Otherwise, if the Mantel–Fleiss criterion is not met, but the proportion censored is approximately the same in the groups being compared, an exact log rank test [as implemented by the algorithm of Thomas (1975)] is used.

D. Logistic Regression and Extensions to Ordinal Data

Logistic regression can be used to describe the effects of a set of explanatory variables on a dichotomous response variable, such as the occurrence/nonoccurrence of an adverse experience over the treatment period. Extensions of logistic regression can be used for the analysis of polychotomous response variables, such as the severity of adverse experiences. In this section, some aspects of the statistical theory for logistic regression are summarized. The material presented follows the notation and style of Koch and Edwards (1985).

Let Y denote a dichotomous (0, 1) response variable with expected value $\pi = \Pr(Y = 1)$, and let $\mathbf{x} = (x_1, x_2, \ldots, x_t)'$ be a vector of t categorical or continuous explanatory variables. We are interested in modeling π as a function of $\mathbf{x}$. The linear logistic model has the form

$$\pi(\mathbf{x}) = \exp(\alpha + \mathbf{x}'\boldsymbol{\beta})/[1 + \exp(\alpha + \mathbf{x}'\boldsymbol{\beta})] \tag{2.9}$$

where α is the intercept parameter and $\boldsymbol{\beta} = (\beta_1, \beta_2, \ldots, \beta_t)'$ is a vector of regression parameters. An important property of this model is that the regression curve is S-shaped; as $\mathbf{x}'\boldsymbol{\beta}$ approaches $+\infty$, $\pi(\mathbf{x})$ approaches 1.0, and as $\mathbf{x}'\boldsymbol{\beta}$ approaches $-\infty$, $\pi(\mathbf{x})$ approaches 0.0. The curve is nearly linear for $0.2 \leq \pi(\mathbf{x}) \leq 0.8$. With a logistic transformation of $\pi(\mathbf{x})$, the model becomes

$$\operatorname{logit} \pi(\mathbf{x}) = \ln\{\pi(\mathbf{x})/[1 - \pi(\mathbf{x})]\} = \alpha + \mathbf{x}'\boldsymbol{\beta}$$

Estimates for α and $\boldsymbol{\beta}$ are usually obtained by maximum likelihood methods. Let $i = 1, 2, \ldots, s$ index the s subpopulations corresponding to distinct vectors of explanatory variables $\mathbf{x}_i = (x_{i1}, x_{i2}, \ldots, x_{it})'$. Let n_{i1} denote the number of patients in the i-th subpopulation for whom the value of the response variable Y_i is 1 rather than 0, and let $n_i = (n_{i1}, n_{i2})'$ denote the distribution of responses from the $n_{i+} = n_{i1} + n_{i2}$ patients in the i-th subpopulation. If each i corresponds to an individual patient, then $n_{i+} = 1$ for all i. Assuming a product binomial distribution for the responses, the likelihood for the data is

$$L = \prod_{i=1}^{s} [n_{i+}!\,\pi_i^{n_{i1}}(1 - \pi_i)^{n_{i2}}/n_{i1}!\,n_{i2}!]$$

where π_i is the expected value of Y_i. By replacing π_i in L by its model (2.9) counterpart, differentiating $\ln L$ with respect to α and $\boldsymbol{\beta}$, and setting the result equal to 0, one obtains the following series of equations:

$$L = \prod_{i=1}^{s} \left\{ n_{i+}!/(n_{i1}!\,n_{i2}!) \frac{\{\exp(\alpha + \mathbf{x}_i'\boldsymbol{\beta})\}^{n_{i1}}}{\{(1 + \exp(\alpha + \mathbf{x}_i'\boldsymbol{\beta})\}^{n_{i+}}} \right\}$$

$$\ln L = C + \sum_{i=1}^{s} n_{i1}(\alpha + \mathbf{x}_i'\boldsymbol{\beta}) - \sum_{i=1}^{s} n_{i+} \ln\{1 + \exp(\alpha + \mathbf{x}_i'\boldsymbol{\beta})\}$$

$$\frac{\partial \ln L}{\partial \alpha} = \sum_{i=1}^{s} n_{i1} - \sum_{i=1}^{s} n_{i+} \left\{ \frac{\exp(\alpha + \mathbf{x}_i'\boldsymbol{\beta})}{1 + \exp(\alpha + \mathbf{x}_i'\boldsymbol{\beta})} \right\} = \sum_{i=1}^{s} (n_{i1} - n_{i+}\hat{\pi}_i) = 0 \tag{2.10}$$

$$\frac{\partial \ln L}{\partial \boldsymbol{\beta}} = \sum_{i=1}^{s} n_{i1}\mathbf{x}_i' - \sum_{i=1}^{s} n_{i+} \left\{ \frac{\exp(\alpha + \mathbf{x}_i'\boldsymbol{\beta})}{1 + \exp(\alpha + \mathbf{x}_i'\boldsymbol{\beta})} \right\} \mathbf{x}_i' = \sum_{i=1}^{s} (n_{i1} - n_{i+}\hat{\pi}_i)\mathbf{x}_i' = \mathbf{0} \tag{2.11}$$

If we let $\mathbf{x}_{iA} = [1, \mathbf{x}_i']'$ and $\boldsymbol{\beta}_A = (\alpha, \boldsymbol{\beta}')'$ then the likelihood equations (2.10) and (2.11) can be written as

$$\sum_{i=1}^{s} (n_{i1} - n_{i+}\hat{\pi}_i)\mathbf{x}_{iA} = 0$$

where $\hat{\pi}_i = \exp(\mathbf{x}_{iA}'\hat{\boldsymbol{\beta}}_A)/\{1 + \exp(\mathbf{x}_{iA}'\hat{\boldsymbol{\beta}}_A)\}$ are the model-predicted maximum-likelihood estimates of π_i, based on $\mathbf{x}_{iA}$ and $\hat{\boldsymbol{\beta}}_A$, the maximum likelihood estimates of $\boldsymbol{\beta}_A$. The term $\hat{\boldsymbol{\beta}}_A$ must generally be calculated using an iterative procedure such as the Newton–Raphson method. This method involves adjusting a g-th step estimate $\hat{\boldsymbol{\beta}}_{Ag}$ to a $(g+1)$-th step estimate via the algorithm

$$\hat{\boldsymbol{\beta}}_{A,g+1} = \hat{\boldsymbol{\beta}}_{Ag} + \mathbf{V}(\hat{\boldsymbol{\beta}}_{Ag}) \left\{ \sum_{i=1}^{s} (n_{i1} - n_{i+}\hat{\pi}_i)\mathbf{x}_{iA} \right\}$$

where $\mathbf{V}(\hat{\boldsymbol{\beta}}_{Ag}) = \{\sum_{i=1}^{s} n_{i+}\hat{\pi}_i(1 - \hat{\pi}_i)\mathbf{x}_{iA}\mathbf{x}_{iA}'\}^{-1}$ is the negative of the inverse of the matrix of second-order partial derivatives of $\ln L$ evaluated at $\hat{\boldsymbol{\beta}}_{Ag}$. The term $\mathbf{V}(\hat{\boldsymbol{\beta}})$ is the g-th step estimate for the asymptotic covariance matrix of $\hat{\boldsymbol{\beta}}_A$. The maximum-likelihood estimator $\hat{\boldsymbol{\beta}}_A$ approximately has a multivariate normal distribution when the n_{ij} are sufficiently large for the linear functions $\sum_{i=1}^{s} n_{i1}\mathbf{x}_{iA}$ to have an approximately multivariate normal distribution.

If $n_{i+} \geq 10$ for most of the s subpopulations, then either the Pearson chi-square statistic

$$Q_{\mathrm{P}} = \sum_{i=1}^{s} \sum_{j=1}^{2} (n_{ij} - \hat{m}_{ij})^2 / \hat{m}_{ij}$$

where $\hat{m}_{i1} = n_{i+}\hat{\pi}_i$ and $\hat{m}_{i2} = n_{i+}(1 - \hat{\pi}_i)$, or the log-likelihood ratio chi-square statistic

$$Q_{\mathrm{L}} = \sum_{i=1}^{s} \sum_{j=1}^{2} 2n_{ij} \ln(n_{ij} / \hat{m}_{ij})$$

can be used to assess goodness of fit. Both statistics are asymptotically equivalent, and both have approximate chi-square distributions with $(s-t-1)$ degrees of freedom. If many of the n_{ij} are small, Q_{P} and Q_{L} should be viewed cautiously.

An alternative strategy for assessing goodness of fit when the n_{ij} are small is to fit an expanded model and then verify that the contribution of effects not in the original model is nonsignificant. Let the specification matrix for the original model be denoted by $\mathbf{X}_A$ where $\mathbf{x}'_{iA}=[1,\mathbf{x}'_i]$ are the rows of $\mathbf{X}_A$. The expanded model, $[\mathbf{X}_A, \mathbf{W}]$, contains the t original variables, the intercept, and w additional explanatory variables, and must have full rank $(1+t+w)$. The significance of the contribution of $\mathbf{W}$ to $\mathbf{X}_A$ may be evaluated by the difference of the log-likelihood ratio chi-square statistics for $\mathbf{X}_A$ and $[\mathbf{X}_A, \mathbf{W}]$, that is,

$$Q_{\mathrm{LR}} = \sum_{i=1}^{s} \sum_{j=1}^{2} 2n_{ij}[\ln(\hat{m}_{ij,w}/\hat{m}_{ij})]$$

where the $\hat{m}_{ij,w}$ are the predicted values for model $[\mathbf{X}_A, \mathbf{W}]$.

An alternative statistic that does not require the fitting of the expanded model is the Rao score statistic

$$Q_{\mathrm{S}} = (\mathbf{n}_{*1}-\hat{\mathbf{m}}_{*1})'\mathbf{W}\{\mathbf{W}'[\mathbf{D}_{\hat{\mathbf{v}}}^{-1} - \mathbf{D}_{\hat{\mathbf{v}}}^{-1}\mathbf{X}_A(\mathbf{X}'_A\mathbf{D}_{\hat{\mathbf{v}}}^{-1}\mathbf{X}_A)^{-1}\mathbf{X}'_A\mathbf{D}_{\hat{\mathbf{v}}}^{-1}]\mathbf{W}\}^{-1} \times \mathbf{W}'(\mathbf{n}_{*1}-\hat{\mathbf{m}}_{*1})$$

where $\mathbf{n}_{*1}=(n_{11}, n_{2i}, \ldots, n_{s1})$, $\hat{\mathbf{m}}=(\hat{m}_{11}, \hat{m}_{21}, \ldots, \hat{m}_{s1})$, and $\mathbf{D}_{\hat{\mathbf{v}}}$ is the diagonal matrix with diagonal elements $\hat{\mathbf{v}}_i=[n_{i+}\hat{\pi}_i(1-\hat{\pi}_i)]^{-1}$. Both Q_{LR} and Q_{S} have approximate chi-square distributions with w degrees of freedom under the hypothesis that the coefficients for the w additional variables are all zero.

In this chapter, computations for logistic regression were performed primarily with the SAS procedure LOGIST of Harrell (1986a). For example, in Section VI, a contingency table is constructed for the occurrence/nonoccurrence of adverse experiences by treatment for a set of investigators, and the score statistic capability of LOGIST is used to assess the significance of the treatment by investigator interaction. LOGIST is also used for case-record data, that is, one subject per observation. In Sections IV and V, the stepwise variable selection capability of LOGIST is used to identify important predictors of selected adverse experiences and to evaluate the importance of treatment relative to other explanatory variables. The LOGIST procedure uses Rao score statistics for variable selection, as proposed by Bartolucci and Fraser (1977).

The LOGIST procedure can also be used to fit a logistic regression model to an ordinal response variable by the method described in Walker and Duncan (1967, section 6, as referenced by Harrell, 1986a). McCullagh (1980) refers to this model as the proportional odds model. If the response variable Y_i has levels $0, 1, \ldots, r$, the model statement for the proportional odds model is

$$\Pr(Y_i \geq j) = \exp(\alpha_j + \mathbf{x}_i'\boldsymbol{\beta})/\{1 + \exp(\alpha_j + \mathbf{x}_i'\boldsymbol{\beta})\}$$

for $j = 1, 2, \ldots, r$. This model thus uses all response categories for each logit.

An alternative logit model for ordinal data for which there is available software for maximum likelihood estimation is the equal adjacent odds ratio model, described by Imrey et al (1981, 1982) and Koch, Amara et al. (1982). As its name implies, this model uses only adjacent response levels in the formation of the logits. Other logit models are reviewed in Agresti (1983) and Cox and Chuang (1984).

As noted by Koch, Amara, and Singer (1985), the proportional odds model is more appropriate than the equal adjacent odds model when the response categories can be viewed as falling along an underlying continuum. In Section IV, the proportional odds model is used to assess the association of explanatory variables with the severity of the most severe occurrence of drowsiness during the treatment period.

E. Weighted Least-squares Methods

The weighted least-squares (WLS) methods of Grizzle, Starmer, and Koch (GSK) (1969) can be used for modeling counts and rates of adverse experiences when the subpopulations (typically defined by treatment groups and possibly other explanatory variables) are moderately large, for example, greater than 20. The GSK strategy involves three stages: (1) construction of appropriate functions of the responses, (2) fitting of regression models to these functions with WLS estimation, and (3) testing hypotheses about linear combinations of the model parameters. An advantage of this modeling strategy over logistic regression is that the response functions for WLS may be more general than the dichotomous or polychotomous response variables required for logistic regression. However, the inclusion of covariables is much more awkward with WLS because each covariable must be incorporated in the stratification used to produce subpopulations, thus increasing the sample size requirements. In this section, aspects of the WLS method are summarized using notation similar to that of Johnson et al. (1981). The data structure of Section IV is used as a context for discussion. In that section, WLS methods are used to model the average proportion of the eight treatment period assessments at which drowsiness was reported for patients in each of four treatment groups.

The quantities necessary for the implementation of the WLS method are **F** (a vector of functions of the response data), $\mathbf{V_F}$ (a consistent estimator of the covariance matrix of **F**), and **X** (the specification matrix for a linear model for **F**). Let the subpopulations be indexed by $i = 1, 2, \ldots, s$. In Section IV the subpopulations of interest are the four treatment groups, so $s = 4$. The response vector for patient k in subpopulation i (where $k = 1, 2, \ldots, n_i$) is $\mathbf{y}_{ik} = \{y_{ijk}\} = (y_{i1k}, y_{i2k}, \ldots, y_{i8k})'$, since there are eight assessments. Each of the y_{ijk} is an indicator variable with value 1 if the patient had drowsiness at assessment j ($j = 1, 2, \ldots, 8$), and value 0 otherwise. Let the within-subpopulation mean vector be denoted by $\bar{\mathbf{y}}_i = (\bar{y}_{i1}, \bar{y}_{i2}, \ldots, \bar{y}_{i8})'$ where $\bar{y}_{ij} = \sum_{k=1}^{n_i} y_{ijk}/n_i$. The summary measures of interest for this example may be expressed as $\bar{a}_i = \mathbf{A}\bar{\mathbf{y}}_i$ where $\mathbf{A} = [1\ 1\ 1\ 1\ 1\ 1\ 1\ 1]/8$. Thus $\bar{a}_i$ is the average proportion of the assessments at which patients in the i-th treatment group had drowsiness. The vector of functions of interest is $\mathbf{F} = (\bar{a}_1, \bar{a}_2, \bar{a}_3, \bar{a}_4)'$, for which the covariance matrix $\mathbf{V_F}$ is a block diagonal matrix with blocks

$$\mathbf{V}_i = \mathbf{A}\left[\sum_{k=1}^{n_i} (\mathbf{y}_{ik} - \bar{\mathbf{y}}_i)(\mathbf{y}_{ik} - \bar{\mathbf{y}}_i)'\right]\mathbf{A}'/n_i$$

More generally, **F** can be any vector of functions obtained from combinations of linear, logarithmic, or exponential transformations of the response data. The term $\mathbf{V_F}$ can then be obtained using linear Taylor series methods as described by Koch, Imrey, Singer, Atkinson, and Stokes (1985).

A linear model for describing the variation in **F** is

$$E_A(\mathbf{F}) = \mathbf{X}\boldsymbol{\beta}$$

where **X** is the specification matrix, $\boldsymbol{\beta}$ is the vector of parameters to be estimated, and E_A denotes asymptotic expectation. The WLS estimated model parameters **b** and covariance matrix $\mathbf{V_b}$ are

$$\mathbf{b} = (\mathbf{X}'\mathbf{V_F}^{-1}\mathbf{X})^{-1}\mathbf{X}'\mathbf{V_F}^{-1}\mathbf{F}$$

and

$$\mathbf{V_b} = (\mathbf{X}'\mathbf{V_F}^{-1}\mathbf{X})^{-1}$$

The Wald statistic for evaluating the goodness of fit of the model is

$$Q_W = (\mathbf{F} - \mathbf{Xb})'\mathbf{V}_\mathbf{F}^{-1}(\mathbf{F} - \mathbf{Xb})$$

When the subpopulations are moderately large (i.e., $n_i \geq 20$), Q_W has an approximate chi-square distribution with degrees of freedom equal to the difference between the dimensions of **F** and **b**. When model fit is supported, hypotheses regarding linear combinations of model parameters, H_C: $\mathbf{C}\boldsymbol{\beta} = \mathbf{0}$, may be tested using a Wald statistic

$$Q_{W,C} = \mathbf{b}'\mathbf{C}'(\mathbf{C}\mathbf{V}_\mathbf{b}\mathbf{C}')^{-1}\mathbf{C}\mathbf{b}$$

which has an approximate chi-square distribution with degrees of freedom equal to the rank of **C**.

The program MISCAT (documented in Stanish, Koch, and Landis, 1978) has the capability of calculating the mean vectors $\{\bar{a}_i\}$ from case-record data, as well as implementing combinations of linear, logarithmic or exponential functions of the response vectors to form the function vector **F**. The corresponding covariance matrix $\mathbf{V}_\mathbf{F}$ is also estimated. Specified models are fitted with WLS estimation, and Wald statistics are provided for evaluation of model fit and testing of specified hypotheses. MISCAT has the additional capability of providing multivariate ratio estimates of the mean vectors $\{\bar{a}_i\}$ in the case of missing data, as described by Stanish, Gillings, and Koch (1978). When the data are in contingency table format, the CATMOD procedure of SAS Institute, Inc. (1985) may be used for WLS calculations.

F. Cox Regression

With respect to the analysis of time to event data, a widely known model is that of Cox (1972). The Cox model is formulated in terms of the effects of the covariables on the hazard function. Let $\mathbf{x}_i = (x_{i1}, x_{i2}, \ldots, x_{it})'$ denote the vector of covariables for the i-th patient ($i = 1, 2, \ldots, n$), and let $\lambda_i(z)$ denote the corresponding hazard function, which may vary over time. The Cox model has the form

$$\lambda_i(z) = \lambda_0(z)\exp(\mathbf{x}_i'\boldsymbol{\beta})$$

where $\lambda_0(z)$ is the unspecified hazard function of the underlying survival distribution when $\mathbf{x}_i = \mathbf{0}$, and $\boldsymbol{\beta}$ is a $(t \times 1)$ vector of regression parameters to be estimated. The Cox model is an example of a proportional hazards model, so called because the ratio of the hazard functions for any two individuals does not depend on time (given that the $\mathbf{x}_i$ do not depend on time), that is,

$$\lambda_i(z)/\lambda_{i'}(z) = \exp(\mathbf{x}_i - \mathbf{x}_{i'})'\boldsymbol{\beta}$$

Nonproportional hazards models arise when $\lambda_0(z)$ depends on the $\mathbf{x}_i$.

Several authors (including Cox, 1975; Kalbfleisch and Prentice, 1973; Breslow, 1974) have approached the construction of a likelihood function for the Cox model from different perspectives. When there are no ties in the uncensored times to failure, there is a consensus as to the likelihood function. Let z_i be the censored time at risk or the uncensored time to failure for the i-th patient, and let U be the set of patients who failed. Given that there are no ties in the z_i, the likelihood function may be written

$$L = \prod_{i \in U} \left\{ \exp[(\mathbf{x}_i'\boldsymbol{\beta})] \Big/ \sum_{j \in R(z_i)} \exp(\mathbf{x}_j'\boldsymbol{\beta}) \right\}$$

where $R(z_i)$, the risk set at z_i, is the set of patients who have not failed or withdrawn prior to time z_i.

The authors cited above differ with respect to the likelihood function proposed for the case of ties in the uncensored data. The likelihood function proposed by Breslow (1974) is the most tractable from a computational standpoint, and is used in the SAS procedure PHGLM of Harrell (1986b) and the BMD program P2L of Hopkins (1981). If there are q distinct times of failure among the n patients and m_h patients failed at time z_h ($h = 1, 2, \ldots, q$), the Breslow likelihood can be expressed as

$$L = \prod_{h=1}^{q} \left\{ \exp(\mathbf{s}_h'\boldsymbol{\beta}) \Big/ \left[\sum_{j \in R(z_h)} \exp(\mathbf{x}_j'\boldsymbol{\beta}) \right]^{m_h} \right\}$$

where $\mathbf{s}_h$ is the sum of the covariate vectors for the m_h patients who failed at z_h. Extensions of the Cox regression model may be used for the case of grouped times to failure, as discussed by Prentice and Gloeckler (1978) and in Section III.G.

In this chapter, the procedure PHGLM is used for Cox model regression. This program has stepwise capabilities for variable selection, through the use of Rao score statistics. Stratified analysis [as discussed by Breslow (1979) among others] can also be performed. When group membership is the only covariable in the model, the score statistic for the Cox model is virtually the same as the Mantel–Haenszel (or Mantel–Cox) statistic. This equivalence is used in Section VI where treatment group comparisons of time to first adverse experience are performed, stratifying by investigator, using PHGLM.

An important assumption of the Cox model is the multiplicative relationship between the underlying hazard function, and the function of covariables, which, for our purposes, do not depend on time. This proportionality assumption may be examined graphically [e.g., by checking whether the −ln −ln (estimated survival) curves appear parallel]. Nagelkerke, Oosting, and Hart (1984) proposed the use of a test for proportionality based on the "partial residuals" of Schoenfeld (1982). An alternative test based on these "residuals" has been included in the truncation used to investigate the proportionality assumption in Section VI.

G. Poisson Regression and Piecewise Exponential Models

Poisson regression is a method for assessing the relationship between observed counts that are assumed to have independent Poisson distributions and a set of explanatory variables. The most common form of Poisson regression is the log-linear model. In this section, this model is described along with several auxiliary statistics that are useful in assessing model fit. The applicability of Poisson regression computing procedures for fitting piecewise exponential models to survival data is also described. The notation and style of the presentation follows that of Koch, Atkinson, and Stokes (1986) and also Atkinson (1984).

The log-linear model has the form

$$E(\mathbf{n}) = \boldsymbol{\mu} = \mathbf{D}_N \,\mathbf{exp}(\mathbf{X}\boldsymbol{\beta})$$

for which $\mathbf{n} = (n_1, n_2, \ldots, n_s)'$ is an $s \times 1$ vector of observed counts for the respective s subpopulations, $\boldsymbol{\mu}$ is the corresponding $s \times 1$ vector of expected values, $\mathbf{N}$ is the $s \times 1$ vector of known exposure measures (e.g., person-days of treatment), $\mathbf{D_N}$ is an $s \times s$ diagonal matrix with the elements of $\mathbf{N}$ down the main diagonal, $\mathbf{X}$ is the $s \times t$ model specification matrix, $\boldsymbol{\beta}$ is the $t \times 1$ vector of model parameters to be estimated, and **exp** is the operation that exponentiates the elements of a matrix. Each μ_i is assumed to be the product $N_i\lambda_i$ where λ_i is the rate at which the events counted in $\mathbf{n}$ accumulate per unit N_i; thus $\lambda_i = \exp(\mathbf{x}_i'\boldsymbol{\beta})$, where $\mathbf{x}_i'$ is the row of $\mathbf{X}$ corresponding to the i-th subpopulation.

The likelihood function of the counts $\{n_i\}$ is

$$L = \prod_{i=1}^{s} \mu_i^{n_i}[\exp(-\mu_i)]/n_i!$$

After substituting $N_i \exp(x'_i\beta)$ for μ_i in L, differentiating $\ln L$ with respect to β, and equating the result of 0, the resulting set of nonlinear equations has the form

$$\mathbf{X'n} = \mathbf{X'}\hat{\boldsymbol{\mu}} = \mathbf{X'D_N}[\exp(\mathbf{X}\hat{\boldsymbol{\beta}})]$$

Since these equations usually do not have an explicit solution, an iterative procedure, such as the Newton–Raphson procedure, is necessary to solve for $\boldsymbol{\beta}$. In order for $\hat{\boldsymbol{\beta}}$ to have approximately a multivariate normal distribution with a covariance matrix that can be estimated by

$$\mathbf{V}(\boldsymbol{\beta}) = (\mathbf{X'D}_{\hat{\mu}}\mathbf{X})^{-1}$$

the observed counts **n** must be sufficiently large for the linear functions **X'n** to have approximately a multivariate normal distribution from central limit theory.

Two measures of goodness of fit for the model **X** are the Pearson chi-square criterion

$$Q_{\mathrm{P}} = \sum_{i=1}^{s} (n_i - \hat{\mu}_i)^2/\hat{\mu}_i$$

and the log-likelihood chi-square criterion

$$Q_{\mathrm{L}} = \sum_{i=1}^{s} 2n_i \ln(n_i/\hat{\mu}_i)$$

Both of these statistics have $(s-t)$ degrees of freedom when the n_i are sufficiently large (e.g., all $n_i \geq 5$), and both address the compatibility of the observed counts with the model-predicted counts.

As in Section III.D, the goodness of fit of the model may also be evaluated by assessing the contribution of columns **W** (as $s \times w$ matrix) to the matrix **X** (which is $s \times t$) via the log-likelihood ratio statistic

$$Q_{\mathrm{LR}} = \sum_{i=1}^{s} 2n_i \ln(\hat{\mu}_{i,w}/\hat{\mu}_i)$$

where $\hat{\mu}_{i,w}$ are the predicted counts for the expanded model $[\mathbf{X}, \mathbf{W}]$ and $\hat{\mu}_i$ are the predicted counts for the original model **X**. An asymptotically equivalent statistic for assessing the effect of **W** that requires only that the model $\mathbf{X}$ be fit is the Rao score statistic

$$Q_S = (\mathbf{n} - \hat{\boldsymbol{\mu}})'\mathbf{W}\{\mathbf{W}'[\mathbf{D}_{\hat{\mu}} - \mathbf{D}_{\hat{\mu}}\mathbf{X}(\mathbf{X}'\mathbf{D}_{\hat{\mu}}\mathbf{X})^{-1}\mathbf{X}'\mathbf{D}_{\hat{\mu}}]\mathbf{W}\}^{-1}\mathbf{W}'(\mathbf{n} - \hat{\boldsymbol{\mu}})$$

Both Q_{LR} and Q_S have approximate chi-square distributions with w degrees of freedom under the hypothesis that the coefficients for the w additional variables are all zero.

Frome (1983) describes several statistics that may be used to detect influential observations in Poisson regression and outliers from model fit. The two measures to be described in this section and illustrated in Section VI are the diagonal elements of the $\mathbf{H}$ matrix and the adjusted standardized residuals. In Poisson regression the $\mathbf{H}$ matrix has the form

$$\mathbf{H} = \mathbf{W}^{1/2}\mathbf{P}(\mathbf{P}'\mathbf{W}\mathbf{P})^{-1}\mathbf{P}'\mathbf{W}^{1/2}$$

and

$$\mathbf{W} = \mathbf{D}_{\mathbf{N}}\mathbf{D}^{-1}_{\exp(\mathbf{X}\boldsymbol{\beta})} \quad \text{and} \quad \mathbf{P} = \mathbf{D}_{\exp(\mathbf{X}\boldsymbol{\beta})}\mathbf{X}$$

and $\boldsymbol{\beta}$ is evaluated at the maximum-likelihood estimate $\hat{\boldsymbol{\beta}}$. Diagonal elements of $\mathbf{H}$ that exceed $2t/s$ (where s and t are the row and column dimensions of $\mathbf{X}$) are considered to be influential observations, that is, points in the model space that may substantially influence the fitted model (Frome, 1983).

The adjusted standardized residuals are the standardized residuals,

$$(\mathbf{n} - \hat{\boldsymbol{\mu}})/\hat{\boldsymbol{\mu}}^{1/2}$$

divided by their variance, which is shown in Atkinson (1984) to be $\mathbf{I} - \mathbf{H}$. The adjusted standardized residuals

$$\frac{(n_i - \hat{\mu}_i)/(\hat{\mu}_i)^{1/2}}{(1 - h_i)^{1/2}} \qquad i = 1, 2, \ldots, s$$

that deviate from the standard normal distribution may be indicative of outliers from model fit.

In Section VI, Poisson log-linear computing procedures are used to fit piecewise exponential models to survival (time to adverse experience) data. The piecewise exponential likelihood function may be written as

$$L_{PE} = \prod_{i=1}^{s} \prod_{j=1}^{r} \lambda_{ij}^{n_{ij}} [\exp(-\lambda_{ij}N_{ij})]$$

where i indexes the subpopulations formed from the covariates; j indexes the time intervals; and n_{ij}, N_{ij}, and λ_{ij} are respectively the number of patients with the adverse experience, the number of person-days of treatment, and the hazard rate for the i-th group in the j-th interval. As shown by Holford (1980) and independently by Laird and Olivier (1981), L_{PE} is proportional to its Poisson counterpart,

$$L_{PO} = \prod_{i=1}^{s} \prod_{j=1}^{r} (N_{ij}\lambda_{ij})^{n_{ij}}[\exp(-N_{ij}\lambda_{ij})]/n_{ij}!$$

$$= L_{PE}\left[\prod_{i=1}^{s} \prod_{j=1}^{r} N_{ij}^{n_{ij}}/n_{ij}!\right]$$

Therefore, computing procedures that maximize L_{PO} also maximize L_{PE}.

IV. AN ANTIHISTAMINE/DECONGESTANT DRUG TRIAL EXAMPLE

Suzanne Edwards, Gary G. Koch, and William Sollecito

A. Description of the Trial

The data analyzed in this section are from a randomized, double-blind, parallel-designed study of four treatments: a combination drug (AB) for treatment of rhinitis, each of its two components (A, the antihistamine, and B, the decongestant), and placebo (P). One hundred fifty-five patients suffering from nasal congestion associated with allergic rhinitis were enrolled. The study was conducted by a single investigator during three succeeding allergy seasons: fall (ragweed season) 1978, summer (grass season) 1979, and fall 1979. A summary of the demographic characteristics of each treatment group is given in Table 2.1. Randomization appears to have produced treatment groups that are reasonably comparable with respect to the distribution of demographic characteristics; the only departures were tendencies for the placebo-group patients to be a little heavier than patients in other groups, and the females in group B to be somewhat lighter than the females in the other groups. There were no statistically significant treatment differences with respect to any of the demographic variables.

Each patient was studied for one day. Medication was given at 10:00 a.m., 1:00 p.m., and 4:00 p.m. Adverse experiences were assessed at 10:00 a.m. (the baseline assessment) and afterward at hourly intervals, the last assessment being at 6:00 p.m. Four adverse experiences were of primary interest: drowsiness, dizziness, jitteriness, and nausea. Information regarding the occurrence of these symptoms was solicited at each

TABLE 2.1 Summary statistics of demographic characteristics by treatment group

	AB ($n = 40$)	A ($n = 39$)	B ($n = 40$)	Placebo ($n = 36$)	p value[a]
Sex					0.851
Female	12 (30%)	15 (38%)	13 (33%)	11 (31%)	
Male	28 (70%)	24 (62%)	27 (67%)	25 (69%)	
Race					0.191
Caucasian	40 (100%)	35 (90%)	37 (93%)	33 (92%)	
Other	0 (0%)	4 (10%)	3 (7%)	3 (8%)	
Age					0.869
Median	22.0	22.0	23.0	22.0	
Mean	24.1	24.8	23.9	24.6	
Range	18–45	18–54	18–36	18–59	
Weight (lb.)					0.427
All patients					
Median	150.0	147.0	152.5	161.5	
Mean	149.1	151.0	149.1	156.4	
Range	95–190	105–225	96–215	98–200	
Females only					0.387
Median	126.5	131.0	116.0	130.0	
Mean	129.9	132.6	120.3	134.2	
Range	95–170	105–170	96–150	98–185	
Males only					0.373
Median	155.0	162.5	165.0	165.0	
Mean	157.3	162.5	163.0	166.2	
Range	115–190	126–225	125–215	121–200	
Height (in.)					
All patients					0.559
Median	69.5	68.0	69.0	70.0	
Mean	69.1	68.3	68.3	69.1	
Range	62–75	61–78	60–75	61–74	
Females only					0.454
Median	66.5	63.0	66.0	64.0	
Mean	65.8	64.4	64.5	64.4	
Range	62–69	61–71	60–68	61–70	
Males only					0.443
Median	71.0	71.0	70.0	72.0	
Mean	70.6	70.8	70.1	71.1	
Range	65–75	65–78	63–75	65–74	

[a]The p value for sex is from the Pearson chi-square test. The p value for race is from Fisher's exact test. All other p values are from Kruskal–Wallis tests (chi-square approximation).

assessment. Other adverse experiences volunteered by the patients were also recorded. Severity was coded according to a five-point scale: none, mild, moderate, severe, and very severe. The level of severity for all reports of jitteriness, dizziness, and nausea was at most mild. The severity levels of drowsiness ranged from mild to very severe. However, there were very few reports of very severe drowsiness, and so the levels severe and very severe were combined in the analysis.

Since the study was so short, there were very few major protocol violations or missing values; thus the possible bias in treatment comparisons is minimal. Three patients received only two tablets over the 8-h observation period. Two patients slept through one or more assessments; for the purposes of analysis, these two were assigned drowsiness values of severe/very severe for the assessments they missed due to being asleep. One patient did not return after the 11:00 a.m. assessment, and three other patients missed one assessment each due to unknown causes.

This study is unusual in that the direction of the bias due to protocol noncompliance can be assessed, at least for comparisons of group AB with any of the other groups. There were no major protocol violations or missing values in group AB, and the nature of the protocol noncompliance (missed doses, missed assessments) of patients in groups A, B, and P is such as to decrease, rather than increase, the likelihood of those patients reporting adverse experiences. Since the direction of the bias is such as to put group AB, the test drug group, at a disadvantage, statistical comparisons of group AB with any other group are conservative.

Drug A is known to produce drowsiness, and drug B is suspected of producing jitteriness. It is of interest to investigate whether the two components counteract each other so that the combination drug AB produces less drowsiness than drug A or less jitteriness than drug B.

B. Overview of Statistical Analyses

Of the data sets used for illustration of analyses, the data from the antihistamine/decongestant clinical trial is the least complex with respect to the analysis of adverse experiences. This trial was conducted at only one site, the dosing schedule was fixed, only four adverse experiences were of primary interst, and the treatment lasted only one day so the amount of protocol violations and missing data is minimal.

Relatively few patients had any of the four adverse experiences at baseline (see Table 2.2). However, baseline status must be considered in the analysis because the first treatment-period assessment occurs so shortly after the baseline assessment, and thus baseline status is likely to

TABLE 2.2 Number (%) of patients with adverse experiences by treatment group[a]

Group	N	Baseline	Treatment period (all patients included)	Treatment period (those with adverse experience at baseline excluded)
			Drowsiness	
AB	40	4 (10%)	31 (78%)	27 (75%)
A	39	5 (13%)	27 (69%)	22 (65%)
B	40	6 (15%)	21 (53%)	15 (44%)
P	36	0 (0%)	16 (44%)	16 (44%)
			Jitteriness	
AB	40	0 (0%)	5 (13%)	5 (13%)
A	39	0 (0%)	1 (3%)	1 (3%)
B	40	0 (0%)	6 (15%)	6 (15%)
P	36	0 (0%)	0 (0%)	0 (0%)
			Dizziness	
AB	40	1 (3%)	10 (25%)	9 (23%)
A	39	1 (3%)	6 (15%)	5 (13%)
B	40	2 (5%)	6 (15%)	4 (11%)
P	36	0 (0%)	5 (14%)	5 (14%)
			Nausea	
AB	40	1 (3%)	5 (13%)	4 (10%)
A	39	0 (0%)	1 (3%)	1 (3%)
B	40	1 (3%)	2 (5%)	1 (3%)
P	36	0 (0%)	0 (0%)	0 (0%)

[a]There was one assessment at baseline and eight during the treatment period. The p value for an exact test (Pagano and Halvorsen, 1981) of treatment group differences with respect to prevalence of baseline drowsiness is 0.078.

be a much stronger predictor than any of the other variables. All 15 of the patients with baseline drowsiness also had drowsiness one or more times during the treatment period (11 of the 15 had it at the first hourly assessment), three of the four patients with baseline dizziness had treatment-period dizziness, and both patients with baseline nausea had treatment-period nausea. No patients had baseline jitteriness.

In the analyses of dizziness and nausea, patients having either of these respective adverse experiences at baseline are excluded. Too few patients had either of these adverse experiences at baseline for the baseline status to be useful as a stratification variable or covariable in the analysis.

There are also difficulties with the use of baseline status as a stratification variable or covariable in the analysis of the occurrence/nonoccurrence of drowsiness during the treatment period. In logistic regression, since all patients with baseline drowsiness also had treatment-period drowsiness, computational difficulties arise when baseline status is included as a predictor in logistic regression. The problem is that the predicted probability of drowsiness for those with baseline drowsiness is 1, corresponding to an infinite predicted logit. In randomization-based analysis, there are difficulties with the use of baseline status as either a stratification variable or covariable. Using baseline status as a stratification variable produces one uninformative stratum, since all patients with baseline drowsiness had the same response. However, baseline status cannot be used as a covariable in randomization-based analysis because the treatment groups are not comparable with respect to the prevalence of baseline drowsiness (see Table 2.2). Therefore, in the analyses that follow, patients with baseline drowsiness are excluded from the analysis of drowsiness, unless otherwise noted.

In addition to baseline status, other potential explantory variables include time of enrollment (fall 1978, summer 1979, or fall 1979), sex, age, weight, and an indicator of obesity constructed from weight and height, the Quetelet index [100 times the weight (in pounds) divided by the squared height (in inches)]. The age range in this study is somewhat limited; all patients are at least 18 years old and only three are older than 40. There is some confounding between sex and season because the protocol was originally designed to exclude women of child-bearing potential. This restriction was not relaxed until after fall 1978, so very few women were enrolled until spring 1979. Also, as is the case with most studies which enroll both sexes, sex and weight are correlated. Weight may be an important predictor of adverse experiences because the doses were given in milligrams, rather than milligrams per kilogram. Thus, all other factors being equal, lighter patients would have a larger amount of drug in the body, per unit weight, than heavier patients. Since weight and sex are correlated, weight will be nested within sex in the analyses.

The types of analyses undertaken for this study include contingency-table methods, randomization-based analyses with covariable adjustment for the explanatory variables, logistic regression, ans weighted least-squares analyses. The subsections that follow pertain to the analysis of the various aspects of an adverse experience profile, as discussed in Section II. The analysis of the occurrence/nonoccurrence of each of the four adverse experiences is presented in Section IV.C, and the analyses of the severity and frequency of drowsiness is presented in Section IV.E.

Drowsiness is the only adverse experience for which severity levels other than mild were reported. Also, drowsiness is the only adverse experience that occurred with some frequency. Thus analyses of severity and frequency are of interest for drowsiness, although not necessarily for the other adverse experiences. One aspect of the adverse experience profile not previously discussed is the tendency of different adverse experiences to occur together. A correlation analysis of the four adverse experiences is presented in Section IV.D.

C. Analysis of Occurrence/Nonoccurrence

This section pertains to the analysis of the occurrence/nonoccurrence of each of the four adverse experiences via contingency-table analysis, stratified covariance randomization-based analysis, and logistic regression. Here, an adverse experience is classified as having occurred during the treatment period if it was reported for at least one of the eight postdosing assessments.

In Section IV.C.1, contingency-table methods are used to explore the first-order associations of the occurrence/nonoccurrence of the four adverse experiences with treatment and other explanatory variables. Since very few patients had jitteriness or nausea, a contingency-table analysis with exact tests for statistical significance may be the most appropriate means of analysis for these two adverse experiences. Some discussion of the power of the tests is provided, and the effect of using more strict criteria for the classification of the occurrence of drowsiness is also explored in Section IV.C.1.

The results of covariate-adjusted randomization-based analyses of occurrence/nonoccurrence are presented in Section IV.C.2. Treatment comparisons are undertaken, with adjustment for the explanatory variables found in Section IV.C.1 to be associated with the incidence of adverse experiences.

Logistic regression is used to evaluate the relative importance of the explanatory variables to the occurrence/nonoccurrence of adverse experiences. The results of logistic regression analyses are presented in Section IV.C.3.

1. Contingency-Table Analyses

The number and percentage of patients having each of the probed for adverse experiences is presented, by treatment group, in Table 2.2. It was hypothesized that group AB might have lower incidence of drowsiness than group A and lower incidence of jitteriness than group B. However, the incidence of drowsiness is higher for group AB than for group A, which is the reverse of what was hypothesized, and the incidence of jitteriness is only slightly lower for group AB than group B. Group AB has a higher incidence of dizziness and nausea than any of the other groups.

Note the high treatment-period incidence for drowsiness: 42% of the placebo group were drowsy during the treatment period, although none were drowsy at baseline. This may be due to either a high background incidence for drowsiness or a strong placebo effect. No background incidence/placebo effect for jitteriness is apparent in this data; no patients had it at baseline, and none of the placebo group developed it during the treatment period.

The results of all pairwise treatment comparisons for the four adverse experiences are given in Table 2.3. Fisher's (two-sided) exact test is used instead of Pearson's chi-square test because some of the tables have cells with small expected values. For drowsiness, two sets of treatment comparisons are shown: one including all patients, and one in which patients with baseline drowsiness have been excluded. Note that for comparisons involving the placebo group, the p values are much smaller for the set of all patients than for the set of patients with no baseline drowsiness. This is because all patients who had baseline drowsiness also had treatment-period drowsiness, and, whereas at least 10% of the patients in groups AB, A, and B had baseline drowsiness, none of the placebo group had baseline drowsiness. Thus, the A versus P comparison is significant at the 0.05 level for the set of all patients, but not for the more restricted set ($p = 0.10$), and the AB versus P comparison is significant at the 0.01 level for the set of all patients, but significant at the 0.05 level for the more restricted set. The AB versus B comparison is significant at the 0.05 level for both sets of data.

Group B has significantly higher incidence of jitteriness than the placebo group ($p < 0.05$). Group AB also has a higher incidence of jitteriness than the placebo group, and this treatment difference approaches significance ($p = 0.056$). None of the treatment comparisons are statistically significant for dizziness or nausea.

Without a power analysis, the interpretation of the treatment comparisons that showed no statistically significant difference is ambiguous. The lack of significance may be due to inadequate sample size rather than the lack of a treatment difference. An example of one of the nonsignificant comparisons of interest is the AB versus A comparison for drowsiness. One would like to be assured that treatment-induced drowsiness is due to component A alone, and that the combination treatment AB does not produce increased incidence of drowsines. The null hypothesis is that the true population proportions for these two treatments are equal, that is, H_0: $\pi_{AB} = \pi_A$. The formula for power based

TABLE 2.3 Significance tests for treatment comparisons of occurrence of adverse experiences during the treatment period

Adverse experience	Comparison	Fisher's exact test (two-sided) p value
Drowsiness, all patients included	AB vs. P	0.004[b]
	AB vs. A	0.453
	AB vs. B	0.034[a]
	A vs. P	0.037[a]
	B vs. P	0.501
	A vs. B	0.168
Drowsiness, excluding those with baseline drowsiness	AB vs. P	0.016[a]
	AB vs. A	0.437
	AB vs. B	0.014[a]
	A vs. P	0.100
	B vs. P	1.000
	A vs. B	0.144
Jitteriness (none had baseline jitteriness)	AB vs. P	0.056
	AB vs. A	0.201
	AB vs. B	1.000
	A vs. P	1.000
	B vs. P	0.027[a]
	A vs. B	0.108
Dizziness, excluding those with baseline dizziness	AB vs. P	0.381
	AB vs. A	0.567
	AB vs. B	0.224
	A vs. P	1.000
	B vs. P	0.732
	A vs. B	0.736
Nausea, excluding those with baseline nausea	AB vs. P	0.116
	AB vs. A	0.358
	AB vs. B	0.358
	A vs. P	1.000
	B vs. P	1.000
	A vs. B	1.000

[a]Comparisons where $p < 0.05$.
[b]Comparisons where $p < 0.01$.

on the normal approximation to the binomial (see Lachin 1981) requires specification of values for π_{AB} and π_A under the alternative hypothesis H_1. The power $1 - \beta$, is then equal to $\Pr(Z < Z_\beta)$ where Z is a standard normal random variable,

$$Z_\beta = \frac{N^{1/2}|\pi_{AB} - \pi_A| - Z_\alpha[\bar{\pi}(1-\bar{\pi})(Q_{AB}^{-1} + Q_A^{-1})]^{1/2}}{[\pi_{AB}(1-\pi_{AB})Q_{AB}^{-1} + \pi_A(1-\pi_A)Q_A^{-1}]^{1/2}}$$

such that $N = N_{AB} + N_A$ is the total sample size, π_{AB} and π_A are the incidence proportions for groups AB and A, respectively, under H_1, Z_α is the standard normal deviate at significance level α, Q_{AB} and Q_A are the sample fractions N_{AB}/N and N_A/N, and $\bar{\pi} = Q_{AB}\pi_{AB} + Q_A\pi_A$.

Power calculations for various alternative hypotheses are shown in Table 2.4. In this table, π_c refers to the hypothesized incidence in the control group (group A in this example), and π_e refers to the hypothesized incidence in the experimental drug group (group AB). Power calculations are not shown for $\pi_c < 0.10$ because the normal approximation to the binomial does not hold for moderate sample sizes when π is close to zero. A rule of thumb is that $n\pi$ should be at least 5; this rule is not satisfied even for $\pi_c = 0.10$.

If group A is hypothesized to have drowsiness incidence of 65% (the sample value when those with baseline drowsiness are excluded), then the power to detect an increase of 10% in group AB via a chi-square test is approximately 0.24. This is actually a generous estimate of the power because the calculations in the table are based on $N = 76$ (38 per group) and $Z_\alpha = 1.645$ (for $\alpha = 0.10$, two-sided). With so little power to detect a difference of the magnitude that occurred in the sample, the result of the significance test for AB versus A is still inconclusive. About all that can be said is that the incidence difference between the two groups is probably less than 30%, since the power to detect a 30% change from 65% is 0.96. A similar type of conclusion could alternatively be reached by usage of a confidence interval for the incidence difference.

Since $\bar{\pi}(1-\bar{\pi})$ is maximized at $\bar{\pi} = 0.50$, for incidence differences of a given magnitude, the farther $\bar{\pi}$ is from 0.50, the greater the power. Thus there is a greater probability of detecting differences of a given magnitude for adverse experiences with low control-group (background) incidence than those that commonly occur spontaneously. As can be seen in Table 2.4, however, with a total sample size of 76, the power to detect an incidence difference of 20% is above 0.70 only for $\pi_c = 0.10$.

A heuristic approach to the analysis of adverse experiences with high background incidence (e.g., drowsiness) is to explore whether using more strict criteria for the classification of occurrence results in more pronounced treatment differences. The original criterion for classifying a patient as having treatment period drowsiness is the report of drowsiness for at least one of the eight treatment-period assessments. The alternative criteria should be selected so that treatment-related instances of drowsiness are still counted, but spontaneously occurring instances of

TABLE 2.4 Power calculations for two independent proportions under various specifications of the alternative hypothesis (for 2 groups of 38 each and $Z_\alpha = 1.645$)

π_c	π_e	$\lvert\pi_e - \pi_c\rvert$	$\bar{\pi}$	Z_β	Power
0.10	0.20	0.10	0.15	−0.428	0.334
	0.30	0.20	0.20	0.552	0.710
	0.40	0.30	0.25	1.466	0.929
0.20	0.30	0.10	0.25	−0.643	0.260
	0.40	0.20	0.30	0.264	0.604
	0.50	0.30	0.35	1.155	0.876
0.30	0.40	0.10	0.35	−0.735	0.231
	0.50	0.20	0.40	0.137	0.555
	0.60	0.30	0.45	1.032	0.849
0.40	0.50	0.10	0.45	−0.773	0.220
	0.60	0.20	0.50	0.101	0.540
	0.70	0.30	0.55	1.032	0.849
0.50	0.60	0.10	0.55	−0.773	0.220
	0.70	0.20	0.60	0.137	0.555
	0.80	0.30	0.65	1.155	0.876
0.60	0.70	0.10	0.65	−0.735	0.231
	0.80	0.20	0.70	0.264	0.604
	0.90	0.30	0.75	1.466	0.929
0.65	0.75	0.10	0.70	−0.698	0.243
	0.85	0.20	0.75	0.379	0.647
	0.95	0.30	0.80	1.752	0.960

drowsiness are more likely not to be counted. The investigator's opinion as to causality is not available for this data. However, one might expect that treatment-related drowsiness would occur with more frequency and consistency than spontaneously occurring drowsiness. Hence, patients were classified as having treatment-period drowsiness according to three increasingly strict criteria, and treatment comparisons were performed for each criterion. The criteria are as follows:

1. having at least two reports of drowsiness during the eight hours
2. reporting drowsiness after at least two of the three doses
3. reporting drowsiness for at least 50% of the assessments

The patient who did not return after the 11:00 a.m. assessment was excluded from all these analyses because it would be impossible for this patient to meet either criterion 1 or 2.

The number of patients satisfying each of these criteria in each treatment group, the estimated risk ratio and risk difference, and the results of Fisher's exact tests for all treatment comparisons (except B versus P; neither B nor P is suspected of producing drowsiness) are shown in Table 2.5. Under criterion 1, and again under criterion 3, an

TABLE 2.5 Number (%) with drowsiness by various criteria[a] and treatment comparisons

Treatment group or comparison	Original criterion	Criterion 1	Criterion 2	Criterion 3
	Number (%) with drowsiness			
AB ($N = 36$)	27 (75%)	21 (58%)	21 (58%)	16 (44%)
A ($N = 33$)	22 (67%)	17 (52%)	16 (48%)	12 (36%)
B ($N = 34$)	15 (44%)	9 (26%)	9 (26%)	6 (18%)
P ($N = 36$)	16 (44%)	12 (33%)	8 (22%)	6 (17%)
	Estimated risk ratios			
AB vs. P	1.69	1.75	2.63	2.67
AB vs. A	1.13	1.13	1.20	1.22
AB vs. B	1.70	2.20	2.20	2.52
A vs. P	1.50	1.55	2.18	2.18
A vs. B	1.51	1.95	1.83	2.06
	Estimated risk differences			
AB vs. P	0.31	0.25	0.36	0.28
AB vs. A	0.08	0.07	0.10	0.08
AB vs. B	0.31	0.32	0.32	0.27
A vs. P	0.22	0.18	0.26	0.20
A vs. B	0.23	0.25	0.22	0.19
	p Values for treatment comparisons by Fisher's exact (two-sided) tests			
AB vs. P	0.016[b]	0.058	0.004[c]	0.020[b]
AB vs. A	0.596	0.633	0.474	0.625
AB vs. B	0.014[b]	0.009[c]	0.009[c]	0.021[b]
A vs. P	0.090	0.149	0.026[b]	0.099
A vs. B	0.087	0.047[b]	0.080	0.104

[a]*Criteria:* The original criterion for classifying a patient as having treatment period drowsiness is that he reported drowsiness at at least one of the eight assessments. Three alternative criteria are as follows:

1. having at least two reports of drowsiness,
2. reporting drowsiness after at least two of the three doses, or
3. reporting drowsiness at at least 50% of the assessments.

Patients with baseline drowsiness are excluded from all analysis. One patient who did not return after the 11:00 a.m. assessment is also excluded.

[b]$p < 0.05$.

[c]$p < 0.01$.

appreciable percentage of each treatment group becomes no longer classified as having treatment-period drowsiness. Criteria 1 and 2 differ mainly in their effect on the placebo group. For each of the criteria, the estimated risk ratio for each treatment comparison (except A versus B, criterion 2) is at least as large as it was for the less strict criteria. However, the estimated risk differences do not necessarily increase with increasingly strict criteria. The risk differences are generally greatest under criteria 2, and the p values for treatment comparisons are generally smallest for criterion 2. Thus, increasing the strictness of the criteria for drowsiness with the expectation of strengthening the treatment comparisons did not prove to be totally successful for this data set.

Another area of interest with respect to contingency-table analysis of

TABLE 2.6 Significance tests[a] for association of explanatory variables other than treatment with occurrence of adverse experiences

	Drowsiness	Jitteriness	Dizziness	Nausea
Age (25 or less vs. >25)	0.716	0.043[b]	0.464	0.360
Sex	0.588	0.211	0.636	0.016[c]
Weight by sex				
Females (125 or less vs. >125)	0.232	0.191	0.725	0.350
Males (165 or less vs. >165)	0.675	0.669	0.160	1.000
Quetelet index (3.2 or less vs. >3.2)	0.306	0.765	1.000	1.000
Season	0.844	0.747	0.015[d]	0.879

[a]With the exception of season, the p values for the variables are from Fisher's two-sided exact tests. The p values for season are from an exact test for $r \times c$ tables (Pagano and Halvorsen, 1981).

[b]Seven (15%) of the 46 patients over 25 years of age had jitteriness, as opposed to 5 (5%) of the 109 patients less than or equal to 25.

[c]Five (10%) of the 51 females had nausea, as opposed to one (1%) of the males.

[d]Two (4%) of the 47 patients in spring 1979 had dizziness, as opposed to 8 (18%) of the 45 patients in fall 1978 and 14 (24%) of the 59 patients in fall 1979. Since season and sex are confounded, contingency tables were also constructed for season stratified by sex. The permutation test p values for these tables are for females, $p = 0.042$, and for males, $p = 0.250$. Thus, the association of season and dizziness is only evident for females. Neither of the two females enrolled in fall 1978 had dizziness, one (4%) of the 23 females enrolled in spring 1979 had it, and 8 (33%) of the 24 females enrolled in fall 1979 had it.

adverse experiences is the association between the occurrence of adverse experiences and explanatory variables other than treatment. The results of significance tests for the association of adverse-experience incidence with each of the variables age, sex, weight, Quetelet index, and season of enrollment are shown for all treatment groups combined in Table 2.6. The explanatory variables are dichotomized with the cutpoints being the overall medians (the overall mean is used for age since the median age, 22, is very close to the minimum age, 18). None of these explanatory variables are significantly associated with drowsiness. Having age greater than 25 is positively associated with jitteriness, and being female is positively associated with nausea ($p < 0.05$ by Fisher's two-sided exact test for both comparisons). Note that five of the six patients with nausea were female. Season of enrollment is significantly associated with dizziness; only 4% of the patients enrolled in spring 1979 had dizziness, as opposed to 18% of those enrolled in fall 1978 and 24% of those enrolled in fall 1979. Also, as explained in the footnote of Table 2.6, the season association is only evident for females. Since a different set of patients was enrolled at each season, the apparent season difference may be due to random subpopulation differences, rather than to changes occurring over time.

Since age is significantly associated with jitteriness, more refined and possibly more powerful treatment comparisons can be obtained by stratifying for age category. This was done using the program documented in Thomas (1975), which produces exact one-sided p values for stratified comparisons. The p values for treatment comparisons of jitteriness, stratified by age category (i.e., 25 or less versus over 25), are as follows:

Comparison	p value
AB vs. P	0.051
AB vs. A	0.128
AB vs. B	0.402
A vs. P	0.571
B vs. P	0.017
A vs. B	0.043

Since these p values are one-sided, they cannot be directly compared with the two-sided Fisher's exact test p values in Table 2.3. The most appropriate way to relate the results of a one-sided test to a two-sided test is to compare the p value from the one-sided test to one-half the significance level used for the two-sided test. If the two-sided test is considered significant at $p < 0.05$, and of borderline significance at $0.05 < p < 0.10$, then the one-sided test would be considered significant at $p < 0.025$, and of borderline significance at $0.025 < p < 0.05$. Thus, the B versus P treatment comparison for jitteriness would be considered significant by both the unstratified and stratified tests. The AB versus P comparison is of borderline significance by the unstratified test, although not (barely) by the stratified test, and the A versus B comparison is of borderline significance by the stratified test, although not (barely) by the unstratified test.

Stratified treatment comparisons could also be carried out for nausea, stratified by sex, and dizziness, stratified by season. However, since only one male had nausea, stratification by sex would produce a degenerate table (i.e., at least one of the marginals equal to zero), resulting in a loss of information. For dizziness, since none of the treatment comparisons are even close to borderline significance, conducting a stratified analysis would not be expected to produce a gain in power sufficient to result in significant treatment differences.

2. Covariate-Adjusted Randomization Statistics Analysis

In this section, a randomization statistics analysis is carried out for jitteriness covariate-adjusted for age, and for nausea covariate-adjusted for sex. The covariates chosen are the ones found in Section IV.C.1 to be significantly associated with the respective adverse experiences. The results of this analysis are shown in Table 2.7. Calculations were performed using the procedure described in Amara and Koch (1980). For each treatment comparison, two-sided p values are shown for each of three statistics: $Q(Y)$, the unadjusted statistic for comparison of treatments with respect to incidence of the adverse experience; $Q(X)$, the statistic for comparison of treatments with respect to the covariable; and $Q_G(Y|X)$, the covariate-adjusted statistic for comparison of treatments with respect to incidence of the adverse experience.

In order for the $Q_G(Y|X)$ statistic to be valid, the treatment groups must be comparable with respect to the distribution of the covariable. Thus, the $Q(X)$ statistic should not be significant, and none of the $Q(X)$ p values in Table 2.7 approach significance. The covariate-adjusted statistic is not guaranteed to be more significant than the unadjusted statistic. However, for the treatment comparisons performed for jitteriness and nausea, the adjusted statistics tend to be slightly more significant than the unadjusted statistics.

An advantage of covariate-adjusted randomization statistics analysis compared to stratified contingency-table analysis is that the covariables may include variables that if used for stratification would result in degenerate tables (e.g., sex in the case of nausea, or continuous variables

TABLE 2.7 Covariate-adjusted randomization statistics analysis of jitteriness and nausea

Adverse experience	Covariable	Comparison	$Q(Y)^a$ p value	$Q(X)^b$ p value	$Q_G(Y\|X)^c$ p value
Jitteriness	Age (continuous)	AB vs. P	0.029^d	0.742	0.027^d
		AB vs. A	0.098	0.655	0.089
		AB vs. B	0.747	0.892	0.714
		A vs. P	0.337	0.917	0.339
		B vs. P	0.016^d	0.623	0.011^d
		A vs. B	0.053	0.536	0.037^d
Nausea	Sex	AB vs. P	0.050^d	0.984	0.044^d
		AB vs. A	0.168	0.478	0.108
		AB vs. B	0.168	0.810	0.134
		A vs. P	0.337	0.475	0.391
		B vs. P	0.337	0.798	0.352
		A vs. B	1.000	0.639	0.917

[a] $Q(Y)$ is the unadjusted statistic for comparison of treatments with respect to incidence of the adverse experience.
[b] $Q(X)$ is the statistic for comparison of treatments with respect to the covariable.
[c] $Q_G(Y|X)$ is the statistic for comparison of treatments with respect to incidence of the adverse experience, adjusted for the covariable.
[d] $p < 0.05$.

like age). Multiple covariates may also be used. A disadvantage of randomization statistics analysis is that, for all practical purposes, asymptotic tests must be used rather than exact tests. Thus the $Q(Y)$ p values in Table 2.7 are smaller than the corresponding Fisher's exact test p values in Table 2.3. Also, the sample size requirements for covariate-adjusted randomization statistics with dichotomous response variables have not been thoroughly studied. The asymptotics for covariate-adjusted randomization statistics are likely to be better than for the Pearson chi-square because they are based on variables with more than two possible values (i.e., the residuals of the regression of Y on X; see Section III.A.2). Therefore, if the sample size requirements for a Pearson chi-square test are satisfied, then the requirements for a covariance randomization statistics test should also be satisfied (Koch, Imrey, Singer, Atkinson, and Stokes, 1985). A common requirement for the Pearson chi-square is that at least 80% of the cells have expected values of at least 5. This requirement is not satisfied for any of the nausea treatment comparisons or for most of the jitteriness comparisons. Thus, for this data, an exact contingency table analysis with stratification for significant explanatory variables is probably more appropriate than a randomization statistics analysis with covariance adjustment.

3. Logistic Regression

Logistic regression of occurrence/nonoccurrence of the four adverse experiences was used to supplement the results of randomization-based

TABLE 2.8 Final logistic regression models[a]

Drowsiness (80/140 had drowsiness)

Variable	$\hat{\beta}$	se($\hat{\beta}$)	p value	COMP A	Estimated probability of adverse experience: Model predicted	Sample proportion
Intercept	−0.230	0.241	0.340	No	0.443	0.429
COMP A	1.077	0.355	0.002	Yes	0.700	0.700

Jitteriness (12/155 had jitteriness)

Variable	$\hat{\beta}$	se($\hat{\beta}$)	p value
Intercept	−4.874	1.076	<0.001
COMP B	2.478	1.064	0.020
AGECAT	1.331	0.636	0.036

See Figure 2.1

Dizziness (24/151 had dizziness)

Variable	$\hat{\beta}$	se($\hat{\beta}$)	p value	SEASON2	Estimated probability of adverse experience: Model predicted	Sample proportion
Intercept	−1.316	0.240	<0.001	No	0.211	0.212
SEASON2	−1.798	0.761	0.018	Yes	0.043	0.043

Nausea (6/153 had nausea)

Variable	$\hat{\beta}$	se($\hat{\beta}$)	p value	SEX	TRT AB	Estimated probability of adverse experience: Model predicted	Sample proportion
Intercept	−5.652	1.217	<0.001	M	No	0.004	0.000
SEX	2.587	1.134	0.023	M	Yes	0.027	0.037
TRT AB	2.080	0.925	0.025	F	No	0.045	0.051
				F	Yes	0.272	0.250

[a]Variable definitions:

COMP A, COMP B:	indicator variables for component A, component B
TRT AB:	indicator variable for treatment AB
AGE:	continuous age
AGECAT:	1 if age greater than 25, 0 otherwise
SEX:	1 if female, 0 if male
QUET:	continuous Quetelet index
WEIGHT F:	continuous weight for females, 0 for males
WEIGHT M:	continuous weight for males, 0 for females
SEASON2:	1 if spring 1979, 0 otherwise
SEASON3:	1 if fall 1979, 0 otherwise

analyses presented in previous sections. For drowsiness, stepwise logistic regression was used to assess treatment effects simultaneously with the effects of other explanatory variables. For jitteriness, dizziness, and nausea, however, due to the small numbers of patients having these adverse experiences, logistic regression modeling was used more for descriptive purposes than for variable selection. When there are m observations in the least frequent category of a dichotomous response variable, Harrell (1986a) recommends considering no more than $m/10$ explanatory variables in the analysis in order to derive a somewhat reliable model. Since only 12 patients had jitteriness and only six had nausea, simultaneous consideration of several explanatory variables must be undertaken with extreme caution for these two adverse experiences.

The parameter estimates and predicted values for the logistic regression models derived are shown in Table 2.8, and the definitions of the candidate variables for inclusion are shown in the footnote at the bottom of this table. The treatment candidate variables reflect the factorial nature of the study design; there are indicator variables for components A and B, and an indicator variable for the combination treatment AB. Other candidate variables include two age variables (continuous age and an indicator for age greater than 25), sex, a variable for the Quetelet index, two variables for weight nested within sex, and two indicator variables for season. Calculations were performed using the SAS procedure LOGIST. The significance level to enter the models was 0.15, and the significance level to stay was 0.10.

For drowsiness, the only variable to enter the model was the indicator for component A. This agrees with all the analysis done thus far, in that the difference between treatment AB and treatment A is not significant, nor are any of the nontreatment variables significant. One way to assess the power to detect an increase in drowsiness due to treatment AB is to include the indicator variables for component A and treatment AB in a logistic model, and use the estimated standard error for the coefficient of treatment AB in a power calculation. For such a model, the coefficient for treatment AB is 0.492, and the standard error is 0.526. Therefore, under the assumption that the coefficient is normally distributed with known variance, the power to detect a two-sided alternative like 1:3 odds ratio (e.g., 50% in group A versus 75% in group AB, or vice versa) is

$$
\begin{aligned}
\text{Power} &= 1 - \Pr\left\{-1.96 - \frac{\ln(0.333)}{0.526} \leq Z \leq 1.96 - \frac{\ln(0.333)}{0.526}\right\} \\
&= 1 - \Pr\{0.131 \leq Z \leq 4.051\}
\end{aligned}
$$

Alternatively, the results from logistic regression can be used to construct the 95% confidence interval $\exp\{0.492 \pm 1.96(0.526)\} = (0.58, 4.89)$ for the odds ratio; its wide range further clarifies the limitations of the available sample size for supporting conclusions about the similarity of treatment A and treatment AB.

For jitteriness, a similar stepwise regression was conducted, and the indicator variables for component B and for age greater than 25 were the only variables to enter the model. It is impossible to assess the interaction of these two variables because none of the patients whose age is less than or equal to 25 and who did not receive component B had jitteriness. However, a second model was computed using continuous age (AGE) instead of the age indicator variables, and for this model the interaction between age and component B (COMP B) was not significant. This second model, without the interaction term, was used to produce a graphical display of the predicted probabilities of jitteriness for treatment group (component B versus no component B) by age. The parameter estimates for this model are shown below, and a plot of predicted values is given in Figure 2.1.

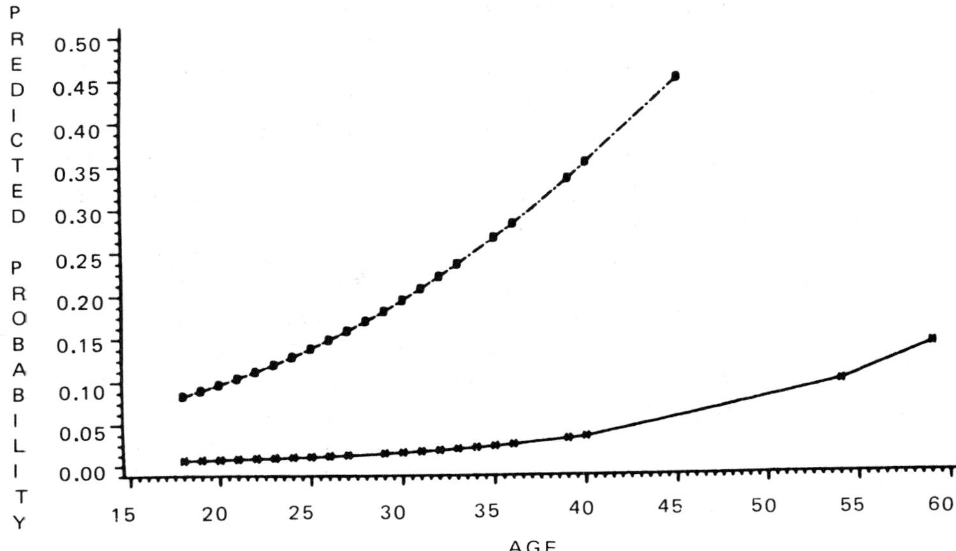

FIGURE 2.1 Predicted probabilities of jitteriness by age and treatment for sample observations. The top curve is for treatments containing component B, and the bottom curve is for treatments not containing component B. (Please note that only three patients are older than 40.)

Variable	$\hat{\beta}$	se($\hat{\beta}$)	Q	p value
Intercept	−6.600	1.712	14.86	<0.001
COMP B	2.737	1.116	6.02	0.014
AGE	0.081	1.041	3.88	0.049

The only variable to enter the stepwise regression for dizziness was an indicator variable for season. For nausea, stepwise variable selection was not used. Instead, the model was forced to include only the indicator variables for sex and treatment AB. For both dizziness and nausea, the model-predicted probabilities of the adverse experience are very close to the sample proportions.

D. Correlation Analysis

A correlation analysis was undertaken in order to describe the extent to which different adverse experiences tend to occur simultaneously. For example, it would not be expected that patients would experience both drowsiness and jitteriness simultaneously. However, many of the patients with jitteriness might also have nausea or dizziness. Since the dosing and assessments times were at regular intervals, and since very few patients missed assessments, the proportion of assessments at which a patient reported a given adverse experience is a meaningful variable for this study. This proportion was used in calculating a Spearman rank correlation coefficient for each pair of adverse experiences. These correlations are shown in Table 2.9 for the pooled group of patients and by treatment group. Also shown are the p values for testing whether the correlations differ from zero. The p values were obtained by noting that $(n-1)r^2$ is approximately distributed as a chi-square with one degree of freedom, where r is the sample Spearman correlation and n is the sample size (Landis et al., 1979). Because baseline occurrence of adverse experiences appears to be strongly associated with treatment-period occurrence, patients having any of the four adverse experiences at baseline are excluded from the correlation analysis.

For the pooled group of patients, the only correlation that is significant at the 0.05 level is the correlation between jitteriness and nausea, which is based on only a few cases. Thirteen of the 137 patients had either jitteriness of nausea, and only two patients had both (one in group A and one in group B). The group A patient with both nausea and jitteriness is solely responsible for the perfect correlation between nausea and jitteriness in group A, and the group B patient with both is respon-

TABLE 2.9 Spearman rank correlations between adverse experiences[a]

	Adverse experience (number with adv. exp.)	Jitteriness		Dizziness		Nausea	
		r	p value	r	p value	r	p value
Pooled group of pts. ($n = 137$)	Drowsiness (77)	−0.033	(0.699)	0.130	(0.130)	0.144	(0.093)
	Jitteriness (9)			−0.039	(0.648)	0.241	(0.005)
	Dizziness (22)					0.104	(0.225)
	Nausea (6)						
Group AB ($n = 34$)	Drowsiness (25)	0.161	(0.354)	0.319	(0.067)	0.448	(0.010)
	Jitteriness (3)			0.050	(0.775)	−0.113	(0.515)
	Dizziness (8)					0.228	(0.191)
	Nausea (4)						
Group A ($n = 34$)	Drowsiness (22)	−0.200	(0.250)	−0.060	(0.729)	−0.200	(0.250)
	Jitteriness (1)			−0.080	(0.645)	1.000	(0.000)
	Dizziness (6)					−0.080	(0.645)
	Nausea (1)						
Group B ($n = 33$)	Drowsiness (14)	−0.114	(0.520)	0.100	(0.572)	−0.145	(0.412)
	Jitteriness (5)			−0.133	(0.452)	0.447	(0.012)
	Dizziness (3)					−0.056	(0.752)
	Nausea (1)						
Group P ($n = 36$)	Drowsiness (16)			0.131	(0.438)		
	Jitteriness (0)						
	Dizziness (5)						
	Nausea (0)						

[a]Patients with any of the four adverse experiences at baseline are excluded from the analysis.

sible for the high correlation in group B. The only other correlation worthy of note is the drowsiness–nausea correlation, which is of borderline significance for the pooled group of patients, and highly significant for group AB. There were four patients with nausea in group AB, and all four also had drowsiness.

E. Analysis of Severity and Frequency of Drowsiness

The analysis so far has shown that drowsiness is associated with component A, and that treatments AB and A do not differ significantly with respect to whether or not patients had drowsiness during the treatment period. However, the failure to detect a difference between treatments AB and A may be due to the power of the tests being low, rather than to the lack of a treatment difference.

It is also of interest to compare treatments AB and A with respect to the severity and frequency of drowsiness. However, the power of statistical tests for treatment differences with respect to these two variables would also be low, and thus nonsignificant results would also be inconclusive. Although an in-depth analysis of the severity and frequency of drowsiness is probably not warranted for this study, the data set provides a useful context for discussion of the issues pertaining to the analysis of such variables. Several approaches are illustrated by examples.

Severity is an ordinal variable with four categories: none, mild, moderate, and severe (which includes very severe). A reasonable choice for a summary variable is the severity of the most severe episode of drowsiness during the treatment period. The frequency of drowsiness can be represented, as in Section IV.D, by the proportion of assessments at which the patient reported drowsiness. Since almost all patients had eight treatment period assessments, frequency is essentially a discrete ratio-scale variable with nine levels.

Several methods of analysis are possible. Randomization-based analysis, as described in Section III.A, can be used for either severity or frequency or a multivariate analysis of both variables. The randomization-based analysis can employ the variables as described above, or a variety of scores constructed from the variables. For example, it may be that mild drowsiness is considered tolerable in the treatment of nasal congestion, whereas moderate or severe drowsiness is not. In this case, dichotomous variables for severity would be appropriate.

Logistic regression can also be used for analysis of dichotomous variables. Extensions of logistic regression can be used for ordinal variables (e.g., severity) or grouped continuous variables (e.g., frequency, if grouped into three or four categories). Two well-known models for multiple response logistic regression are the proportional odds model and the equal adjacent odds model. As discussed in Section III.D, the equal adjacent odds model is appropriate for the analysis of a fixed set of categories, whereas the proportional odds model can be used when the responses are viewed as falling along an underlying continuum (Koch, Amara, and Singer, 1985). For the analysis of severity and frequency, the proportional odds model is probably more appropriate than the equal adjacent odds model.

Weighted least-squares methods can also be used in the analysis of either severity or frequency. Since there must be at least a moderate sample size in each subpopulation (e.g., at least 20), treatment groups can be used as subpopulations, but the study size is not large enough for further stratification.

In addition to choosing the method of analysis, one must also decide how to incorporate the baseline data. The simplest method is to exclude the patients with baseline drowsiness. There are too few patients with baseline drowsiness to use baseline status as a stratification variable. However, the difficulties that arose with using baseline status as a covariable in the analysis of occurrence/nonoccurrence do not apply to the analysis of severity or frequency. Baseline status (either occurrence/nonoccurrence or severity) can be used as a covariable with either logistic regression or randomization-based analysis. Another way to incorporate the baseline data in the analysis of severity is to use the change from baseline as a response variable.

A graphical display of the severity of drowsiness by treatment group is presented in Figure 2.2. Although groups AB and A have about the same proportion of patients with severe drowsiness, group AB has a somewhat higher proportion with moderate drowsiness. The results of randomization-based analysis of severity are shown in Table 2.10. The AB versus P and AB versus B comparisons are the only ones significant at the 0.05 level. Also shown in this table are the results of a randomization-based analysis of frequency, and a randomization-based multivariate analysis of both severity and frequency. The AB versus P and AB versus B comparisons are the only significant ones here also. The p values for the multivariate analysis are generally larger than the p values for either of the univariate analyses.

A stepwise logistic regression using the proportional odds model was carried out for severity of drowsiness, and the results of this analysis are shown in Table 2.11. Calculations were performed using the SAS procedure LOGIST. As might be expected, the indicator variable for component A was the only variable to enter the model.

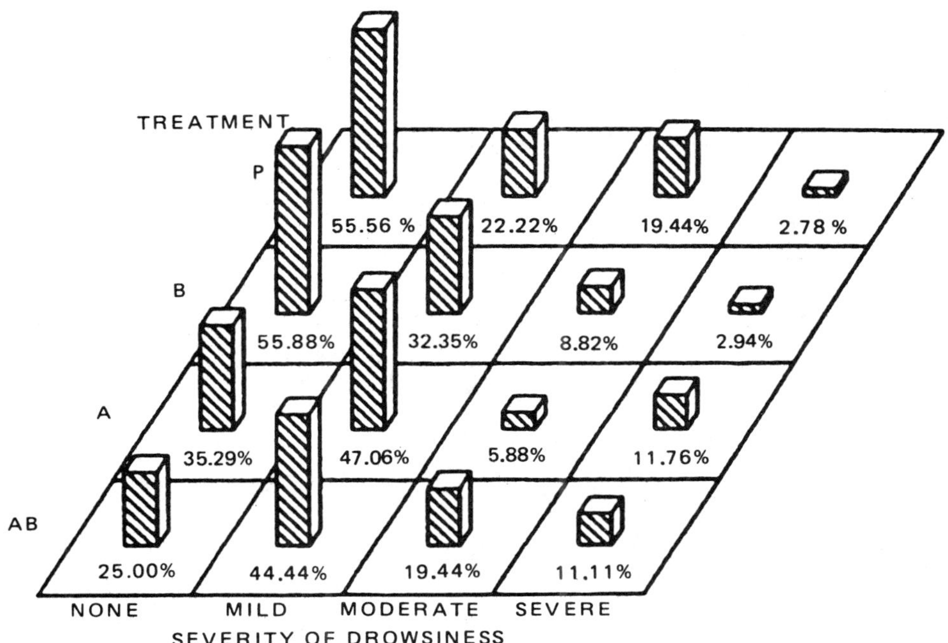

FIGURE 2.2 Summary of severity of drowsiness by treatment group. Patients with baseline drowsiness are excluded.

TABLE 2.10 Randomization-based analysis of severity[a] and frequency[b] of drowsiness

	p Values for treatment comparisons		
Treatment comparison	Severity	Frequency	Multivariate analysis of severity and frequency
AB vs. P	0.033[c]	0.002[d]	0.010[c]
AB vs. A	0.319	0.198	0.436
AB vs. B	0.008[d]	0.007[d]	0.019[c]
A vs. P	0.263	0.063	0.174
B vs. P	0.595	0.830	0.600
A vs. B	0.099	0.119	0.226

[a]Severity: 0 = none, 1 = mild, 2 = moderate, 3 = severe.
[b]Frequency: (assessments where drowsiness reported)/(assessments made).
[c]$p < 0.05$.
[d]$p < 0.01$.

TABLE 2.11 Stepwise logistic regression for severity of drowsiness[a]

Parameter estimates Variable[a]	$\hat{\beta}$	se($\hat{\beta}$)	Q	p value
Intercept1	−0.167	0.238	0.49	0.483
Intercept2	−1.861	0.288	41.85	<0.001
Intercept3	−3.099	0.387	64.00	<0.001
COMP A	0.908	0.323	7.90	0.005

[a]The response variable is the severity of drowsiness (0 = none, 1 = mild, 2 = moderate, 3 = severe). Patients with baseline drowsiness were excluded. Sixty patients had no drowsiness, 51 had mild, 19 had moderate, and 10 had severe.
[b]Candidate variables:

COMP A: indicator variable for component A
TRT AB: indicator variable for treatment AB
SEX: 1 if female, 0 if male
AGE: continuous age
AGECAT: 1 if age greater than 25, 0 otherwise

A weighted least-squares analysis of frequency was carried out using the program MISCAT (documented in Stanish et al., 1978). The functions to be modeled were the average proportion of assessments at which drowsiness was reported for each treatment group. These functions were calculated by first submitting to MISCAT an array of patient by assessment indicator variables: 1 if the patient reported drowsiness at the assessment, 0 if no drowsiness, or missing. A ratio estimator was used to calculate the mean of the observations present, and the covariance matrix was estimated via the delta method (see Stanish et al., 1978). The functions modeled were the means of these means (i.e., for each treatment group, the sum of the means divided by eight). A four by four identity matrix was used as the design matrix, and contrast matrices were used for pairwise comparisons of the treatments. The methodology of MISCAT is only recommended if the missing data occur randomly and with low probability. Since there are very few missing values, one may assume that this assumption is met.

The results of this weighted least squares analysis are shown in Table 2.12. The p values for treatment comparisons are smaller than the corresponding p values from the randomization-based analysis. However, as pointed out in Johnson et al. (1981), these two methods have different orientations. The weighted least-squares analysis uses all observations simultaneously in all treatment comparisons, whereas the randomization-based analyses use only the two treatment groups to be compared.

TABLE 2.12 Results of weighted least-squares analysis of frequency of drowsiness[a]

Estimated model parameters (with standard errors):

$$\mathbf{X} = \mathbf{I}_4 \qquad \begin{bmatrix} 0.417\ (0.060) \\ 0.315\ (0.056) \\ 0.188\ (0.051) \\ 0.171\ (0.043) \end{bmatrix} = \begin{bmatrix} \text{average proportion for group AB} \\ \text{average proportion for group A} \\ \text{average proportion for group B} \\ \text{average proportion for group P} \end{bmatrix}$$

Treatment comparison	Contrast matrix	Q	p value
AB vs. P	[1 0 0 −1]	11.05	0.001[b]
AB vs. A	[1 −1 0 0]	1.52	0.217
AB vs. B	[1 0 −1 0]	8.39	0.004[b]
A vs. P	[0 1 0 −1]	4.15	0.042[c]
B vs. P	[0 0 1 −1]	0.07	0.797
A vs. B	[0 1 −1 0]	2.80	0.095

[a]Patients with baseline drowsiness are excluded. The functions (and model parameters) are the average proportion of assessments at which drowsiness was reported for each treatment group.

[b]$p < 0.01$.

[c]$p < 0.05$.

V. AN ANTIDEPRESSANT DRUG TRIAL EXAMPLE

Suzanne Edwards, Gary G. Koch, and William Sollecito

A. Description of the Trial

The data analyzed in this chapter are from a parallel-designed, randomized, double-blind clinical trial of an experimental antidepressant drug versus placebo control. The main objective of the study was to evaluate the efficacy and chronic dose tolerance of the experimental drug in initially hospitalized nonpsychotic depressed patients. The study was conducted in two centers, and the treatment phase was to last a maximum of 28 days.

Following a washout period, patients were randomized to receive daily doses of either the antidepressant drug or a placebo. The antidepressant was given according to an ascending dosage schedule, with an increase in dosage at day 5 and another at day 8. If the treatment was not adequately tolerated, however, dosage could be adjusted downward to not less than a minimum dose, and subsequently upward, as deemed necessary by the investigator.

A patient was considered to have completed the study if the patient either (1) received at least 3 weeks of treatment or (2) showed substantial improvement and a Hamilton Depression Score of less than 10, in which case termination from treatment could occur after 2 weeks. Forty-seven of the 117 patients enrolled did not complete the study. Of these, four dropped out before the first treatment-period assessment, so only 113 patients provide data for safety analyses.

Adverse experiences were to be assessed once during the baseline period, at 5, 8, 11, 14, 21, and 28 days after the start of treatment, and at 1 and 7 days posttreatment. The treatment-phase assessments were not always made on the scheduled day, so an assignment of observed assessment days to scheduled assessment days was made for the purposes of analysis. The investigators used an adverse-experience check list to record the severity (not present, mild, moderate, or severe), drug relationship (none, remote, possible, probable, or definite), and action taken with respect to 34 potential adverse experiences. Space was also provided for the investigator to write in other adverse experiences.

The two centers differed appreciably with respect to a number of factors that could influence either the occurrence or reporting of adverse experiences. Center 1 was a private psychiatric hospital, and Center 2 was a Veterans Administration hospital. As can be seen in Table 2.13 the two centers differed substantially with respect to sex composition: 73% of the patients in Center 1 were female, as opposed to 8% of the patients in Center 2. In addition, most of the patients in Center 1 were married, whereas most of the patients in Center 2 were single, especially those randomized to receive the active drug. The two centers also differed with respect to the patients' psychiatric diagnoses (mainly manic depressive in Center 1 versus mainly neurotic depressive in Center 2) and duration of the current episode of depression (generally longer in Center 2).

In addition to the differences in the demographic and medical characteristics of the study patients, the centers also differed with respect to several aspects of study management. In Center 1, the doses were adjusted more on an individual patient basis, whereas in Center 2, most patients received the same regimen. The mean daily dose was higher for Center 2. However, the dosage was in milligrams rather than milligrams per kilogram, and, since most of the patients in Center 2 were male, the mean plasma concentration may not have been higher. The use, or at least the reporting, of all types of concomitant medications was substantially higher in Center 1. This included the use of psychoactive medications, which were forbidden by the protocol. Another difference between the centers concerned an unofficial protocol amendment allowing patients to be discharged from the hospital and continue in the study

TABLE 2.13 Summary statistics of demographic characteristics

	Center 1		Center 2	
Characteristic	Placebo	Active	Placebo	Active
N	21	43	17	32
Sex				
Female	18 (86%)	29 (67%)	3 (18%)	1 (3%)
Male	3 (14%)	14 (33%)	14 (82%)	31 (97%)
Race				
Caucasian	20 (95%)	41 (95%)	14 (82%)	28 (88%)
Other	1 (5%)	2 (5%)	3 (18%)	4 (12%)
Age (years)				
Mean	50.2	44.0	43.9	49.8
Median	47.0	43.0	41.0	51.0
Range	22–78	20–70	19–86	20–84
Marital status[a]				
Married	12 (57%)	23 (53%)	8 (47%)	3 (9%)
Single	9 (43%)	20 (47%)	9 (53%)	29 (91%)

[a]Single defined as never married, separated, divorced, or widowed.

as outpatients if the investigator believed they had improved enough. Twenty-one (33%) of the patients in Center 1 did this, as compared with 2 (14%) of the patients in Center 2.

All of the 113 patients evaluated for safety had at least one adverse experience during the treatment period. However, only 57 patients had adverse experiences that were considered by the investigator to be possibly to definitely drug-related. Table 2.14 shows the number of patients having none versus at least one treatment-phase adverse experience, where only those considered to be possibly to definitely drug-related are counted. In Center 1, 67% of the patients in the active drug group had at least one such adverse experience, as compared to 33% of the placebo group. This treatment difference is statistically significant ($p = 0.015$, Fisher's exact test, two-sided) for Center 1, but no treatment difference is apparent for Center 2 ($p = 0.999$). Thus the two centers also differed in the extent to which a treatment effect is apparent for adverse experiences considered possibly to definitely drug-related. It is interesting to note that the two centers also differed with respect to demonstration of treatment efficacy. In Center 1, the drug was significantly more efficacious than placebo, whereas in Center 2 no statistically significant treatment difference in efficacy was found.

TABLE 2.14 Number of patients having possibly to definitely drug-related adverse experiences during the treatment phase by center and treatment

		No. poss. to def. related adverse experiences	At least one	Total	p value[a]
Center 1	Placebo	14 (67%)	7 (33%)	21	$p = 0.015$
	Active	14 (33%)	29 (67%)	43	
				64	
Center 2	Placebo	10 (59%)	7 (41%)	17	$p = 0.999$
	Active	18 (56%)	14 (44%)	32	
				49	

[a]The *p* values are from two-sided Fisher's exact tests.

B. Overview of Statistical Analyses

The first type of analysis undertaken for this data set is a contingency-table analysis for the comparison of treatments within centers with respect to the occurrence/nonoccurrence of each of the adverse experiences during the treatment period. Refinements to this analysis are then considered. The refinements in Section V.C involve restricting attention to a subset of the adverse experiences that are more likely to be treatment-induced. Treatment comparisons with respect to two commonly used subsetting criteria are undertaken and the results are compared. The first criterion involves the investigator's opinion of the causality of the adverse experience, and the second involves the severity of the adverse experience relative to its baseline severity.

In Section V.D, selected treatment comparisons from Section V.C are further refined by using randomization statistics with stratification by center and covariate adjustment for baseline and number of assessments. In any study where there is an appreciable dropout rate, the binary occurrence/non-occurrence variable is likely to depend on some measure of time on study, for example, the number of assessments. In this study it is particularly important to adjust in some way for time on study because the investigators were to follow an ascending dose schedule, and thus the patients in the active drug group were exposed to higher single doses, as well as higher cumulative doses, as the study progressed. A randomization statistics analysis is also carried out for two other summary response variables, a measure of severity and a measure of frequency/duration, and these results are compared to the results for the binary response measure.

Descriptive analyses via logistic regression modeling are undertaken in Section V.E for selected adverse experiences. The explanatory variables considered include center, treatment, baseline severity, number of assessments, sex, age, efficacy of treatment, and concomitant medication usage.

C. Comparison of Adverse Experience Patterns for Various Criteria

The percent of patients having at least one treatment-period adverse experience, regardless of drug relationship, is shown for 31 of the adverse experiences by center and treatment in Table 2.15. The only adverse experiences not shown in this table are sex-related adverse experiences (menstrual disturbance and impotence) and dystonia (no patients had it). The adverse experiences appear under the same headings as were used in the data collection forms, that is, psychological/behavioral, neurological, autonomic, cardiovascular, and other. The treatment groups within centers were compared with respect to each of the adverse experiences by Fisher's exact tests. Due to the large number of tests performed, each of the individual p values in this table must be viewed cautiously. If all 31 adverse experiences were independent, which is not the case, one would expect about three of the comparisons to be significant at the 0.10 level due to chance alone.

Six of the treatment comparisons in Table 2.15 are significant at the 0.10 level. Of these, the significantly higher incidence of increased appetite, rigidity, and dry mouth for the placebo group in Center 2 can be at least partially explained by differences between the treatment groups at baseline. The Center 2 placebo group had a higher incidence of increased appetite ($p = 0.116$) at baseline, and a significantly higher incidence of rigidity ($p < 0.05$) and dry mouth ($p < 0.01$) at baseline. The treatment differences for Center 1, on the other hand, cannot be explained by baseline treatment differences. The active drug group had a higher incidence of both tiredness and decreased appetite at baseline. The fact that the placebo group has a significantly higher incidence of these two adverse experiences during the treatment period may be evidence of the efficacy of active drug, since both tiredness and decreased appetite are symptoms of depression. The other significant treatment comparison in Center 1 is the higher incidence of tremor in the active group. The active group also had higher incidence of tremor at baseline, but the difference did not approach significance.

In Table 2.15, little agreement is shown between the two centers with

TABLE 2.15 Percent of patients having adverse experiences during the treatment period by center and treatment[a]

Adverse experience	Center 1				Center 2			
	Placebo ($n = 21$) %	Active ($n = 43$) %	>%	p Value	Placebo ($n = 17$) %	Active ($n = 32$) %	>%	p Value
Psychological/behavioral								
Hallucinations	0	0	—		6	0	P	
Euphoria	0	5	A		0	3	—	
Agitation/excitement	100	88	P		82	97	A	
Irresponsible behavior	24	23	—		6	19	A	
Inapprop. aggression	19	19	—		6	16	A	
Insomnia	100	98	—		94	97	—	
Tiredness	100	84	P	0.085	94	81	P	
Drowsiness	33	16	P		41	47	A	
Decreased appetite	95	60	P	0.003	53	69	A	
Increased appetite	5	7	—		24	3	P	0.043
Headache	76	58	P		76	72	—	
Neurological								
Myoclonus	0	5	A		0	0	—	
Cramps	5	2	—		6	3	—	
Rigidity	0	5	A		18	0	P	0.037

Tremor	10	42	A	0.010	41	22	P	
Akathisia	0	2	—		0	0	—	
Paresthesia	5	7	—		12	9	—	
Dyskinesia	0	0	—		0	3	—	
Autonomic								
Blurred vision	19	14	P		29	41	A	
Dry mouth	52	58	A		71	25	P	0.005
Increased salivation	5	5	—		6	0	P	
Constipation	71	51	P		41	28	P	
Urinary retention	5	7	—		12	3	P	
Nocturia	19	9	P		24	22	—	
Diarrhea	5	9	—		24	9	P	
Sweating	14	30	A		29	22	P	
Nausea/vomiting	57	49	P		24	31	A	
Cardiovascular								
Fainting/dizziness	71	65	P		47	28	P	
Palpitations	52	49	—		65	50	P	
Other								
Dermatologic	5	9	—		18	3	P	
Joint pain/stiffness	14	14	—		24	22	—	

[a]The column headed ">%" shows the group having higher percentage of patients with adverse experiences during the treatment period. It is shown only if the two groups differ by at least 5 percentage points. The p values are from Fisher's (two-sided) exact tests, and are shown only if $p < 0.10$.

respect to which treatment group has higher incidence of each of the adverse experiences. The treatment comparisons may be refined by restricting attention to a subset of adverse experiences that are more likely to be treatment-induced. Two commonly used subsetting criteria are (1) using only adverse experiences that are considered by the investigator to be at least possibly drug-related, and (2) using only adverse experiences that are treatment-emergent, that is, new or exacerbated relative to baseline. The second criterion is the same as that proposed by Metzler and Schooley (1981) as a way to differentiate the potential side effects of the drug from the symptoms of the underlying disease in trials of psychoactive drugs (see Section II.B.1). In this section, treatment comparisons using each of these criteria are presented, and the advantages of each approach are discussed.

The criterion of treatment emergence is the more objective of the two criteria. However, the patient's status at baseline is not always a relevant consideration. Baseline status is less relevant for adverse experiences that often occur spontaneously (e.g., headache or drowsiness), especially if these adverse experiences occur several weeks after the baseline assessment, and if they are not reported at the intervening assessments. Theoretically, the investigator takes the baseline status into consideration, along with other factors, in deciding drug relationship, so the criterion of being at least possibly drug-related should generally provide a more relevant subset. However, although guidelines are usually provided for determining drug relationship, some subjectivity on the part of the investigator is inevitable, particularly if there is any lack of blindedness in the study. The choice of using adverse experiences considered at least *possibly* drug-related is also subjective. One could easily have decided to choose those considered at least remotely drug-related. In view of the arguments of Skegg and Doll (1977; see Section I.F.), it may not be advisable to make this criterion any more strict, such as to choose only those adverse experiences at least probably drug-related.

Treatment comparisons for adverse experiences considered at least possibly drug-related are shown in Table 2.16. The pattern of incidence shown in this table is much more coherent than in Table 2.15 where all adverse experiences are considered. Within both centers, the active group has a higher incidence than the placebo group of all adverse experiences for which the incidence difference is at least 5%.

Treatment comparisons for the treatment-emergent adverse experiences are shown in Table 2.17. Note that the sample sizes of the treatment groups are not shown in this table. This is because for each adverse experience the patients with a baseline intensity of "severe" were excluded, since exacerbation from baseline is not possible in this case.

For many of the adverse experiences in Table 2.17, the effective sample sizes were smaller than the true sample sizes, thus reducing the power to detect treatment differences. This is particularly true for the adverse experiences that are also symptoms of depression. For insomnia, the reduction in sample size was substantial: 56% of the patients had severe insomnia at baseline.

The incidence patterns shown in Tables 2.16 and 2.17 are very different. In Table 2.17, the placebo group has higher incidence for many of the adverse experiences, and there is little agreement between the centers. In Table 2.16, on the other hand, the active group has higher incidence for all adverse experiences for which the incidence difference was at least 5%. In view of the lack of agreement between Tables 2.16 and 2.17, the consistency of the higher incidence for the active group in Table 2.16 raises the suspicion, at least, that blindedness may have been violated.

The only adverse experience for which a significant treatment difference was shown in both Tables 2.16 and 2.17 (and also in Table 2.15) was tremor: the active group in Center 1 had significantly higher incidence. However, this difference is not supported by the Center 2 data. Although the Center 2 active group has a slightly higher incidence than the placebo group of at least possibly drug-related tremor (Table 2.16), the Center 2 placebo group has a higher incidence than the active group of treatment-emergent tremor (Table 2.17).

The criterion of at least possible drug relationship appears to be the more stringent of the two criteria. For each of the adverse experiences except insomnia, tiredness, drowsiness, decreased appetite, and constipation in the Center 1 active group, the number of patients per center and treatment who met the criterion for Table 2.17 is at least as large as the corresponding number in Table 2.16 (note that only the percentages, not the numbers, are shown in the tables).

Four of the treatment-emergent adverse experiences for which the Center 1 placebo group has a significantly higher incidence than the active group are insomnia, tiredness, drowsiness, and decreased appetite. Since all four of these are symptoms of depression, these results may provide evidence of the efficacy of the active drug, although they are not supported by the Center 2 data. The other significant treatment differences in Table 2.17 are the higher incidence in the Center 1 placebo group of nocturia ($p = 0.085$) and fainting/dizziness ($p < 0.01$). The higher incidence of headache for the Center 1 placebo group is also close to borderline significance ($p = 0.120$).

The only adverse experiences, other than tremor, for which a significant treatment difference was shown in Table 2.16 were constipation in

TABLE 2.16 Percent of patients having possibly to definitely drug-related adverse experiences during the treatment period by center and treatment[a]

	Center 1				Center 2			
Adverse experience	Placebo ($n = 21$) %	Active ($n = 43$) %	>%	p value	Placebo ($n = 17$) %	Active ($n = 32$) %	>%	p value
Psychological/behavioral								
Hallucinations	0	0	—		0	0	—	
Euphoria	0	2	—		0	3	—	
Agitation/excitement	14	28	A		0	22	A	0.080
Irrespons. behavior	5	2	—		0	0	—	
Inapprop. aggression	5	5	—		0	3	—	
Insomnia	10	26	A		0	13	A	
Tiredness	10	14	—		0	9	A	
Drowsiness	0	12	A		0	3	—	
Decreased appetite	10	26	A		0	9	A	
Increased appetite	0	7	A		0	0	—	
Headache	10	16	A		6	19	A	
Neurological								
Myoclonus	0	2	—		0	0	—	
Cramps	0	0	—		0	0	—	
Rigidity	0	0	—		0	0	—	

Tremor	5	28	A	0.045	0	6	A
Akathisia	0	2	—		0	0	—
Paresthesia	0	5	A		0	0	—
Dyskinesia	0	0	—		0	0	—
Autonomic							
Blurred vision	0	9	A		0	9	A
Dry mouth	5	21	A		12	13	—
Increased salivation	5	2	—		0	0	—
Constipation	0	26	A	0.012	0	3	—
Urinary retention	0	2	—		0	3	—
Nocturia	5	2	—		0	3	—
Diarrhea	0	5	A		0	3	—
Sweating	5	19	A		0	3	—
Nausea/vomiting	10	23	A		6	13	A
Cardiovascular							
Fainting/dizziness	14	28	A		6	6	—
Palpitations	5	23	A	0.085	0	6	A
Other							
Dermatologic	0	5	A		6	3	—
Joint pain/stiffness	0	2	—		0	0	—

[a]The column headed ">%" shows the group having higher percentage of patients with adverse experiences during the treatment period. It is shown only if the two groups differ by at least 5 percentage points. The p values are from Fisher's (two-sided) exact tests, and are shown only if $p < 0.10$.

TABLE 2.17 Percent of patients having treatment-emergent adverse experiences during the treatment period by center and treatment[a]

Adverse experience	Center 1 Placebo %	Center 1 Active %	Center 1 >%	Center 1 p value	Center 2 Placebo %	Center 2 Active %	Center 2 >%	Center 2 p value
Psychological/behavioral								
Hallucinations	0	0	—		6	0	P	
Euphoria	0	5	A		0	3	—	
Agitation/excitement	43	32	P		25	40	A	
Irrespons. behavior	24	21	—		0	3	—	
Inapprop. aggression	19	16	—		0	6	A	
Insomnia	33	4	P	0.038	25	45	A	
Tiredness	41	10	P	0.010	23	19	—	
Drowsiness	29	7	P	0.050	24	20	—	
Decreased appetite	24	5	P	0.039	13	21	A	
Increased appetite	5	7	—		12	3	P	
Headache	35	17	P		21	30	A	
Neurological								
Myoclonus	0	5	A		0	0	—	
Cramps	5	2	—		6	0	P	
Rigidity	0	2	—		0	0	—	

Tremor	10	37	A	0.036	18	9	P
Akathisia	0	2	—		0	0	—
Paresthesia	5	7	—		0	3	—
Dyskinesia	0	0	—		0	0	—
Autonomic							
Blurred vision	19	9	P		13	16	—
Dry mouth	24	21	—		24	16	P
Increased salivation	5	5	—		6	0	P
Constipation	19	21	—		0	13	A
Urinary retention	5	7	—		6	3	—
Nocturia	19	5	P	0.085	12	3	P
Diarrhea	0	9	A		18	6	P
Sweating	14	19	A		6	16	A
Nausea/vomiting	33	35	—		24	25	—
Cardiovascular							
Fainting/dizziness	67	28	P	0.006	6	19	A
Palpitations	29	26	—		12	6	P
Other							
Dermatologic	5	5	—		12	3	P
Joint pain/stiffness	5	14	A		0	7	A

[a]The column headed ">%" shows the group having higher percentage of patients with adverse experiences during the treatment period. It is shown only if the two groups differ by at least 5 percentage points. The p values are from Fisher's (two-sided) exact tests, and are shown only if $p < 0.10$.

Center 1 ($p = 0.012$), palpitations in Center 1 ($p = 0.085$), and agitation/excitement in Center 2 ($p = 0.080$). The active group had higher incidence of each of these adverse experiences. None of the treatment comparisons from the other center in Table 2.16 or the comparisons from Table 2.17 strongly contradict these results, although there are some minor contradictions (the Center 2 placebo group has slightly higher incidence of treatment-emergent palpitations and the Center 1 placebo group has slightly higher incidence of treatment-emergent agitation/excitement).

In summary, the two criteria produce substantially different results. When only the possibly to definitely drug-related adverse experiences are considered, the active group has a higher incidence of all adverse experiences for which the treatment difference is significant. However, the placebo group has a higher incidence than the active group for most of the treatment-emergent adverse experiences in which a significant treatment difference was shown. For only one adverse experience in one center, namely tremor in Center 1, is there a significant treatment difference by both criteria.

D. Stratified Covariate-Adjusted Randomization Statistics Analysis

In this section randomization statistics are used to compare the treatments with respect to four of the adverse experiences (agitation/excitement, tremor, constipation, and palpitations), stratifying by center and covariate-adjusting for baseline severity and number of treatment period assessments. These four adverse experiences are the only ones for which the active group had significantly ($p < 0.10$) higher incidence than the placebo group in the treatment comparisons of Section V.C. The analysis is restricted to the adverse experiences considered at least possibly drug-related, since, except for tremor in Center 1, the significantly higher incidences for the active group occurred with this criterion only. Calculations are performed using the methods described in Amara and Koch (1980). Two specifications are used for the dependent variable: a dichotomous variable for the occurrence/nonoccurrence of the adverse experience during the treatment period, and an integer score for the severity of the most severe occurrence of the adverse experience during the treatment period.

The dichotomous variable analysis is shown in Table 2.18. For each of the adverse experiences, the unadjusted and covariate-adjusted randomization statistics for treatment comparisons within the individual centers are shown, as well as the unadjusted and covariate-adjusted stratification statistics. Strictly speaking, the covariate-adjusted statistics

TABLE 2.18 Randomization statistics for treatment comparisons of occurrence of adverse experiences with stratification by center and covariate adjustment for baseline severity and number of assessments

Adverse experience	Statistic[a]	Center 1 Q	Center 1 p value	Center 2 Q	Center 2 p value	Stratification statistic Q_G	Stratification statistic p value
Agitation/ excitement	Unadjusted	1.44	0.231	4.25	0.039	4.78	0.029
	Cov.-adj.	1.08	0.298	5.03	0.025	4.70	0.030
Tremor	Unadjusted	4.60	0.032	1.09	0.298	5.67	0.017
	Cov.-adj.	3.92	0.048	1.40	0.236	5.27	0.022
Constipation	Unadjusted	6.39	0.012	0.53	0.466	6.91	0.009
	Cov.-adj.	6.63	0.010	0.47	0.493	7.07	0.008
Palpitations	Unadjusted	3.34	0.068	1.09	0.298	4.39	0.036
	Cov.-adj.	3.53	0.060	0.85	0.358	4.38	0.036

[a]The covariate-adjusted statistic is adjusted for both baseline severity (0 = none, 1 = mild, 2 = moderate, 3 = severe) and number of treatment-period assessments. The randomization statistic for the covariates is significant for constipation in Center 2 ($p = 0.024$).

are only valid when there is no difference between the treatment groups with respect to the covariables, or, if there is a difference, it is with respect to covariables that are known prior to treatment randomization (e.g., baseline severity, age, sex). The randomization statistic for the covariates is significant for constipation in Center 2 ($p = 0.024$). This is partly due to the Center 2 active group tending to have more treatment period assessments than the placebo group; a randomization statistic for the Center 2 treatment difference with respect to number of asessments is close to borderline significance [$Q_h(\mathbf{X}) = 2.27$, d.f. = 1, $p = 0.131$]. Since the treatment groups in Center 2 vary somewhat with respect to a covariate that is not available prior to randomization, the covariate-adjusted statistics for Center 2 must be viewed cautiously. However, there is little difference between the unadjusted and covariate-adjusted statistics for any of the adverse experiences.

Treatment comparisons with respect to the severity of the most severe occurrence of the adverse experiences are shown in Table 2.19. The covariates adjusted for in this table are the same as in the previous table. However, almost all of the p values in Table 2.19 are larger than their counterparts in Table 2.18. One might expect the integer score analysis to result in more significant p values than the dichotomous variable analysis since in dichotomizing one loses information. The fact that the dichotomous variable analysis results in smaller p values in-

TABLE 2.19 Randomization statistics for treatment comparisons of severity of adverse experiences with stratification by center and covariate adjustment for baseline severity and number of assessments

Adverse experience	Statistic[a]	Center 1		Center 2		Stratification statistic	
		Q	p value	Q	p value	Q_G	p value
Agitation/ excitement	Unadjusted	0.65	0.418	3.94	0.047	3.62	0.057
	Cov.-adj.	0.18	0.667	4.79	0.029	3.10	0.078
Tremor	Unadjusted	3.35	0.067	1.04	0.307	4.36	0.037
	Cov.-adj.	2.64	0.104	1.19	0.275	3.82	0.051
Constipation	Unadjusted	5.38	0.020	0.53	0.466	5.90	0.015
	Cov.-adj.	5.57	0.018	0.47	0.493	6.01	0.014
Palpitations	Unadjusted	1.77	0.183	0.97	0.324	2.69	0.101
	Cov.-adj.	1.84	0.176	0.93	0.335	2.72	0.099

[a]The covariate-adjusted statistic is adjusted for both baseline severity (0 = none, 1 = mild, 2 = moderate, 3 = severe) and number of treatment period assessments. The randomization statistic for the covariates was significant for constipation in Center 2 ($p = 0.024$).

dicates that there may be measurement error or other "noise" in the severity variable.

In the preceding analyses the number of assessments is adjusted for by using it as a covariable. One could also have categorized the number of assessments into two or more levels and used it, along with center, as a stratification variable. This may be more appropriate than covariate adjustment when there is a strong tendency for one treatment group to stay in the study longer than the other treatment group. Another way to adjust for the number of assessments is by incorporating it into the response variable. In Table 2.20 the treatments are compared using as the response variable the sum of the lengths of the intervals during which a patient had an adverse experience divided by the time until the last assessment. For example, if a patient did not report an adverse experience at the day 5 assessment, reported it on the day 8 assessment, then dropped out of the study, the response measure for this patient is 3/8. As discussed in Section II.B.2, this measure is a crude surrogate for both the frequency and duration of the adverse experience. In this study, since dosage was adjusted according to patient tolerance, the analysis of frequency/duration is not as meaningful as for the antihistamine/decongestant study of Section IV, where the doses were fixed, and within each treatment group, almost all patients got the same dose over the same length of time.

TABLE 2.20 Randomization statistics for treatment comparisons of proportion of the treatment period with adverse experience, with stratification by center and number of assessments and covariate adjustment for baseline severity

		Stratification[a] statistic	
Adverse experience	Statistic	Q_G	p value
Agitation/excitement	Unadjusted	3.55	0.060
	Cov.-adj.	2.12	0.146
Tremor	Unadjusted	3.40	0.065
	Cov.-adj.	2.19	0.139
Constipation	Unadjusted	3.94	0.047
	Cov.-adj.	4.72	0.030
Palpitations	Unadjusted	1.78	0.182
	Cov.-adj.	1.85	0.174

[a]The stratification is by center and number of assessments (at most four versus five or more). This corresponds to at most 2 weeks versus 3 or more weeks. The differences were in the same direction in all strata for all adverse experiences.

The interpretation of the response variable used in Table 2.20 depends somewhat on the time on study; for example, a response of 28/28 is more serious than a response of 5/5. Therefore, the analysis is stratified by number of assessments (at most four versus five or more) as well as center. This stratification approximately corresponds to at most 2 weeks on study versus 3 or more weeks. The p values in Table 2.20 are all appreciably less significant than those for the binary response measure in Table 2.18.

E. Logistic Regression

Stepwise logistic regression is used to supplement the randomization-based analysis of the previous section for four of the adverse experiences of interest (possibly to definitely drug-related agitation/excitement, tremor, constipation, and palpitations). The objective of the analysis is to evaluate the importance of treatment relative to other explanatory variables. Also, since for each of the four adverse experiences a significant treatment difference is shown in Table 2.16 for only one of the two centers, it is of interest to see whether the center difference is significant, and if so whether it can be explained by other variables for which the centers differ, notably sex. An analysis of center by treatment interaction is not possible with this data set because for each of the four adverse experiences there is a zero frequency in Table 2.16 for at least one of the treatment groups within centers.

The candidate variables used for the initial stepwise regressions are treatment, baseline severity, number of assessments, sex, age, percent improvement from baseline in the Hamilton Depression Score (an efficacy measure), and indicator variables for each of three classes of concomitant medications (nonnarcotic analgesics, sedatives/hypnotics, and gastrointestinal preparations). Center is not a candidate variable for the initial regressions; however, it is considered in the follow-up analyses. The number of patients having each of the adverse experiences of interest is small relative to the number of candidate variables, and thus the logistic regressions are undertaken more from a descriptive than an inferential perspective. As noted in Section IV.C.3, the recommended number of variables to consider as candidate variables should not exceed $m/10$ where m is the number of observations in the least frequent category of the dichotomous response variable (Harrell, 1986a). For the four adverse experiences of interest, m ranges from 12 to at most 22.

Although associations of adverse experiences with concomitant medication usage are of interest to note, they are difficult to interpret. An apparent association may be due to the concomitant medication causing the adverse experience, either directly or through an interaction with the active treatment, or because the concomitant medication was given to *counteract* the adverse experience of interest (e.g., headaches and aspirin, hypnotics and insomnia) or to counteract a closely related adverse experience. The concomitant medications must often be grouped in order to have a sufficient number to use in statistical analysis. Thus adverse experiences due to a specific concomitant medication or due to interactions with the active treatment would rarely be detected by logistic regression, particularly in a data set this small. In this example, the three classes of concomitant medications that were used by at least 15 patients were selected as explanatory variables. Each of these classes comprises several different chemical entities. Since there is a greater tendency for all three classes of concomitant medications to be given in Center 1 than in Center 2, any association of the concomitant medications with the adverse experiences may be partially due to center.

The results of the initial stepwise logistic regressions for each of the four adverse experiences are shown in Table 2.21. The candidate variables, shown in the footnote at the bottom of the table, are the same for each of the regressions. Calculations were performed using the SAS procedure LOGIST with the significance level to enter the model and the significance level to stay in the model both set to 0.10.

TABLE 2.21 Stepwise logistic regression models for four possibly to definitely drug-related adverse experiences

Adverse experience	Number with adv. exp.	Variable[a]	$\hat{\beta}$	se($\hat{\beta}$)	p value
Agitation/ excitation	22	Intercept	−3.01	0.80	<0.001
		Efficacy	0.04	0.01	<0.001
		Treatment	2.91	0.85	<0.001
		Sex	1.65	0.65	0.011
Tremor	15	Intercept	−7.95	1.98	<0.001
		Treatment	2.87	1.13	0.011
		Sex	2.45	0.78	0.002
		Age	0.04	0.02	0.047
		Baseline	1.10	0.58	0.057
Constipation[b]	12	Intercept	−4.22	0.92	<0.001
		Efficacy	−0.04	0.01	0.003
Palpitations	13	Intercept	−20.40	7.19	0.005
		Sex	4.67	1.68	0.005
		Treatment	7.19	2.25	0.001
		Efficacy	0.11	0.04	0.003
		Number of assess.	2.07	1.02	0.043
		Sedatives	2.92	1.76	0.097

[a]Candidate variables:

Treatment (1 = active, 0 = placebo)
Baseline severity (0 = none, 1 = mild, 2 = moderate, 3 = severe)
Number of assessments (1 to 6)
Sex (1 = female, 0 = male)
Age (continuous)
Efficacy {% improvement from baseline Hamilton Depression Score, i.e., [(final HDS − baseline HDS)/baseline HDS] × 100}
Usage of nonnarcotic analgesics, sedatives/hypnotics, gastrointestinal medications (1 = yes, 0 = no for each)

[b]Treatment is not included in the candidate variables because only the active group had constipation.

For the agitation/excitement regression, the variables that entered the model were the efficacy variable, and variables for active treatment and female sex. The higher the Hamilton Depression Score, the more severe the depression, so negative values for the efficacy variable are indicative of improvement from baseline. The coefficient for the efficacy variable in this model is positive, so patients in whom the drug was not efficacious were more likely to have agitation/excitement. A follow-up regression was done in which the three variables for efficacy, treatment, and sex were forced to be included in the model, and center was allowed as a candidate variable (1 = Center 1, 0 = Center 2). The variable for center did enter the model, and after the center variable entered, the sex variable was no longer significant ($p > 0.25$). So it appears that the previous significant difference for sex was due more to the center difference and the sex difference between the center than to the effect of sex on response.

For tremor, the variables that entered the regression model were treatment, sex, age, and baseline, all with positive coefficients. If the strategy of stopping the model building when the Rao efficient score chi-square statistic for the joint significance of all variables not in the model is nonsignificant had been followed [as recommended by Bartolucci and Fraser (1977), and referenced in Harrell (1986a)], then sex would have been last variable to enter the model. A follow-up regression similar to the one above was done in which treatment, sex, age, and baseline were forced into the model, and center was considered as a candidate variable. Center did not enter this model. However, in a regression in which all candidate variables, including center, were allowed to compete, center, treatment, and baseline entered the model, but sex and age did not. So for tremor, although center appears to explain more of the variation than sex, the preference for center is not as strong as in the regression for agitation/excitement.

The logistic regression for constipation is not as interesting because treatment could not be included as a candidate variable, since all patients who had possibly to definitely drug-related constipation received the active treatment. The only variable to enter the model was the efficacy variable, which is highly correlated with treatment, at least in Center 1. The negative coefficient for the efficacy variable indicates that those patients for whom the treatment was efficacious had greater tendency to have constipation. When center was allowed as a candidate variable, it also entered the model ($p = 0.094$).

The variables that entered the model for palpitations were sex, treatment, efficacy, number of assessments, and the indicator variable for use of sedatives/hypnotics. If the Bartolucci and Fraser (1977) strategy for stopping had been followed, the number of assessments would have been the last variable entered. For palpitations, sex explains more of the variation than center. When all candidate variables, including center, are allowed to compete for entry, center does not enter the model.

One other set of logistic regressions was done. This was for the four psychological/behavioral treatment-emergent adverse experiences for which the placebo group had significantly higher incidence than the active group in Table 2.17 (i.e., insomnia, tiredness, drowsiness, and decreased appetite). It was conjectured that the significantly higher incidence in the placebo group for these four adverse experiences might be evidence of the efficacy of the active treatment. Therefore it is of interest to see whether the patients in whom the drug was efficacious, according to the Hamilton Depression Score, also tended to have favorable status with respect to the occurrence of these adverse experiences. The response variable for a patient was defined as favorable if the severity throughout the treatment period was less than the baseline severity or if the patient never had the adverse experience. If the treatment-period severity was ever the same as or worse than the baseline status, the response was defined as unfavorable. A stepwise regression was conducted for each of the four adverse experiences using the following candidate variables: clinic, treatment, efficacy, number of assessments, sex, and age. The efficacy variable was the first variable to enter all four of the regressions. The association between efficacy and favorable adverse experience status was significant at the 0.01 level for insomnia, tiredness, and decreased appetite, and at the 0.05 level for drowsiness. The only other variables to enter any of the models were number of assessments (negatively associated with favorable status of tiredness and decreased appetite), and age (positively associated with favorable status of drowsiness).

VI. AN EXAMPLE USING A SERIES OF ANALGESIC DRUG TRIALS

Suzanne Edwards, Gary G. Koch, and William Sollecito

A. Description of the Data

A series of clinical trials was performed in support of a New Drug Application (NDA) for a new analgesic. The trials differed with respect to analgesic indication of the patients, length of trial, treatment given the controls, and dose regimens for the treatment groups. For the purposes of this example, all trials that lasted longer than one day and in which the control group received aspirin (ASA) were selected for analysis. There were six such trials: two single-center 14-day trials, two single-center 28-day trials, and two multi-center 84-day trials.

The data for this example differs from those in previous examples in a number of respects. The exact days of the adverse experiences (based on patient recall) are recorded, rather than just the intervals of occurrence. No baseline or severity data are available. The control treatment, ASA, is active rather than placebo, so the relative occurrence of adverse experiences within trials depends on the relative doses of the test drug and ASA. Most importantly, the data are from multiple protocols with

TABLE 2.22 Summary of protocols selected for analysis

		Length of trial				Sex		Age	
Protocol[a]	Indication[b]	(days)	Treatment	Dose[c]	N	F	M	Median	Range
1	RA	14	Test	High	10	6	4	60	50–68
			ASA	High	10	8	2	53	39–71
2	RA	28	Test	High	20	14	6	48	27–60
			ASA	High	20	14	6	49	19–64
3	RA	28	Test	Low	5	4	1	59	48–69
			ASA	High	5	5	0	65	61–70
4	RA	84	Test	Low	46	34	12	57	18–78
			ASA	Low	47	36	11	57	20–81
5	misc.	14	Test	Low	2	0	2	28	25–30
			ASA	Low	3	0	3	31	27–37
6	misc.	84	Test	Low	28	23	5	56	23–83
			ASA	Low	22	17	5	54	26–77
Total					218	161	57		

[a]Protocols 4 and 6 are multicenter studies. The counts and summary statistics shown are for all centers pooled together.
[b]RA is rheumatoid arthritis; the other indication is miscellaneous pain.
[c]High dose refers to the highest dose of either the test drug or aspirin (ASA) given to patients in any of the protocols. Low dose refers to all lower doses.

different lengths and possibly different admission criteria and patient management procedures.

A profile of the major characteristics of the protocols selected for analysis is given in Table 2.22. Four trials are in rheumatoid arthritis patients, and two trials are in patients with miscellaneous pain. The only patient characteristic variables available for this data are age and sex. Most of the study patients are female, and the median age for all protocols except Protocol 5 is at least 48 years. The patients in Protocol 5 are all relatively young males, but there are only five patients in this protocol. The only dose levels coded were the doses for patients on the days of their adverse experiences, or if a patient had no adverse experiences, the dose on the last day of treatment. The interpretation of this continuous dose variable is unclear. However, from the doses that were recorded, it appears that all patients received either "high" doses or "low" doses of their respective treatments. High dose refers to the highest dose of the treatment recorded for patients in any of the protocols, and low dose refers to all lower doses. Within protocols, all patients in the same treatment group received the same dose level (see Table 2.22), and therefore any comparisons of dose groups within treatments must be done across protocols. Only the patients in the rheumatoid arthritis trials received high doses of either treatment.

An area of interest for this set of trials is whether the test drug is associated with a higher incidence of digestive-system side effects than ASA, which is known to affect the digestive system, and also whether the pattern of first occurrence differs for the two drugs. All digestive-system adverse experiences (DSAEs) were considered together in the analysis as one composite variable. The component adverse experiences include nausea, abdominal discomfort, gastrointestinal pain, diarrhea, and dyspepsia.

B. Overview of Statistical Analyses

In Section VI.C, contingency-table methods are used to compare the treatments within and across protocols with respect to whether or not patients had any digestive-system adverse experiences (DSAEs) while on study. Treatment by protocol interactions are assessed with logistic regression. Although contingency-table methods are of interest, they may be misleading if the patients receiving a particular treatment tended to stay in their respective studies longer than patients receiving the other treatment. Thus methods that account for time on study are also of interest. The rest of the section focuses on survival data analysis methods for comparison of treatment groups with respect to time to first DSAE.

Some of the issues related to survival data analysis of a set of trials with different protocols and different study lengths are discussed in Section VI.D. Of particular interest are the effect of censoring by the end of study, and the implications of combining results from different protocols. In Section VI.E, preliminary analyses are carried out to examine the first-order associations of dose group and pain indication with time to first DSAE. A treatment comparison of survival curves is then carried out based on these findings.

Regression-type approaches for the analysis of adverse experience data are also of interest for several purposes. One is the comparison of subgroups in a setting for which the effects of other variables with strong associations with the occurrence of adverse experiences are taken into account. Another is the evaluation of the homogeneity of the effects of important variables (e.g., treatment) across subgroups. Several types of regression analyses of time to DSAE are carried out. Piecewise exponential model fitting via Poisson regression is presented in Section VI.F. This method is used to fit both proportional hazards and non-proportional hazards models, and diagnostic measures are used to assess model fit. Cox regression models are fit in Section VI.G, and parallel themes are noted between Cox regression and piecewise exponential model fitting. The assumption of proportional hazards is investigated using the method of successive truncation. In Section VI.H, the analogies between proportional hazards regression and logistic regression are illustrated.

It must be emphasized that DSAEs are recurrent events, and since for this data set all DSAEs were recorded, analysis pertaining to only the first DSAE does not make full use of the data. Often, however, data are collected on a per assessment basis: that is, only one record is entered per adverse experience per assessment, regardless of the frequency of the adverse experience in the interval since the last assessment. In that case, analysis of time to first adverse experience (although it must be estimated) is more straightforward than analysis of frequency. It may be argued, however, that for chronic diseases, such as rheumatoid arthitis, which require chronic administration of treatment, the frequency of an adverse experience is more important than its time to onset. Thus an analysis of the frequency of DSAEs is presented in Section VI.I.

In the final section, VI.J, the DSAE data are used to provide the context for a discussion of alternative summary measures that might be used in the package insert.

C. Treatment-Group Comparisons of Proportion Having Digestive-System Adverse Experiences

Treatment group comparisons of the proportion of patients having at least one DSAE while on study were performed for each protocol using two-sided Fisher's exact tests. The results are shown in Table 2.23. Although the incidence of DSAE's is higher for the test drug than for ASA for all but two of the centers within protocols, the difference is statistically significant ($p < 0.05$) only for Protocol 2, where the patients in both treatment groups were given high doses for 28 days. The Mantel–Haenszel statistic for the comparison of treatment groups stratified by center is $Q = 6.57$, which is statistically significant ($p < 0.010$) with respect to the chi-square distribution with one degree of freedom. However, when the contribution of Protocol 2 is removed from the Mantel–Haenszel statistic, it is no longer significant at the 0.05 level ($Q = 2.83$, $p = 0.093$).

Because the treatment difference is so much more pronounced in Protocol 2 than in any of the other protocols, a logistic regression was

TABLE 2.23A Treatment group comparisons[a] of proportion having digestive-system adverse experiences (DSAES)

		Proportion with DSAE				
		Test drug		ASA		Fisher's exact test (two-sided)
Protocol	Number of patients	Number	(%)	Number	(%)	p value
1	20	3/10	(30%)	1/10	(10%)	0.334
2	40	10/20	(50%)	3/20	(15%)	0.041
3	10	0/5	(0%)	2/5	(40%)	0.444
4	8	4/4	(100%)	2/4	(50%)	0.429
	29	10/14	(71%)	10/15	(67%)	0.999
	20	4/10	(40%)	2/10	(20%)	0.629
	16	3/8	(38%)	4/8	(50%)	0.999
	20	6/10	(60%)	2/10	(20%)	0.170
5	5	0/2	(0%)	0/3	(0%)	—
6	26	2/15	(13%)	0/11	(0%)	0.492
	24	4/13	(31%)	3/11	(27%)	0.999

[a]The Mantel–Haenszel statistic for treatment comparisons over all centers is $Q = 6.57$, $p = 0.010$. When Protocol 2 is excluded, the Mantel–Haenszel statistic over the remaining centers is $Q = 2.83$, $p = 0.093$.

TABLE 2.23B Results of logistic regression for assessment of treatment by protocol interaction[a]

Model specification matrix	Interpretation of parameters
$$\mathbf{X} = \begin{bmatrix} 1 & 0 & 0 & 0 & 0 & 0 \\ 1 & 0 & 0 & 0 & 0 & 1 \\ 1 & 1 & 0 & 0 & 0 & 0 \\ 1 & 1 & 0 & 0 & 0 & 1 \\ 1 & 0 & 1 & 0 & 0 & 0 \\ 1 & 0 & 1 & 0 & 0 & 1 \\ 1 & 0 & 0 & 1 & 0 & 0 \\ 1 & 0 & 0 & 1 & 0 & 1 \\ 1 & 0 & 0 & 0 & 1 & 0 \\ 1 & 0 & 0 & 0 & 1 & 1 \end{bmatrix}$$	β_1 is the reference value for Protocol 1, ASA treatment. β_2 is the increment due to Protocol 2. β_3 is the increment due to Protocol 3. β_4 is the increment due to Protocol 4. β_5 is the increment due to Protocol 6. β_6 is the increment due to the test drug.

[a]Model goodness of fit is supported by the nonsignificance of the Pearson criterion ($Q_P = 6.56$, 4 d.f., $p = 0.161$) and the likelihood ratio criterion ($Q_L = 7.15$, 4 d.f., $p = 0.128$). The vector $\mathbf{W} = (0\ 0\ 0\ 1\ 0\ 0\ 0\ 0\ 0\ 0)'$ was used to compute the Rao score statistic for testing the Protocol 2 by treatment interaction. This interaction was nonsignificant ($Q = 2.07$, 1 d.f., $p = 0.150$).

carried out to test the significance of the treatment by protocol interaction. These results are shown in Table 2.23B. A logistic modelling procedure was used to fit a model to a contingency table of the frequencies of DSAEs for patients in each protocol (pooling across centers for the two multicenter protocols and excluding Protocol 5 in which no DSAEs occurred). The model appears to provide an adequate fit; the Pearson chi-square for goodness of fit is 6.56, which with 4 degrees of freedom has p value 0.161. This goodness-of-fit statistic is equivalent to the Rao score statistic for testing protocol by treatment interaction, and thus this interaction is nonsignificant. However, the goodness-of-fit statistic needs to be viewed cautiously due to the small counts for several of the protocols. A Rao score statistic was also used to separately test the significance of the Protocol 2 by treatment interaction, as shown in the footnote to Table 2.23. No significant difference was found. The protocol by treatment interaction was further tested with an exact test [using the algorithm of Thomas (1975)] and was not found to be significant ($p = 0.21$).

The logistic model presented in Table 2.23 does not take account of study-to-study variation within the multicenter studies. One other test of

Protocol 2 by treatment interaction was also conducted by fitting a model similar to the model in Table 2.23 except that the columns corresponding to protocol effects are replaced with columns corresponding to individual center effects. For this model, the Rao score statistic corresponding to Protocol 2 by treatment interaction was also not found to be significant.

2. Survival Data Analysis Issues

This section focuses on issues related to survival analysis methods for estimation of probability of first DSAE and hypothesis testing of treatment differences in time to first DSAE. Before conducting a survival data analysis, it is important to consider the potential effects of censoring. For example, if subjects withdraw from a study because they are at high risk of having the adverse experience (or if they have the adverse experience and then withdraw before reporting it), the life-table estimates of the probability of a DSAE will be too small. If this phenomenon tends to occur more often in one treatment group than another, then the statistical comparison of survival curves for the treatment groups will not be valid.

Two assumptions are often made in survival data analysis (Lachin, 1982b):

1. The unobserved experience of the censored observations is equivalent to the experience of the uncensored observations, that is, the censored observations are unbiased.
2. The censoring mechanism acts on each of the treatment groups in the same way, that is, censoring is not related to treatment.

The first assumption is necessary for life-table estimation to be valid. If this assumption is met within each of the treatment groups to be compared, then the statistical comparison of survival curves is also valid. Even if the first assumption is not met, treatment comparisons may still be valid if the second assumption is met.

Lachin points out that, although neither of these assumptions can be tested directly, they may be examined by indirect methods. With respect to the first assumption, one may examine whether the proportion and timing of censored observations differ between the levels of covariables that are potentially associated with the failure event. If, for example, females tend to withdraw earlier or at a higher rate than males, and females are also more likely than males to develop the adverse experience, then the first assumption would not hold. A way to evaluate whether the censoring pattern differs between levels of potential prognostic covariables is by using life-table methods where withdrawal is treated as the failure event and occurrence of a DSAE is treated as the censoring event. The second assumption can be examined in a similar fashion by comparing the censoring pattern between the treatment groups. A significant difference between treatments may suggest a violation of the assumption.

The issues related to censoring become more complex when considering survival data analysis of a set of trials with different lengths. If life-table estimates are obtained by pooling data from more than one study [as recommended by Idanpaan-Heikkila (1983)], censoring by the end of study becomes an issue. One must assume (assumption 1 above) that patients censored by the end of study are at the same risk of adverse experiences as the uncensored patients, that is, that patients in the shorter studies and patients in the longer studies have similar prognostic characteristics. This is unlikely to be true for the data in this example or in general. The studies in which high doses are used are shorter than the lower-dose studies. Also, the lengths of studies may depend on the indications, although in this example there are short and long studies for both indications. Further consideration of the problems of providing overall estimates of the risk of adverse experiences with the test drug is given in Section VI.J.

With respect to hypothesis testing for treatment differences in time to first DSAE, it is advantageous to combine the results from several studies. A combined-study analysis enables one to present more general conclusions. Also, since the power of within-study tests may be low due to small sample sizes and low DSAE rates, combining results leads to increased power to detect treatment differences, and also results in more effective use of the data from the small studies.

The easiest and most obvious way to perform an overall test of treatment differences is to pool all the data together and perform a censored data rank test. If the data from the six protocols in this example are pooled, the test drug group has significantly earlier DSAEs [$p < 0.05$ by both the Breslow (1970) generalized Wilcoxon and the Mantel–Cox tests]. However, since the studies pooled differ with respect to patient indications and dose levels used, and since both dose and indication may well be associated with the incidence of DSAEs, this result is not readily interpretable.

Elashoff (1978) discusses combining results of clinical trials with different protocols in the context of efficacy hypothesis testing. Her recommendation is to combine results only for studies with similar values of the variables potentially associated with the outcome measure. She also recommends methods, such as the Mantel–Haenszel test, that are based on study-by-study differences, rather than simply pooling the data.

These recommendations are implemented in the next section. The association of both indication and dose with DSAE occurrence is investigated, and then, based on these results, study results are combined to test for treatment differences.

E. Analysis of First-Order Associations

In this section censored data rank tests are used to compare the two dose levels for each treatment, the two indications, and finally the two treatments with respect to time to first DSAE. Comparisons between the indications and between the dose levels must be carried out across protocols, and thus the results of such comparisons must be interpreted cautiously since apparent differences between doses or indication may also be due to other unknown differences between the protocols.

A comparison of high dose with low dose within each treatment group involves the following protocols:

Test drug	
High dose	Low dose
1. 14-day, RA, 10 patients	3. 28-day, RA, 5 patients
2. 28-day, RA, 20 patients	4. 84-day, RA, 46 patients
	5. 14-day, misc. pain, 2 patients
	6. 84-day, misc. pain, 28 patients
ASA	
High dose	Low dose
1. 14-day, RA, 10 patients	4. 84-day, RA, 47 patients
2. 28-day, RA, 20 patients	5. 14-day, misc. pain, 3 patients
3. 28-day, RA, 5 patients	6. 84-day, misc. pain, 22 patients

So as not to confound indication and dose, the dose groups were compared within treatment groups for the RA (rheumatoid arthritis) studies only. Thus, for the test drug, the comparison is between Protocols 1 and 2 and Protocols 3 and 4, and for ASA, the comparison is between Protocols 1, 2, and 3 and Protocol 4. Problems involving differential censoring by the end of study can be avoided by initially considering only the first 14 days of treatment. The data from all four RA protocols were included, and if a patient had the first DSAE or was censored after 14 days, then the patient was treated as censored at 14 days. Similarly, the dose groups were also compared over the first 28 days by including only the three protocols that lasted at least 28 days (Protocols 2, 3, and 4), and considering only the first 28 days of treatment. It is impossible to compare the dose groups after 28 days because high doses were only given in studies lasting 28 days or less.

The results of the dose comparisons described above are presented in Table 2.24. The top half of this table shows the comparisons when only the first 14 days of treatment are considered. The Kaplan–Meier estimated probabilities of no DSAE by 4 and 14 days are shown, along with

TABLE 2.24 Dose-level comparisons within treatment group

Consideration of time to DSAE limited to first 14 days						
			Kaplan–Meier[a] estimated probability of no DSAE		p values for[b] group comparisons	
Subset	Dose group	Proportion with DSAE	4 days	14 days	GW-B	M-C
RA, test drug	High	13/30	0.733 (0.081)	0.567 (0.091)	0.077	0.095
	Low	14/51	0.902 (0.042)	0.725 (0.063)		
RA, ASA	High	6/35	0.886 (0.054)	0.827 (0.064)	0.860	0.834
	Low	9/47	0.914 (0.041)	0.806 (0.058)		

Consideration of time to DSAE limited to first 28 days[c]							
			Kaplan–Meier[a] estimated probability of no DSAE			p values for[b] group comparisons	
Subset	Dose group	Proportion with DSAE	4 days	14 days	28 days	GW-B	M-C
RA, test drug	High	10/20	0.650 (0.107)	0.500 (0.112)	0.500 (0.112)	0.046	0.079
	Low	18/51	0.902 (0.042)	0.725 (0.063)	0.642 (0.068)		
RA, ASA	High	5/25	0.880 (0.065)	0.800 (0.080)	0.800 (0.080)	0.591	0.526
	Low	13/47	0.914 (0.041)	0.806 (0.058)	0.718 (0.066)		

[a]The numbers in parentheses are the standard errors for the estimates.
[b]The p values are from Breslow's (1970) generalized Wilcoxon test (GW-B) and the Mantel–Cox (M–C) test, and are generated by program BMDP1L.
[c]Includes only RA studies that lasted at least 28 days (i.e., studies 2, 3, and 4).

p values from both the Breslow and Mantel–Cox tests. Patients receiving high doses of the test drug tend to have earlier DSAEs than patients receiving low doses, and this difference approaches significance ($p < 0.10$ by both tests). No difference between dose groups is apparent for ASA. The bottom half of Table 2.24 shows the dose comparisons over the first 28 days of treatment. Although the sample size is somewhat smaller, the p values from the dose comparison for the test drug are slightly more significant than for the 14-days analysis. As can be seen by examining the Kaplan–Meier estimates, this increased significance is not due to dose group differences in DSAE incidence between 14 and 28 days, but rather to the exclusion of Protocol 1, a high-dose study in which relatively few DSAEs occurred.

The results of a comparison of the RA and miscellaneous pain indications are shown in Table 2.25. So as not to confound indication with treatment and dose, the comparison was made within the low-dose group for each treatment (recall that no miscellaneous pain patients received high doses of either treatment). Also, since the 84-day studies predominate in terms of sample size, only these two studies were included in the comparison. The RA indication patients tended to have earlier DSAEs than the miscellaneous pain patients for both treatments. This difference is highly significant for the test drug group ($p < 0.01$ by both tests), and approaches significance for the ASA group ($p < 0.10$ by both tests).

The interpretation of the comparison of indications is less than straightforward because the pattern of censoring is markedly different for the two indications. In the test drug group, 4% of the RA patients were censored before the end of study, as opposed to 54% of the miscellaneous pain patients, and in the ASA group, 21% of the RA patients were censored, as opposed to 59% of the miscellaneous pain patients. A life-table comparison (with early withdrawal as the failure event and having a DSAE or reaching the end of study as the censoring events) was used to test the difference between the censoring patterns for the two indications. The miscellaneous pain patients had significantly ($p < 0.01$ by both the Breslow and Mantel–Cox tests) earlier times to withdrawal for both treatment groups.

One possible explanation for the censoring rate being so much lower in the RA group is that the RA patients may have had DSAEs before they had a chance to withdraw. However, in a life-table comparison similar to the previous one except that DSAEs were no longer considered censoring events, the miscellaneous pain patients still withdrew significantly ($p < 0.001$) earlier than the RA patients, so this explanation is insufficient.

TABLE 2.25 Comparisons of indication within low dose of each treatment group

		Low-dose test drug group (84-day studies only)						
		Kaplan–Meier estimated probability[a] of no DSAE					p values for[b] group comparisons	
Indication	Proportion with DSAE	4 days	14 days	28 days	56 days	84 days	GW-B	M-C
RA	27/46	0.891 (0.046)	0.696 (0.068)	0.609 (0.072)	0.473 (0.074)	0.406 (0.073)	0.004	0.008
Misc. pain	6/28	0.963 (0.036)	0.963 (0.036)	0.923 (0.053)	0.771 (0.092)	0.706 (0.104)		
		Low-dose ASA groups (84-day studies only)						
		Kaplan–Meier estimated probability[a] of no DSAE					p values for[b] group comparisons	
Indication	Proportion with DSAE	4 days	14 days	28 days	56 days	84 days	GW-B	M-C
RA	20/47	0.914 (0.041)	0.806 (0.058)	0.719 (0.066)	0.572 (0.075)	0.545 (0.076)	0.057	0.054
Misc. pain	3/22	0.952 (0.047)	0.952 (0.047)	0.905 (0.064)	0.823 (0.098)	0.823 (0.098)		

[a]The numbers in parentheses are the standard errors for the estimates.
[b]The p values are from Breslow's (1970) generalized Wilcoxon test (GW-B) and the Mantel–Cox (M–C) test, and are generated by the program BMDPIL.

In view of the apparent association of both indication and dose level of test drug with DSAE incidence, the results of treatment comparisons should probably be presented separately for the RA patients who received high-dose test drug (Protocols 1 and 2), the RA patients who received low-dose test drug (Protocols 3 and 4), and the miscellaneous pain patients (Protocols 5 and 6). A way to combine the results of treatment comparisons of time-to-event data, based on study-by-study differences, is to use stratified censored data rank tests [as presented in Breslow (1979) and elsewhere] using center as the stratification variable. Differences between centers with respect to explanatory variables are thus accounted for, as well as differences in study lengths.

The SAS procedure PHGLM was used to obtain a stratified Mantel–Cox statistic (see Harrell, 1986b) for high-dose test drug versus high-dose ASA for RA patients (Protocols 1 and 2). Protocol (or center, since both are single-center studies) was used as the stratification variable, and treatment was the only independent variable. A significant difference ($p = 0.029$) was found between the high doses for the two treatments, with DSAEs occurring earlier for the high-dose test drug patients.

The treatment comparison for the RA indication, low-dose test drug protocols (3 and 4) is complicated by the fact that in Protocol 3 and in one of the centers in Protocol 4, the ASA group had higher incidence of DSAEs than the test drug group, whereas in the other centers in Protocol 4, the test drug group had higher incidence. For this reason, the results from the two protocols were not combined. An exact test analogous to the Mantel–Cox test was carried out for Protocol 3 using the algorithm of Thomas (1975). No significant treatment difference was found ($p = 0.22$). The results from all five centers were combined for Protocol 4 in spite of the fact that in one of the centers the ASA group had slightly higher incidence of DSAEs than the test drug group. A stratified Mantel–Cox test was conducted, stratifying by center, using PHGLM. The treatment difference was close to borderline statistical significance ($p = 0.118$).

For the miscellaneous pain protocols, no DSAEs occurred in Protocol 5, so attention was restricted to Protocol 6. A Mantel–Cox test was carried out to test for treatment differences after stratification on center for Protocol 6. No significant difference was found ($p = 0.61$). Although Protocol 6 does not satisfy the Mantel–Fleiss (1980) criterion for the Mantel–Cox test, an exact test was not considered necessary for this comparison because the asymptotic result is far from statistical significance.

F. Piecewise Exponential Model Fitting via Poisson Regression

In this section log-linear Poisson regression computing procedures are used to fit piecewise exponential models to the DSAE data. A piecewise type of approach is particularly well suited for modeling this data set because the lengths of the various studies form a natural partition of the time axis: 1–14 days, 15–28 days, and 29–84 days. Within each of these intervals it is assumed that the DSAEs have independent exponential distributions.

Computations are performed using the SAS macro CATMAX documented in Stokes and Koch (1983). In this macro, maximum-likelihood parameter estimates are calculated by applying Newton–Raphson iteration to a set of initial estimates based on weighted least squares. Goodness-of-fit statistics are produced, and hypotheses regarding model parameters may be tested using contrast matrices. The CATMAX macro can also provide Rao score statistics for assessing the contribution of effects not in the model, and residual measures for detecting points of extreme influence or outliers, as documented in Atkinson (1984). Several of these tools are used to derive, validate, and compare various models for describing the relationship of treatment, dose level, and indication with time to the first occurrence of a DSAE.

TABLE 2.26 Frequency table of time to DSAE by treatment, dose level, and indication

Treatment	Dose level	Indication	Time (days)	Number with DSAEs	Person days of exposure	Incidence density within interval
ASA	Low	Misc. pain	1–14	1	313	0.003
			15–28	1	238	0.004
			29–84	1	563	0.002
ASA	Low	RA	1–14	9	573	0.016
			15–28	4	502	0.008
			29–84	7	1309	0.005
ASA	High	RA	1–14	6	421	0.014
			15–28	0	252	0.000
Test	Low	Misc. pain	1–14	1	374	0.003
			15–28	1	310	0.003
			29–84	4	766	0.005
Test	Low	RA	1–14	14	616	0.023
			15–28	4	473	0.008
			29–84	9	1141	0.008
Test	High	RA	1–14	13	291	0.045
			15–28	0	84	0.000

A frequency table of the times to first DSAE, cross-classified by treatment, dose level, and indication, is given in Table 2.26. Also shown for each interval are the number of person-days of exposure to treatment and the ratio of the number of individuals with DSAEs to the number of person-days [Kleinbaum, Kupper, and Morgenstern (1982) and Miettinen (1976) call this quantity the incidence density]. The initial model applied to this data is a model with a proportional hazards structure—that is, the effects of the explanatory variables are assumed to be constant across the time intervals. The model is specified by

$$\mathbf{X}_1 = \begin{bmatrix} 1 & 1 & 1 & 1 & 1 & 1 & 1 & 1 & 1 & 1 & 1 & 1 & 1 & 1 & 1 & 1 \\ 0 & 0 & 0 & 1 & 1 & 1 & 1 & 1 & 0 & 0 & 0 & 1 & 1 & 1 & 1 & 1 \\ 0 & 0 & 0 & 0 & 0 & 0 & 0 & 0 & 1 & 1 & 1 & 1 & 1 & 1 & 1 & 1 \\ 0 & 0 & 0 & 0 & 0 & 0 & 0 & 0 & 0 & 0 & 0 & 1 & 1 & 1 & 1 & 1 \\ 0 & 0 & 0 & 0 & 0 & 0 & 0 & 0 & 0 & 0 & 0 & 0 & 0 & 0 & 1 & 1 \\ 0 & 1 & 0 & 0 & 1 & 0 & 0 & 1 & 0 & 1 & 0 & 0 & 1 & 0 & 0 & 1 \\ 0 & 0 & 1 & 0 & 0 & 1 & 0 & 0 & 0 & 0 & 1 & 0 & 0 & 1 & 0 & 0 \end{bmatrix}'$$

for which the parameter estimates $\hat{\boldsymbol{\beta}} = (\hat{\beta}_1, \hat{\beta}_2, \ldots, \hat{\beta}_7)'$, their estimated standard errors, and associated p values are as follows:

$\hat{\beta}$	se($\hat{\beta}$)	p value	Interpretation
−5.34	0.59	<0.001	Reference value for miscellaneous pain, low-dose ASA, days 1–14
1.11	0.61	0.070	Increment due to RA for ASA group
0.45	0.71	0.520	Increment due to test drug for miscellaneous pain
−0.05	0.76	0.945	Increment due to low dose test drug and RA interaction
0.62	0.35	0.079	Increment due to high-dose test drug over low-dose test drug for RA
−1.04	0.35	0.003	Increment due to days 15–28
−0.91	0.28	0.001	Increment due to days 29–84

The increment due to high-dose test drug over low-dose test drug for RA patients is actually only applicable to the first 28 days of treatment because the high-dose studies were at most 28 days long. The goodness-of-fit of model $\mathbf{X}_1$ is supported by the nonsignificance of the Pearson and likelihood ratio criteria with respect to the chi-square distribution with 9 degrees of freedom ($Q_P = 7.12$, $p = 0.62$ and $Q_L = 9.47$, $p = 0.39$).

Note that an increment for the high dose of ASA was not included in the model. The fact that the model appears to fit well, regardless, provides some evidence that this effect is superfluous. A Rao score statistic was used to explicitly test the effect of high-dose ASA; it was nonsignificant ($Q = 0.41$, d.f. $= 1$, $p = 0.52$).

Treatment comparisons were carried out by testing the significance of linear combinations of the parameters. For the miscellaneous pain patients, a comparison of test drug and ASA is equivalent to the test of the significance of β_3, which is nonsignificant ($p = 0.520$). However, the power to detect a treatment difference for miscellaneous pain patients is not very high. Assuming that $\hat{\beta}_3$ is normally distributed with standard error 0.707, the power to detect a two-sided alternative like $\beta_3 = \ln(2) = 0.693$ (i.e., an increment sufficient to double the hazard rate), using a significance level of 0.10, is

$$\begin{aligned} \text{Power} &= 1 - \Pr\left\{-1.645 - \frac{0.693}{0.707} \leq Z \leq 1.645 - \frac{0.693}{0.707}\right\} \\ &= 0.26 \end{aligned}$$

Alternatively, the limitations of the available sample size for this comparison can be seen in the wide range of the 90% confidence interval $\exp\{0.45 \pm 1.645(0.707)\} = (0.49, 5.02)$ for β_3.

A comparison of low-dose test drug versus ASA for RA patients is equivalent to a test of the hypothesis H_0: $\beta_3 + \beta_4 = 0$. The result from this test is suggestive ($p = 0.145$). The power for this test is also greater than the power for the previous test. The power to detect a two-sided alternative like $\beta_3 + \beta_4 = 0.693$, using a significance level of 0.10, is

$$\begin{aligned} \text{Power} &= 1 - \Pr\left\{-1.645 - \frac{0.693}{0.276} \leq Z \leq 1.645 - \frac{0.693}{0.276}\right\} \\ &= 0.81 \end{aligned}$$

A comparison of high-dose test drug versus ASA is equivalent to a test of the significance of the hypothesis H_0: $\beta_3 + \beta_4 + \beta_5 = 0$. This quantity is significantly different from zero ($p < 0.01$).

The nonsignificance of the increment due to low-dose test drug for RA in model $\mathbf{X}_1$ and the similarity of the two time effects suggest a reduction to the following main effects model:

$$\mathbf{X}_2 = \begin{bmatrix} 1 & 1 & 1 & 1 & 1 & 1 & 1 & 1 & 1 & 1 & 1 & 1 & 1 & 1 & 1 & 1 \\ 0 & 0 & 0 & 1 & 1 & 1 & 1 & 1 & 0 & 0 & 0 & 1 & 1 & 1 & 1 & 1 \\ 0 & 0 & 0 & 0 & 0 & 0 & 0 & 0 & 1 & 1 & 1 & 1 & 1 & 1 & 1 & 1 \\ 0 & 0 & 0 & 0 & 0 & 0 & 0 & 0 & 0 & 0 & 0 & 0 & 0 & 0 & 1 & 1 \\ 0 & 1 & 1 & 0 & 1 & 1 & 0 & 1 & 0 & 1 & 1 & 0 & 1 & 1 & 0 & 1 \end{bmatrix}'$$

The parameter estimates for this model, their standard errors, and associated p values are:

$\hat{\beta}$	se($\hat{\beta}$)	p Value	Interpretation
−5.30	0.39	<0.001	Reference value for misc. pain, low-dose ASA, days 1–14
1.07	0.36	0.003	Increment due to RA
0.41	0.26	0.107	Increment due to low-dose test drug
0.61	0.35	0.081	Increment due to high-dose test drug over low-dose test drug for RA
−0.96	0.25	<0.001	Increment due to days 15–84

Since model $\mathbf{X}_2$ is a main-effects model, β_2 is the increment due to RA for both the ASA and test drug groups, rather than the increment due to RA for the ASA group only as in model $\mathbf{X}_1$. Thus the p value for β_2 in model $\mathbf{X}_2$ is smaller than the p value for β_2 in model $\mathbf{X}_1$. Similarly, the increment due to the low-dose drug, β_3, applies to both the RA and miscellaneous pain indications, rather than just the miscellaneous pain indication, and thus this effect is more nearly significant in model $\mathbf{X}_2$ than in model $\mathbf{X}_1$. Also, the effect for days 15–84 in model $\mathbf{X}_2$ is more significant than either of the separate time effects in model $\mathbf{X}_1$.

The goodness of fit of model $\mathbf{X}_2$ is supported by the nonsignificance of the Pearson and likelihood ratio criteria ($Q_P = 6.98$, $p = 0.80$, and $Q_L = 9.57$, $p = 0.57$; 11 d.f. for both statistics) and by the nonsignificance of the likelihood ratio chi-square statistic for the reduction of model $\mathbf{X}_1$ to model $\mathbf{X}_2$ [$Q_L(\mathbf{X}_2) - Q_L(\mathbf{X}_1) = 9.57 - 9.47 = 0.10$, 2 d.f., $p = 0.99$].

Table 2.27 shows the expected counts under $\mathbf{X}_2$ for each subpopulation and interval. These expected counts may be compared with the observed counts to provide a qualitative evaluation of the fit of the model. Two diagnostic measures are also shown in Table 2.27: the adjusted standardized residuals and the diagonal elements from the **H** matrix (see Section III.G). The adjusted standardized residual is approximately distributed as a standard normal variable, so large values

TABLE 2.27 Diagnostic measures for model $\mathbf{X}_2$

Treatment	Dose	Indication	Time (days)	Observed count	Expected count	Diagnostic measures: Diagonals of H	Diagnostic measures: Adj. std. residuals
ASA	Low	Misc. pain	1–14	1	1.56	0.24	−0.51
			15–28	1	0.45	0.07	0.84
			29–84	1	1.07	0.17	−0.08
ASA	Low	RA	1–14	9	8.31	0.40	0.31
			15–28	4	2.80	0.15	0.78
			29–84	7	7.29	0.40	−0.14
ASA	High	RA	1–14	6	6.11	0.29	−0.05
			15–28	0	1.40	0.08	−1.23
Test	Low	Misc. pain	1–14	1	2.81	0.38	−1.37
			15–28	1	0.89	0.12	0.12
			29–84	4	2.21	0.29	1.43
Test	Low	RA	1–14	14	13.51	0.67[a]	0.24
			15–28	4	3.98	0.20	0.01
			29–84	9	9.60	0.48	−0.27
Test	High	RA	1–14	13	11.70	0.91[a]	1.24
			15–28	0	1.30	0.16	−1.24

[a]Exceeds 0.625 and is thus an influential observation.

may be indicative of outliers from model fit. All of the adjusted standardized residuals for model $\mathbf{X}_2$ are within the range -2 to 2, and thus the fit of this model is further supported. Values of the diagonal of $\mathbf{H}$ greater than $2 \times t/s = 2 \times 5/16 = 0.625$ (where s and t are the respective row and column dimensions of $\mathbf{X}_2$) are considered influential observations. For model $\mathbf{X}_2$ there are two influential observations, one for low dose of the test drug in RA patients for days 1–14, and one for high dose of the test drug in RA patients for days 1–14. The adjusted standardized residuals for these two observations are equivalent to Rao score statistics for the effects of the respective vectors,

$$\mathbf{W} = (0 \quad 0 \quad 0 \quad 0 \quad 0 \quad 0 \quad 0 \quad 0 \quad 0 \quad 0 \quad 0 \quad 1 \quad 0 \quad 0 \quad 0 \quad 0)'$$

and

$$\mathbf{W} = (0 \quad 0 \quad 0 \quad 0 \quad 0 \quad 0 \quad 0 \quad 0 \quad 0 \quad 0 \quad 0 \quad 0 \quad 0 \quad 0 \quad 1 \quad 0)'$$

Since both adjusted standardized residuals are nonsignificant with respect to the standard normal distribution, there is no need to augment model $\mathbf{X}_2$ with these vectors.

Since the two influential observations are both for days 1–14, and since the incidence densities shown in Table 2.26 are greater for days 1–14 than for either of the other two intervals, at least for the RA patients, it is of interest to fit a model where most of the variation due to indication and treatment is assumed to occur within the first 14 days. This type of model is also intuitively appealing because if the DSAEs produced by the test drug and ASA are pharmacological in nature, then one would expect them to occur early. The model $\mathbf{X}_3$ shown below is a nonproportional hazards model:

$$\mathbf{X}_3 = \begin{bmatrix} 1 & 0 & 0 & 1 & 0 & 0 & 1 & 0 & 1 & 0 & 0 & 1 & 0 & 0 & 1 & 0 \\ 0 & 0 & 0 & 1 & 0 & 0 & 1 & 0 & 0 & 0 & 0 & 1 & 0 & 0 & 1 & 0 \\ 0 & 0 & 0 & 0 & 0 & 0 & 0 & 0 & 1 & 0 & 0 & 1 & 0 & 0 & 1 & 0 \\ 0 & 0 & 0 & 0 & 0 & 0 & 0 & 0 & 0 & 0 & 0 & 0 & 0 & 0 & 1 & 0 \\ 0 & 1 & 1 & 0 & 1 & 1 & 0 & 1 & 0 & 1 & 1 & 0 & 1 & 1 & 0 & 1 \end{bmatrix}'$$

The parameter estimates for this model are:

$\hat{\beta}$	se($\hat{\beta}$)	p Value	Interpretation
−6.06	0.74	<0.001	Reference value for misc. pain, low-dose ASA, days 1–14
1.88	0.73	0.010	Increment due to RA, days 1–14
0.37	0.36	0.301	Increment due to low dose test drug, days 1–14
0.70	0.38	0.070	Increment due to high-dose test drug over low-dose test drug for RA, days 1–14
−5.20	0.18	<0.001	Reference value for days 15–84

The goodness-of-fit statistics indicate that model $\mathbf{X}_3$ fits better than model $\mathbf{X}_1$ or $\mathbf{X}_2$ ($Q_P = 6.33$, $p = 0.85$, and $Q_L = 8.43$, $p = 0.67$, 11 d.f. for both statistics). None of the adjusted standardized residuals are significant, and Rao score statistics for the effect of indication in days 15–84, the effect of test drug in days 15–84, and the joint significance of these two effects were all nonsignificant. So there is no evidence for the need of additional columns to model DSAE experience in days 15–28.

Model $\mathbf{X}_3$ can be further reduced by eliminating the nonsignificant effect for (low-dose) test drug in days 1–14. The resulting model,

$$\mathbf{X}_4 = \begin{bmatrix} 1 & 0 & 0 & 1 & 0 & 0 & 1 & 0 & 1 & 0 & 0 & 1 & 0 & 0 & 1 & 0 \\ 0 & 0 & 0 & 1 & 0 & 0 & 1 & 0 & 0 & 0 & 0 & 1 & 0 & 0 & 1 & 0 \\ 0 & 0 & 0 & 0 & 0 & 0 & 0 & 0 & 0 & 0 & 0 & 0 & 0 & 0 & 1 & 0 \\ 0 & 1 & 1 & 0 & 1 & 1 & 0 & 1 & 0 & 1 & 1 & 0 & 1 & 1 & 0 & 1 \end{bmatrix}'$$

has the following parameter estimates, all of which differ significantly ($p < 0.05$) from zero:

$\hat{\beta}$	se($\hat{\beta}$)	Interpretation
−5.84	0.71	Ref. value for misc. pain, low-dose ASA or low-dose test drug, days 1–14
1.82	0.73	Increment due to RA, days 1–14
0.91	0.33	Increment due to high-dose test drug for RA, days 1–14
−5.20	0.18	Reference value for days 15–84

The p values from the goodness-of-fit statistics are only slightly smaller for this model than for model $\mathbf{X}_3$ ($Q_P = 7.42$, $p = 0.83$, and $Q_L = 9.49$, $p = 0.66$, 12 d.f. for both).

The model-predicted probabilities of no DSAE by the end of the intervals can be calculated for a piecewise exponential model as

$$s_{ij} = \prod_{h=1}^{j} \exp[-a_h \exp(\mathbf{x}'_{ih}\hat{\boldsymbol{\beta}})]$$

TABLE 2.28 Model-predicted probabilities of no DSAEs by the end of the intervals

				Model $\mathbf{X}_2$		Model $\mathbf{X}_4$	
Treatment	Dose	Indication	Time (days)	Est.	(se)	Est.	(se)
ASA	Low	Misc. pain	1–14	0.933	(0.025)	0.960	(0.028)
			15–28	0.908	(0.033)	0.889	(0.028)
			29–84	0.816	(0.062)	0.653	(0.049)
ASA	Low	RA	1–14	0.816	(0.036)	0.777	(0.036)
			15–28	0.755	(0.041)	0.720	(0.035)
			29–84	0.553	(0.064)	0.529	(0.044)
ASA	High	RA	1–14	0.816	(0.036)	0.777	(0.036)
			15–28	0.755	(0.041)	0.720	(0.035)
Test	Low	Misc. pain	1–14	0.900	(0.035)	0.960	(0.028)
			15–28	0.865	(0.044)	0.889	(0.028)
			29–34	0.736	(0.078)	0.653	(0.049)
Test	Low	RA	1–14	0.736	(0.050)	0.777	(0.036)
			15–28	0.654	(0.054)	0.720	(0.035)
			29–84	0.408	(0.069)	0.529	(0.044)
Test	High	RA	1–14	0.569	(0.089)	0.535	(0.093)
			15–28	0.459	(0.100)	0.496	(0.086)

where i indexes the subpopulations; $a_h = 14$, 14, and 56 are the respective lengths of the three intervals ($h = 1, 2, 3$); and $\mathbf{x}'_{ih}$ is the row of $\mathbf{X}$ corresponding to the i-th subpopulation and h-th interval. These estimated probabilities for models $\mathbf{X}_2$ and $\mathbf{X}_4$ are shown in Table 2.28, along with their estimated standard errors, which were calculated using linear Taylor series methods.

G. Cox Regression

There are several advantages of Cox regression over piecewise exponential model fitting. With the availability of computer programs, such as the SAS procedure PHGLM, that take advantage of Breslow's (1974) modification for tied data, Cox regression with variable selection procedures is readily implemented. Cox regression can accommodate continuous covariables, whereas the piecewise exponential model covariables usually need to be categorical. Also, in Cox regression, time to event is treated as a continuous, rather than discretized, variable. However, this is not necessarily an advantage in adverse-experience data analysis because often only the interval of occurrence of the adverse experience is known. Piecewise exponential models can accommodate grouped data easily.

Cox models and piecewise exponential models with proportional hazards structure differ only with respect to the specification of the underlying hazard rate (i.e., the hazard rate for a population in which the value of all covariables is zero). For a piecewise exponential proportional hazards model, the underlying hazard is constant within each of the time intervals considered, whereas for the Cox model, the underlying hazard is unspecified.

Since the two models are structurally so similar, it is of interest to compare the regression coefficients from the two procedures. In Table 2.29, the coefficients from the piecewise exponential proportional hazards model $\mathbf{X}_1$ are shown alongside the coefficients from an analogous Cox model. The coefficient corresponding to the underlying hazard and the coefficients for the time effects are not estimated in Cox regression. The coefficients and standard errors for the other effects are very similar for the two procedures.

From a computational standpoint, it is not as straightforward to accommodate a nonproportional hazards situation with Cox regression as with piecewise exponential models. However, in a data set consisting of observations from patients enrolled in different protocols for different lengths of time, the assumption that the effect of important covariables is constant over time merits some scrutiny. One way to investigate this

TABLE 2.29 Comparison of coefficients from piecewise exponential model $\mathbf{X}_1$ with analogous Cox model regression coefficients

Piecewise exponential model $\mathbf{X}_1$				Cox model[a] coefficients	
		Coefficients			
$\mathbf{X}_1$	Interpretation of coefficients	$\hat{\beta}$	se($\hat{\beta}$)	$\hat{\beta}$	se($\hat{\beta}$)
1 0 0 0 0 0 0	Reference value	−5.34	0.59		
1 0 0 0 0 1 0	RA	1.11	0.61	1.12	0.61
1 0 0 0 0 0 1	Test drug	0.45	0.71	0.44	0.71
1 1 0 0 0 0 0	Low-dose test for RA	−0.05	0.76	−0.03	0.76
1 1 0 0 0 1 0	High dose over low for RA	0.62	0.35	0.55	0.36
1 1 0 0 0 0 1	15–28 Days	−1.04	0.35		
1 1 0 0 0 0 0	29–84 days	−0.91	0.28		
1 1 0 0 0 1 0					
1 0 1 0 0 0 0					
1 0 1 0 0 1 0					
1 0 1 0 0 0 1					
1 1 1 1 0 0 0					
1 1 1 1 0 1 0					
1 1 1 1 0 0 1					
1 1 1 1 1 0 0					
1 1 1 1 1 1 0					

[a]Cox model coefficients were estimated using the SAS procedure PHGLM.

proportionality assumption is to perform what may be called Cox regression with successive truncation. Several data sets are formed by successively truncating the data at consecutive time intervals of interest. Cox regression is performed for each of the individual data sets using the same independent variables, and then the coefficients from the regressions are compared. If the coefficients for any of the covariables differ significantly, this provides evidence that the effects of these covariables vary over time, and thus the assumption of proportional hazards does not hold.

This method was used to examine the effects of indication and treatment over the time intervals 1–14 days, 15–28 days, and 29–84 days. Since patients who received high-dose test drug only had DSAEs during days 1–14, the possibility of differential effects of high-dose test drug over time cannot be tested using these intervals. Moreover, the incidence of DSAEs with high doses of test drug has been shown to be significantly greater than with low doses. Therefore the analysis to be carried out, in which the two dose groups are combined, is not totally relevant in view of the preceding analyses. It is intended more to illustrate the use of the method of successive truncation with Cox regression and further parallels between this method and the piecewise exponential approach.

Three data sets were formed, one for each of the three intervals of interest. The first data set (for days 1–14) includes all 218 patients, of whom 44 had their first DSAE within 14 days. If a patient's time (censored or uncensored) to first DSAE was greater than 14 days, this time was considered censored at 14 days. The only patients also eligible to be in the second data set are the 141 patients who had their first DSAE or were censored after day 14. If a patient's time to DSAE was greater than 28, it was considered censored at day 28. Only 10 patients had their first DSAE in the interval 15–28 days, so the proportional hazards regression for this data set should be viewed cautiously. The last data set includes only the 96 patients who had their first DSAE or were censored after day 28. Twenty-one patients had their first DSAE in this interval.

A Cox regression was carried out for each of these data sets using the SAS procedure PHGLM. The fact that there is a lag time of 14 days for the second data set and 28 days for the third data set before any events occur has no effect on the computation of the regression coefficients. The coefficients are the same as if one had, in effect, started the clock over by subtracting 14 days (28 days) from all the times in the second (third) data set. The cofficients for the independent variables indication (1 = RA, 0 = miscellaneous pain) and treatment (1 = test drug, 0 = ASA) are shown below along with their covariance matrices:

Data set	Time frame	Variable	$\hat{\boldsymbol{\beta}}$	$\hat{\mathbf{V}}$	
1	1–14 days	Indication	2.053	0.524	0.006
		Treatment	0.619	0.006	0.098
2	15–28 days	Indication	0.560	0.633	0.056
		Treatment	0.202	0.056	0.405
3	29–84 days	Indication	0.673	0.266	0.024
		Treatment	0.524	0.024	0.204

The only coefficients that were significant at the 0.10 level were those for indication ($p < 0.01$) and treatment ($p < 0.05$) in the data set for days 1–14.

A Wald statistic was used to compare the coefficients using the following formula:

$$Q = \hat{\boldsymbol{\beta}}'\mathbf{C}'[\mathbf{C}\hat{\mathbf{V}}\mathbf{C}']^{-1}\mathbf{C}\hat{\boldsymbol{\beta}}$$

where $\hat{\boldsymbol{\beta}}$ is the concatenated vector of coefficients from the three regressions, $\hat{\mathbf{V}}$ is a 6×6 block diagonal matrix with the three 2×2 blocks being the covariance matrices, and

$$\mathbf{C} = \begin{bmatrix} 1 & 0 & -1 & 0 & 0 & 0 \\ 0 & 1 & 0 & -1 & 0 & 0 \\ 1 & 0 & 0 & 0 & -1 & 0 \\ 0 & 1 & 0 & 0 & 0 & -1 \end{bmatrix}$$

The Wald statistic was not significant with respect to a chi-square distribution with four degrees of freedom ($Q = 3.09$, $p = 0.54$), and thus the effects of indication and treatment were not shown to vary across the intervals.

An analogous test of the proportionality assumption for indication and treatment can be conducted using a piecewise exponential approach. The proportional hazards model,

$$\mathbf{X}_5 = \begin{bmatrix} 1 & 1 & 1 & 1 & 1 & 1 & 1 & 1 & 1 & 1 & 1 & 1 & 1 & 1 & 1 & 1 \\ 0 & 0 & 0 & 1 & 1 & 1 & 1 & 1 & 0 & 0 & 0 & 1 & 1 & 1 & 1 & 1 \\ 0 & 0 & 0 & 0 & 0 & 0 & 0 & 0 & 1 & 1 & 1 & 1 & 1 & 1 & 1 & 1 \\ 0 & 1 & 0 & 0 & 1 & 0 & 0 & 1 & 0 & 1 & 0 & 0 & 1 & 0 & 0 & 1 \\ 0 & 0 & 1 & 0 & 0 & 1 & 0 & 0 & 0 & 0 & 1 & 0 & 0 & 1 & 0 & 0 \end{bmatrix}'$$

is applied to the data shown in Table 2.26. The parameters for this model are the reference value for miscellaneous pain at low-dose ASA, the increment for RA, the increment for test drug, and the increments for days 15–28 and 29–84. The Rao score statistic is then computed for the matrix

$$\mathbf{W} = \begin{bmatrix} 0 & 0 & 0 & 0 & 1 & 0 & 0 & 1 & 0 & 0 & 0 & 0 & 1 & 0 & 0 & 1 \\ 0 & 0 & 0 & 0 & 0 & 1 & 0 & 0 & 0 & 0 & 0 & 0 & 0 & 1 & 0 & 0 \\ 0 & 0 & 0 & 0 & 0 & 0 & 0 & 0 & 0 & 1 & 0 & 0 & 1 & 0 & 0 & 1 \\ 0 & 0 & 0 & 0 & 0 & 0 & 0 & 0 & 0 & 0 & 1 & 0 & 0 & 1 & 0 & 0 \end{bmatrix}'$$

for which the first two columns represent the differential effect of indication in days 15–28 and 29–84, respectively, and the second two columns represent the differential effect of treatment in these two intervals. This score statistic is also nonsignificant ($Q = 3.81$, d.f. $= 4$, $p = 0.43$).

H. Proportional Hazards Regression Compared to Logistic Regression for Days 1–14

Additional regression analysis for the interval from 1 to 14 days is of interest for several reasons. As previously noted, pharmacological adverse experiences tend to occur soon after initiation of treatment. Also, most of the variability in the data appears to occur within the first 14 days, as evidenced by the fit of models $\mathbf{X}_3$ and $\mathbf{X}_4$ in Section VI.F, and the fact that the coefficients for indication and treatment in the Cox regressions in Section VI.G were significant only for the data set pertaining to this interval [however, since most of the DSAEs (44/75) occurred in the first 14 days, the power is also greatest for this interval].

In this section, a stepwise Cox regression is conducted for the data set corresponding to the first 14 days of treatment. Patients with no DSAE as of 14 days were considered censored at 14 days. The candidate variables include indicator variables for indication, treatment, high dose of test drug, sex, dichotomized age, and also a continuous age variable. The indicator variables for indication and high dose of test drug were the only variables to enter the model at significance level 0.10. The coefficients and their standard errors are shown in Table 2.30.

TABLE 2.30 Proportional hazards regression as compared to logistic regression for days 1–14

	Cox regression[b]		Logistic[c] regression		Piecewise exponential model $\mathbf{X}_4$	
Variable[a]	$\hat{\beta}$	se($\hat{\beta}$)	$\hat{\beta}$	se($\hat{\beta}$)	$\hat{\beta}$	se($\hat{\beta}$)
Intercept			−3.277	0.720		
Indication	1.822	0.731	2.000	0.750	1.822	0.731
High-dose test drug (for RA)	0.843	0.335	1.009	0.424	0.908	0.334

[a]Candidate variables for Cox and logistic stepwise regressions:

Indication	(1 if RA, 0 if misc. pain)
Treatment	(1 if test drug, 0 if ASA)
High-dose test drug	(1 if yes, 0 if no)
Sex	(1 if female, 0 if male)
Dichotomized age	(1 if ≥60, 0 otherwise)
Continuous age	

[b]Cox regression computation was done using the SAS procedure PHGLM.
[c]Logistic regression computation was done using the SAS procedure LOGIST.

Based on the theoretical results of Elandt-Johnson (1980), Green and Symons (1983) describe conditions under which the coefficients and standard errors from the logistic model approximate those for a Cox model with constant underlying hazard rate λ [sometimes also called Glasser's (1967) model]. The coefficients from the two models should approximate each other if the function of logistic regression parameters, $\exp(\alpha + \boldsymbol{\beta}'\mathbf{x})$, is small where α is the intercept parameter and $\boldsymbol{\beta}$ is the vector of coefficients for the covariable vector $\mathbf{x}$. The intercept parameter is shown to be a function of the cumulative incidence (λT) over the treatment period T, and thus the approximation is improved for rare failure events and short follow-up periods. Elandt-Johnson (1980) also showed that under these conditions, the standard errors for the coefficients from the two models also approximate each other.

For purposes of comparison, a stepwise logistic regression was conducted for the data set corresponding to the first 14 days of treatment, using the same independent variables and the same entrance criterion as for the Cox regression. Again, indication and high dose of the test drug were the only variables to enter the model. The coefficients and standard errors, shown in Table 2.30, are slightly larger than those for the proportional hazards model. Although the follow-up time is relatively short, the event is not rare: 44 of the 218 patients had a DSAE within the first 14 days. Also, for the logistic coefficients to approximate the proportional hazards model coefficients, it is assumed that all patients are followed for the entire follow-up period. This was not the case: 33 of the patients withdrew before 14 days and before having a DSAE.

As previously discussed, the Cox model does not assume a constant underlying hazard. However, in the piecewise exponential model $\mathbf{X}_4$ of Section IV.F, in which all the variation due to indication and high dose of the test drug is assumed to occur in days 1–14, the underlying hazard for days 1–14 is required to be constant. The coefficients for the increments due to RA (β_2) and the increment due to high-dose test drug for RA (β_3) from model $\mathbf{X}_4$ are also shown in Table 2.30.

I. Weighted Least-Squares Analyses of Frequency

As discussed in Section VI.B for chronic diseases such as arthritis, which require chronic administration of treatment, the frequency of a recurrent adverse experience may be more important than its time to onset. A summary measure for the frequency of a recurrent event is the total incidence, which may be estimated by the total number of occurrences of the event divided by the total number of person-days of exposure (Kleinbaum, Kupper, and Morgenstern, 1982, pp. 101–102). This quan-

TABLE 2.31 Comparison of total incidence for subgroups formed from cross-classification of indication, treatment, and dose

Subpopulation	Indication	Treatment	Dose	Number of patients	Total incidence Est.	Total incidence se
1	Misc. pain	ASA	Low	25	0.0050	0.0030
2	RA	ASA	Low	47	0.0156	0.0038
3	RA	ASA	High	35	0.0165	0.0084
4	Misc. pain	Test	Low	30	0.0067	0.0026
5	RA	Test	Low	51	0.0250	0.0050
6	RA	Test	High	30	0.0567	0.0165

Contrast	Interpretation	*p* Value
(−1 0 0 1 0 0)	Misc. pain: test vs. ASA	0.678
(0 −1 0 0 1 0)	RA; low-dose test vs. low-dose ASA	0.130
(0 0 −1 0 0 1)	RA: high-dose test vs. high-dose ASA	0.030
(0 −1 1 0 0 0)	RA: high-dose ASA vs. low-dose ASA	0.919
(0 0 0 0 −1 1)	RA: high-dose test vs. low-dose test	0.066

tity, along with its standard error, was calculated for each of six subpopulations defined by the cross-classification of indication, treatment, and dose, as shown in Table 2.31. Contrast matrices were used for comparisons of interest and tested with the program MISCAT (documented in Stanish, Koch, and Landis 1978).

The results are similar to the results of all previous analyses of this data. For the RA indication, the total incidence is significantly greater ($p < 0.05$) for high-dose test drug than for high-dose ASA. The comparison of high-dose test drug versus low-dose test drug in RA patients is nearly significant ($p < 0.10$), and the comparison of low-dose test drug versus low-dose ASA in RA patients is also suggestive ($p = 0.13$). No significant difference was found for the comparison of high-dose ASA versus low-dose ASA in RA patients or for the test drug versus ASA in miscellaneous pain patients.

J. The Package Insert

The most important summary of the adverse experience data for a new drug is what appears in the package insert. The results of the entire clinical testing program must be summarized succinctly and in a form easily understandable by nonstatisticians. Hence the current popularity of the "percent patients" format, in which the adverse experiences that occurred in at least a certain percentage of the patients exposed to the drug (or exposed to at most the maximum recommended dose) are listed, along with the percent of patients in whom they occurred. For acute adverse experiences, this crude proportion is a reasonable estimator of the risk of having a particular adverse experience. However, the measure has been justly criticized because, since time on study is ignored, the risk of nonacute adverse experiences is underestimated.

Idanpaan-Heikkila (1983) and O'Neill (1988) recommend the use of life-table estimates as alternative estimates of risk that do account for time on study. Other possible estimates include Kaplan–Meier estimates when the individual times to adverse experiences are available, or estimates from models, such as the piecewise exponential model estimates in Table 2.28. In the appendix to the Idanpaan-Heikkila report, O'Neill advises that in order to pool the data across studies, the definitions used for adverse experience classification, the dosing regimens, the intensity of follow-up, and the study designs should be reasonably comparable for the trials being combined. For the set of trials considered in this chapter, estimates should probably be presented separately for the RA patients receiving high doses of the test drug (if this dose is within the recommended range), the RA patients receiving low doses of the test drug, and the miscellaneous pain patients. It may be difficult to decide which time point to choose as a reference—for example, should one present the estimated probability of an adverse experience by 14 days or by 84 days? Since censoring by the end of study may induce bias in the estimates, as discussed in Section VI.D, it may be best to choose a reference time no longer than the length of the shortest study included. For the DSAE data this is appropriate because the DSAEs tend to occur within the first 14 days.

Other possible summary measures that also take account of exposure time are the average rate of first occurrences of adverse experiences over a given time period (i.e., the incidence density) or for recurrent events, the total incidence as presented in Section VI.I. As with the estimated risk, the estimated rate may differ for different indications and dose levels and over time, so presenting one rate may be an oversimplification. Additional discussion along these lines is given in O'Neill (1988).

VII. A CROSSOVER TRIAL EXAMPLE

Suzanne Edwards, Gary G. Koch, and William Sollecito

The crossover design has power properties that make its usage attractive in the evaluation of pharmaceutical products. The advantages and disadvantages of the use of this design have been reviewed by Brown (1980), who also documents the frequency of its usage in clinical trials.

The methodology for analyzing data from a crossover design has been described for the parametric case by Grizzle (1965); nonparametric approaches have been described by Koch (1972). The primary focus of these methods has been on data that is at least ordinal in scale. A methodology for analyzing measures that are nominal in scale, such as the occurrence of adverse effects, has been described by Gart (1969). All three of the methods referenced above are directed at the two-period crossover design. Another useful application of the crossover design in biopharmaceutical research is the three-period crossover design. It allows for the comparison of three treatments administered sequentially over three different periods and thereby has the desirable feature of possibly including two active treatments and one placebo. In the continuous parametric case, the model described by Grizzle (1965) for the two-period/two-treatment crossover design can be directly extended to three or more periods and treatments; however, this extension is less direct in the case of ordinal or nominal data, as is most frequently encountered in the analysis of adverse events. The subsequent discussion illustrates statistical methods for the analysis of the incidence and number of occurrences of adverse effects in a three-period crossover design through a hypothetical example.

A. Description of the Trial

The example is based on a crossover trial for aspects of cardiovascular function. The study included 12 healthy volunteers who each received a single dose of two active medications (A, B) and placebo (P) over the course of three treatment periods with sufficient washout periods between each. Each of the treatments and placebo were administered according to the six sequences described in Table 2.32.

TABLE 2.32 Example of three-period crossover design

Subject	Sequence	Period 1	Period 2	Period 3
2, 9	1	A	B	P
5, 12	2	B	P	A
6, 7	3	P	A	B
1, 10	4	A	P	B
3, 1	5	B	A	P
4, 8	6	P	B	A

One approach to analyzing adverse events in such a setting involves the consideration of the three treatments and periods in pairs and carrying out pairwise treatment comparisons that take into account the correlation across periods of observations on the same subjects.

B. Analysis of Occurrence/Nonoccurrence

McNemar's test (McNemar, 1947) and Gart's test (Gart, 1969) are applicable for dichotomous outcomes, that is, the occurrence or nonoccurrence of adverse events. McNemar's test is applied by first sorting the data according to treatment received (ignoring period) and then comparing pairs of treatments (e.g., A and B) to determine if a specific adverse event occurred under treatment A only, treatment B only, neither, or both. If an adverse event occurred in neither or both treatments, it is disregarded as a tie. Thus, the analysis is based only on those events that occurred on one treatment but not the other. This approach is most sensitive for detecting events that are expected to be associated with one treatment but not another, such as in comparisons of active treatment with placebo. This methodology can also be extended to comparisons of other measures of adverse events that can be dichotomized, such as related versus not related, or mild or moderate versus severe adverse events.

For the cardiovascular function trial described here, suppose the occurrence of at least one central nervous system (CNS) symptom is recorded as 1 = Yes and 0 = No for each subject; then an assessment of the statistical significance of the difference in incidence among the three treatment groups is shown in Table 2.33.

The number of patients experiencing one or more CNS symptoms is summarized in the total row of Table 2.33; the incidence of adverse effects for placebo is 8/12 (66.7%); for treatments A and B, it is 10/12 (83.3%) and 1/12 (8.3%), respectively. The right hand side of the total row provides McNemar p values summarizing the comparison of each pair of treatments; these are exact p values computed by assessing the binomial probability of the observed number of +1's and −1's in each pairwise treatment column (zeroes representing ties are ignored in this computation). Thus, from these data, treatment B had significantly fewer CNS symptoms than placebo or treatment A (when comparisons are made at the 0.05 level of significance).

This method is easily applied once the data are arrayed as in Table 2.33 and is generalizable to other types of crossover designs. One possible limitation of this approach is that it ignores the period in which adverse events occur. In many crossover trials, period effects are negli-

TABLE 2.33 Number of subjects reporting at least one CNS symptom in crossover study concerning cardiovascular function

Subject	Placebo (P)[a]	A	B	A–P	B–P	A–B
1	1	1	0	0	−1	1
2	1	0	0	−1	−1	0
3	0	1	0	1	0	1
4	1	1	0	0	−1	1
5	1	1	0	0	−1	1
6	1	0	1	−1	0	−1
7	1	1	0	0	−1	1
8	0	1	0	1	0	1
9	1	1	0	0	−1	1
10	0	1	0	1	0	1
11	1	1	0	0	−1	1
12	0	1	0	1	0	1
Total	8	10	1	$p = 0.344$	$p = 0.016$	$p = 0.012$

[a]For placebo, A, B, 1 = yes, 0 = no.

gible. However, some adjustment for period of treatment is feasible with a version of Gart's test (1969). For this test, treatments would be sorted by the period in which they occurred and pairwise comparisons would be carried out by forming a tabulation according to whether the adverse event occurred in the earlier or later period. An illustration of this procedure for the comparison of treatments A and B is shown in Table 2.34.

Another extension of Gart's test would involve the application of the Mantel–Haenszel (1959) test to a set of (2×2) tables like Table 2.34 with stratification according to the period of placebo (i.e., the treatment not

TABLE 2.34 Number of subjects reporting at least one CNS symptom in sequence groups of crossover study concerning cardiovascular function

	Earlier	Later	
Sequence 1, 3, 4 A→B	4	1	($p = 0.015$)
Sequence 2, 5, 6 B→A	0	6	

being compared). For this method, sequences 3 and 6 would comprise the first stratum, sequences 2 and 4 would comprise the second, and sequences 1 and 5 would comprise the third.

C. Analysis of Total Number of Occurrences

The total number of occurrences of CNS symptoms and the number per subject are summarized in Table 2.35. The p values in the bottom row of Table 2.35 are based on sign tests for the pairwise treatment comparisons. They support the same conclusions as were noted for McNemar's test, that is, treatment B had significantly fewer occurrences of CNS symptoms than either placebo or treatment A. The p values for the B versus P and the A versus B comparisons are exactly the same as those produced by McNemar's test, since the patterns of signs in Table 2.35, for them is the same as in Table 2.33. Alternatively, Wilcoxon signed ranks tests (Wilcoxon, 1949) could be applied to the pairwise differences in Table 2.35.

Extensions like those described for Gart's test are also applicable. They can be based on Wilcoxon rank sum tests (Wilcoxon, 1945) to compare sets of sequences like those shown in Table 2.34 for differences between the earlier and later periods for a particular pair of treatments. With stratification for the period of the treatment that is not being

TABLE 2.35 Number of CNS symptoms reported by subjects in crossover study concerning cardiovascular function

Subject	Placebo	A	B	A–P	B–P	A–B
1	1	4	0	3	−1	4
2	2	0	0	−2	−2	0
3	0	6	0	6	0	6
4	2	2	0	0	−2	2
5	2	3	0	1	−2	3
6	1	0	1	−1	0	−1
7	4	2	0	−2	−4	2
8	0	4	0	4	0	4
9	1	4	0	3	−1	4
10	0	1	0	1	0	1
11	1	2	0	1	−1	2
12	0	2	0	2	0	2
Total	14	30	1	$p = 0.227$	$p = 0.016$	$p = 0.012$
No./subject	1.17	2.5	0.08			

compared, methods like those described in Section III.A.3 are applicable. Due to the small sample size in this example, such methods are not illustrated here.

One other possible method that can be considered for crossover studies is weighted regression for (sequence × period) means. This approach, which is not illustrated here, would use extensions of WLS methods as described in Section III.E.

VIII. SUMMARIZATION AND ANALYSIS SUMMARY

Suzanne Edwards, Gary G. Koch, and William Sollecito

Adverse experience data is considered "soft" data, the kind of data that statisticians generally prefer to avoid. Most references dealing with the analysis of clinical trials are devoted almost exclusively to the analysis of efficacy data. Much less attention has been given to the analysis of safety data in general, and adverse experience data in particular (note the formation in 1984–1985 of the American Statistical Association Biopharmaceutical Section Work Group on the topic 'Summarization and Analysis of Adverse Experience Data'). Thus, the aim of this chapter has not been to extend or fill in gaps in the preexisting literature because there are almost no published works on the subject of adverse experience data analysis. Rather, the aim has been to put the subject in perspective from a statistical point of view and to discuss applications of existing methodology to the analysis of adverse experiences, using real data for illustration.

In Section I, adverse experiences were defined, and an introduction to how adverse experiences occur and how this type of data is typically collected in clinical trials was given. The focus of Section II was on the statistical issues involved in the analysis of adverse experience data. The sampling and measurement processes used to obtain the data were discussed, and the implications of these on the generalizability of statistical results and quality of the data were considered. Four attributes of the data were delineated (occurrence/nonoccurrence, severity, frequency/duration, and timing), and the construction of summary variables characterizing each of these attributes was discussed. Also discussed were the relative merits of design-based analysis versus model-based analysis. In view of the sampling process issues and the limitations of both of these analysis frameworks when considered separately, it was concluded to use both in combination.

Some design- and model-based methods appropriate for the analysis of the summary measures given in Section II were presented in some detail in Section III. The design-based tests for treatment (or other group) differences included randomization statistics with covariate adjustment and/or stratification adjustment, exact tests, and nonparametric tests for group comparisons of time to first adverse experience. The model-based methods included logistic regression for dichotomous response variables (e.g., occurrence/nonoccurrence), extensions of logistic regression for ordinal variables (e.g., severity), weighted least-squares methods for analysis of counts and rates, and Cox regression and piecewise exponential modeling for time to first adverse experience.

The methods of Section III are implemented in the example data sets of Sections IV, V, VI, and VII. The data sets in each section are from different clinical trials, each of a different class of drugs, and each differing with respect to aspects of study design, data collection, and (a posteriori) goal of analysis.

The data in Section IV are from a single-center, one-day, fixed-dose trial of a new combination antihistamine/decongestant. The control groups were given either the antihistamine alone, the decongestant alone, or placebo. Only four adverse experiences were of primary interest. The primary analysis goal was to test whether the combination drug group had less drowsiness than the antihistamine group or less jitteriness than the decongestant group. Other research questions were also explored. Contingency-table analysis, covariate-adjusted randomization statistics, and logistic regression were used for analyses pertaining to the occurrence/nonoccurrence of adverse experiences over the treatment period. A power analysis was performed for the contingency-table treatment comparisons. Univariate and multivariate randomization statistics were used for treatment-group comparisons of the severity and frequency/duration of drowsiness. Weighted least-squares methods were also used to compare treatments with respect to frequency/duration. A correlation analysis was used to describe the extent to which different adverse experiences tended to occur simultaneously.

In contrast to the Section IV data, the data in Section V are from a two-center, 28-day, variable-dose trial of a new antidepressant in psychiatric (depressed) patients. Due to the large number of adverse experiences assessed (34) and the "noisiness" of the data, the main focus of this section was strategies for data reduction. Two commonly used criteria for selecting relevant subsets of adverse experiences were evaluated: (1) using only adverse experiences that are considered by the investigator to be at least possibly drug-related, and (2) using only adverse experiences that are new or exacerbated relative to baseline. Surprisingly, these two criteria produced substantially different results. There were significant treatment differences with respect to several adverse experiences for each of the criteria, but for only one of the adverse experiences in one of the centers was there a significant treatment difference by both criteria.

Other issues that arose from this data set include the need to account in the analysis for baseline status and number of assessments. In Section IV, almost all patients were present for the entire length of the study, and there were so few patients with baseline adverse experiences that the strategy for dealing with these patients in most cases was to exclude them from the analysis. In Section V, on the other hand, many of the patients withdrew early, and many had baseline adverse experiences, especially adverse experiences that are also symptoms of depression. Randomization statistics, with covariate adjustment for baseline and number of assessments and stratification by center, were used for the analysis of occurrence/nonoccurrence and severity of selected adverse experiences. The number of assessments was also used as a stratification variable, along with center in a randomization statistics analysis (covariate-adjusted for baseline) of a measure of frequency/duration. The randomization statistic analyses were supplemented by stepwise logistic regression analysis for descriptive purposes.

In Section VI, the data are from a series of trials of a new analgesic versus aspirin control, and the objective of investigation was the comparison of these two treatments with respect to incidence and pattern of occurrence of digestive system adverse experiences (DSAEs). The main analysis issue here was how to summarize and analyze adverse experience data from different protocols. The protocols differed with respect to pain indication of patients enrolled, dose levels used, and study length, among other attributes. Most of the analysis effort was devoted to the use of survival data methods for the analysis of time to first DSAE.

The Breslow generalized Wilcoxon and Mantel–Cox tests were used to assess the association of dose and indication with time to first DSAE. Both variables were found to be important predictors, and so results were presented separately for different levels of these variables. A stratified Mantel–Cox test, stratifying by center, was used to compare treatments with respect to time to first DSAE.

The model-based methods used for this data included piecewise exponential modeling and Cox regression. Parallels were drawn between Cox models and piecewise exponential models with proportional hazards structure, and between both of these kinds of models and the logistic model. The use of the method of successive truncation as a way of checking the proportional hazards assumption in Cox regression was also discussed.

Because DSAEs are recurrent events, the analysis of time to first

DSAE does not make full use of the data. Thus weighted least-squares methods were used to compare treatments with respect to the frequency of DSAEs relative to time on study. The section concluded with a discussion of possible summary measures which might be used in the package insert.

Section VII introduced methodology for a crossover design using a hypothetical example of a three period/treatment crossover trial. This type of design, which is common in biopharmaceutical studies, allows for the comparison of two active treatments and placebo in a setting where subjects serve as their own controls. The analysis strategies described take into account the correlation structure of the data and, in particular, the lack of independence among treatments administered to the same patients over time. The McNemar test (McNemar, 1947) and the Wilcoxon signed ranks test (Wilcoxon, 1949) are identified for pairwise comparisons for data that have nominal and ordinal scale; both procedures ignore treatment order and possible period effects. Extensions of Gart's test (Gart, 1969) are suggested as methods to account for period of treatment.

The main emphasis throughout this chapter has been on how the analysis of safety data (adverse experience data in particular) differs from the analysis of efficacy data in clinical trials of new drugs. To paraphrase Friedman, Furberg, and DeMets (1981), it is better to wrongly attribute side effects to the experimental drug than to miss side effects that the drug may actually cause. Thus, from a statistical point of view, minimizing the Type II error is more important than minimizing the Type I error. Also, exploratory and descriptive analyses are more appropriate for safety data than for efficacy data. This philosophy was carried out in Sections IV through VII in several ways:

1. A significance level of 0.10 was generally used rather than the usual 0.05.
2. A power analysis was carried out whenever feasible if no treatment difference was shown.
3. The problem of multiple inference was deemphasized. Multiple inference was particularly a problem in Section V where data on 34 adverse experiences were collected. No multiple inference procedures were carried out other than to note the possibility of significant results being due to chance.

Probably one of the most important predictors of adverse experiences is dose. In Section VI, it was possible to distinguish between patients who received "high" and "low" doses of their respective treatments. Usually, when considering data from different protocols, such a simple classification is not possible. Dose is often a time-varying covariate. However, to incorporate it as such makes the analysis more complex than is probably warranted. Other summary measures, such as the maximum dose or the mean dose received prior to the adverse experience, could also be considered.

Another area that deserves further attention is methods for the analysis of adverse experiences as recurrent events. Adverse experiences are usually summarized by whether or not they occur or the time to first occurrence. Neither of these summary measures reflect the recurrent nature of many adverse experiences. In Sections IV–VII, this issue was addressed by the construction and analysis of summary variables for frequency/duration. In Section IV, the summary variable was simply the proportion of assessments at which the patient reported the adverse experience. This measure is appropriate for this data set because the assessments were evenly spaced. In Section V, where the assessments were not evenly spaced, the summary variable was the ratio of the sum of the lengths of the assessment intervals for which the patient reported the adverse experience to the patient's length of time of study. In Section VI, where a separate record was entered for each day the patient had the adverse experience, the summary measure was the ratio of the total number of adverse experiences to the patient's length of time on study.

Bristol and Patel (1985) proposed the use of Markov chains for the analysis of adverse experiences as recurrent events. Two states were defined: reporting the adverse experience at an assessment or not reporting it. Treatment groups were to be compared with respect to the estimated transition probabilities of moving from state to state over a series of assessments. A similar approach is discussed by Leviton et al. (1980), who proposed the use of a four-state (based on severity) Markov chain for modeling the probabilities of headache recurrence.

Another possible method for the analysis of adverse experiences as recurrent events is the multivariate Cox model (Aalen, 1978; Anderson and Gill, 1982). This model can accommodate very general censoring patterns, as well as time-dependent covariates. However, the use of such a mathematically sophisticated model for the analysis of adverse experiences probably falls in the arena of using a "sledge hammer to kill a fly."

Other topics not addressed include the use of interim analyses for safety monitoring (see Canner, 1983; Peace, 1987), and the need for simultaneous assessment of benefit and risk. Safety monitoring is addressed in Section X. Lachin (1982a) gives the hypothetical example of a clinical trial of a drug to dissolve gallstones, in which a patient has his gallstones dissolved but develops cirrhosis of the liver. Thus, for this patient, the trial is a success in terms of efficacy, but a failure in terms of safety.

IX. PRACTICAL CONSIDERATIONS

Suzanne Edwards, Gary G. Koch, and William Sollecito

A. Issues to Consider

The statistical methods presented in this chapter represent a wide range of approaches with varying levels of complexity. It is not proposed that all these methods are applicable to all safety analyses; instead, they are suggested in the spirit of a handbook that might facilitate the planning of an analysis of adverse effect information in a biopharmaceutical clinical trial.

In considering the various approaches that have been presented here, it is important to note that safety analyses are sometimes viewed as a clinical activity for which statistical analyses should be kept to a minimum. If statistical analyses are called for, then three questions need to be addressed to determine the extent of analysis.

The first critical question to consider in deciding on an analysis approach is whether or not formal statistical inference such as that from hypothesis tests or confidence intervals is appropriate. If this is the case, the second question deals with the extent to which inferential methods are applied. Finally, the third question, which is a major topic of this chapter, is concerned with which statistical methods are available for various types of formal statistical analyses of adverse effect information. In making these choices the following points need consideration:

1. Purpose/design of the study
2. Statistical limitations
3. Regulatory considerations

B. Purpose/Design of the Study

Probably the most important issue to consider in choosing an analysis approach is the ultimate purpose of the study; this automatically implies direct consideration of the study design, since studies are usually designed to meet a set of specific objectives. If a study is designed primarily to address efficacy rather than safety, it will most likely be a double-blind study with a parallel group or crossover design. Thus, the methods described in previous sections for these designs may be applicable. However, if the objective of the study is primarily safety, it may not lend itself to inferential statistical analyses. The design of safety-only studies often emphasizes generalizability of results and the ability to detect adverse effects which have low incidence. For example, the design may call for a single treatment, which is administered in a single-blind or open-label fashion. It may be quite sufficient to analyze these types of safety studies with descriptive methods alone.

In the traditional comparative double-blind study, which involves two or more treatments, care should still be taken in choosing the extent of analysis to be carried out. For example, in a crossover study, the primary advantages of the design will most likely be applicable to efficacy parameters that are continuous in nature and thus amenable to powerful parametric analysis techniques which adjust for "nuisance parameters" such as period and carryover effects. Although a methodology was presented in Section VII for analyzing adverse effects in a crossover design, its scope is somewhat limited for situations where period and/or carryover effects are present.

In many crossover trials, sufficient washout periods are included in the design so as to reduce the influence of previous treatments on efficacy assessments in each subsequent treatment period. However, this issue can be more difficult for the evaluation of adverse effects, since there may be phenomena such as withdrawal effects or sensitization of the patients to treatments over time. Thus, if efficacy is the primary purpose of the study and a complex design has been used, inferential analyses may be of less interest for safety parameters.

If safety is the primary purpose of the study, then it can be designed in such a way as to require formal statistical analyses. For example, even in a single-blind or open-label study with a single treatment, such as a postmarketing surveillance study, modeling procedures may be considered appropriate as a way of assessing factors that are significantly associated with the occurrence of adverse effects; these approaches may also be used to evaluate whether higher incidence is observed in one subgroup of the population versus another.

In the next section of this chapter, design issues that should be considered for safety monitoring are further addressed; in regard to choosing an analysis strategy, the point to be considered here is that the purpose and design of the study have a very direct influence on the analysis methodology to be chosen.

C. Statistical Limitations

In addition to study design, other sampling process and measurement process issues directly influence the analysis approach chosen. This point is made relative to general analysis situations in the literature (Koch, Gillings, and Stokes, 1980; Koch and Sollecito, 1984) but also needs special consideration in regard to the analysis of adverse effects in biopharmaceutical trials. The issues that are of greatest concern have to do with the statistical limitations of premarketing trials in regard to sample size and the nature of the data collected to assess adverse effects.

Since most premarketing trials are directed at efficacy, the sample size chosen will generally be too small to provide adequate power for carrying out analyses of adverse effects. This is especially true for adverse effects with low incidence, such as serious adverse effects, which are of the greatest concern for assessing safety in a clinical trial. In this regard, as the incidence of an adverse effect decreases and the corresponding size of the difference to be detected also decreases, the sample size needed to achieve a given level of power increases substantially.

Since most New Drug Applications will include no more than 3000 patients across all studies, it is very unlikely that the sample size in any individual study will be sufficient to provide powerful statistical tests or suitably narrow confidence intervals for adverse effects with low incidence (e.g., less than 1%).

The nature of the data collected in the assessment of adverse effects has a very direct influence on the choice of analysis methodology. First, the measurement scale directly influences this choice, since adverse effect analyses cover the entire range from nominal (incidence) to interval (duration) scale. Second, the reliability of information collected also varies by type of measure.

The primary focus of adverse effect analyses is the summarization of occurrence/nonoccurrence of adverse effects. The measurement of whether or not a patient had an adverse effect is probably the most reliable of all information collected relative to adverse effects. Summarization by body system as well as overall occurrences of any adverse effects will generally provide high enough incidence so that power is sufficient for applying hypothesis testing procedures or related confidence intervals along the lines described in previous sections. The analysis of specific adverse effects is probably better left to purely descriptive procedures due to power considerations and due to the difficulties in classifying verbatim descriptions of adverse effects in a statistically meaningful manner. The use of dictionaries, such as those described in Section I, greatly improves this situation.

In general, the analysis of incidence of adverse effects is most amenable to inferential statistical analysis, and the specific choice as to which method is applied should be based on the degree to which the research issues of interest can be addressed and the degree to which statistical assumptions can be justified. Other related adverse effect indicators may be less amenable to the statistical methods described in this chapter due to reliability and other measurement issues.

The assessment of severity of an adverse effect and the drug relationship of the adverse effect are usually collected on an ordinal scale; thus methods that are applicable to ordinal data are applicable. These measures are generally intended to be clinical descriptors of adverse effects and are most often best summarized through descriptive procedures only. Also worth considering is the fact that these measures are very subjective in nature and are less reliable than occurrence information.

An important class of measures that are often of interest in assessing safety is measures that describe "time to" and/or "duration of" an adverse effect. While it is appealing statistically to analyze these types of measures through the use of survival techniques that have been described here (see Section VI), one should proceed with caution due to the lack of reliability of date and time information in the collection of adverse effect data. Generally, descriptions of adverse effects are elicited at office visits in which a patient is asked to recall when an adverse effect occurred during some time interval between the present visit and last prior visit; this time interval generally ranges from one week and may be up to several months. Thus, details on exact dates, times, and durations of adverse effects, which are the primary focus of survival analysis techniques, may be quite unreliable and may mislead conclusions. However, it should be noted that if these types of data are of special interest, design of a study can include detailed recording of onset and duration of specific adverse effects of interest. In such studies the use of survival analysis techniques to assess "time to" and "duration of" events can provide a very powerful tool for assessing adverse effects.

In summary, sampling and measurement process issues should directly influence the choice of whether or not to perform inferential statistical analyses of data for adverse effects and which methods to apply. The most important of these considerations are the sample size and the nature of the data to be analyzed.

D. Regulatory Considerations

One of the primary purposes of carrying out biopharmaceutical clinical trials is to provide evidence in support of the efficacy and safety of new drugs in order to satisfy regulatory requirements of the Food and Drug Administration (FDA). An important consideration in choosing an analysis approach is the satisfaction of these requirements. While not a statement for how to carry out safety analyses of new products, the recently revised FDA guidelines for the clinical and statistical section of a New Drug Application (FDA, 1988) do provide important guidance in choosing analysis approaches. The primary focus of the guidelines, in regard to summarization of adverse effects, is on clarity of presentation with a clinical rather than statistical emphasis. The guidelines clearly mandate detailed descriptions of all serious or potentially serious adverse events. Certain descriptive summaries are also specifically noted as being of interest. For example, one table that is illustrated (FDA, 1988, p. 72) is a cross-tabulation for each adverse effect of the study drug relationship by severity of the adverse effect.

Where statistical comparisons among treatments are called for, the emphasis is on the rate of occurrence of adverse events and especially important adverse events. The exact methodology for carrying out these analyses is not specified, although some form of inferential analysis is implied. Thus, although the primary focus of a safety analysis may be on descriptive analyses, additional inferential analyses may also be warranted to the extent that they further clarify associations that are noted in descriptive tables and within the limits of the other considerations described above.

In general, the FDA guidelines should be consulted first as part of the process for choosing an analysis approach. In addition, this chapter can provide a guide for choosing methods that are potentially useful for alternative types of analyses of adverse effects.

X. DESIGN, MONITORING, AND OTHER ANALYSIS ISSUES*

Karl E. Peace

A. Designing Trials to Provide Definitive Safety Information

There can be little argument that for drugs for which it is possible to design trials to provide definitive information about aspects of safety, there are few, if any, issues. One would develop the protocol. The protocol would include sections on background, objective, plan of study, data analysis, administrative procedures, and bibliography (see Appendix). The plan of study would include the description of the study population, the description of the study design, and the criteria regarding dealing with problem management. The data analysis section would include criteria for defining safety end points, address statistical design considerations, address early termination considerations, if any, and specify the statistical methods to be used in summarizing and/or analyzing the endpoints. The administration section of the protocol would

*Reprinted, with permission, in part from Peace (1987).

include the review and consent requirements, record keeping, and details regarding monitoring.

There have been several occasions in my pharmaceutical industry experience where it has been possible to design trials to provide definitive information about aspects of safety. For example, in the clinical development of a new antibiotic, a skin rash was observed among several patients at the top dose of a Phase II dose comparison trial. Since the top dose appeared to be more efficacious, a trial was subsequently designed and executed to confirm the rash experience before deciding to terminate the top dose from further clinical development. In designing the follow-up trial, the Phase II dose comparison trial provided estimates for sample size. It consisted of a single arm of the top dose, incorporated sequential procedures as discussed by Armitage (1954), and required 47 patients for confirmation of the skin rash. The decision was subsequently made to terminate the top dose from clinical development.

As another example, a clinical trial was designed and conducted to assess the hypokalemia potential of two doses, 25 mg (B) and 50 mg (C), of hydrochlorothiazide, and 25 mg of hydrochlorothiazide plus 50 mg of triamterene (A). The definition of hypokalemia was serum potassium concentration less than or equal to 3.5 meq/l. The protocol required patients with mild to moderate hypertension to be treated for 6 months. Analyses of the data were to be performed beginning with 6 weeks of treatment. Approximately 171 patients per group were needed to detect a 10% difference in the incidences of hypokalemia among any two regimens with a Type I error rate of 5% and a power of 80%. The outcome of the trial after 6 weeks of treatment is reflected by the ordering $A < B < C$. That is, the combination exhibited a lower incidence of hypokalemia than 25 mg of hydrochlorothiazide alone, which in turn exhibited a lower incidence than the 50-mg dose of hydrochlorothiazide alone.

As a final example, the Phase III clinical development plan for a new antihypertensive compound included a forced-titration, placebo-controlled dose-comparison trial, a trial comparing once versus twice a day administration of the target dose, and a positive control trial against the target dose. Although furnishing antihypertensive efficacy information on the target dose of the new drug relative to the positive control, the aim of the positive control trial was to provide a marketing hook. It was thought that patients on the new drug were less likely to experience "hypertensive rebound" or "blood pressure overshoot" when therapy was withdrawn than patients on the positive control. Very briefly, the design considerations consisted of an initial phase representing treatment for 6 months to control blood pressure, followed by a phase where the antihypertensive compound was withdrawn and blood pressure as subsequently monitored for up to 7 days for overshoot. The number of patients required qualitatively was the number necessary to discriminate between the two regimens in terms of overshoot, inflated to account for the proportions expected to be controlled over the first phase.

B. Premarket Approval Trials—Designing for Efficacy

The previous examples illustrate instances where it is possible to design clinical trials to provide definitive information on aspects of safety. However, for most drugs, particularly premarket approval ones, it is not possible to design trials to provide definitive information about safety.

Some reasons are (1) inadequate information to formulate the objective or question, (2) inadequate information to specify the primary safety end points, and (3) inadequate information to characterize the target population. Even if the end points are specified, the question formulated and the target population identified, (4) it is usually the case that inadequate information on estimates of end points exist for sample size determination. In addition, even if the end points are specified, the question formulated, the target population identified, and sufficient information exists to determine adequate sample sizes, (5) logistical and/or financial dfficulties usually preclude conducting a trial that large.

Therefore, a rational position to take in the development of new drugs is to design trials to provide definitive information about efficacy, to monitor safety and describe the safety profile in each trial, and to accumulate and describe the safety profile across trials. This position is consistent with statutory requirements for new drug, regulatory approval in the United States—which is to provide both clinical and statistical evidence of efficacy and to adequately describe the safety profile. It is thus reasonable to expect that a New Drug Application (NDA) that contains clinical and statistical evidence of the claimed efficacy effects and an adequate description of the safety profile—and which in itself represents no unacceptable safety concerns—would be given regulatory approval to be marketed.

It is interesting to note that regulatory requirements for new drug development allow the sponsor to proceed along the lines indicated by two axioms of drug development.

Axiom 1: Drugs in development are considered nonefficacious until proven otherwise.

Axiom 2: Drugs in development are considered safe until proven otherwise.

From the statistician's point of view, Axiom 1 says that the null hypothesis (HOE) is "the drug is nonefficacious" and that the alternative hypothesis (HAE) is "the drug is efficacious." Axiom 2 says that the null hypothesis (HOS) is "the drug is safe" whereas the alternative hypothesis (HAS) is "the drug is not safe."

In order for a sponsor's drug to be approved as being efficacious, then, enough information must be accumulated to contradict the null hypothesis (HOE). This implies that the Type I error is synonymous with the regulatory decision risk regarding approval for efficacy and that the Type II error is synonymous with the sponsor's risk of failing to detect a truly efficacious drug. In order for the drug to be approved with a decision as to safety, then the null hypothesis (HOS) must not be contradicted by the available safety information. This implies that the Type II error is synonymous with regulatory decision risk regarding approval whereas the Type I error is synonymous with the sponsor's risk.

C. Quality of Safety Information from Efficacy Trials

If new drug development trials are designed to provide definitive information about efficacy rather than safety, it is imperative to consider the quality of safety information from such trials. As a definition, a trial will be regarded as being designed to provide definitive evidence of efficacy if it has a power of 95% to detect a clinically important difference between the primary response measures of the target and reference regimens with a false positive rate of 5%. For discussion purposes, the clinically important difference is taken as 20% and the response variable is assumed to be dichotomous. A dichotomous response variable for efficacy assessment allows a natural connection between the efficacy end point and safety end points such as the proportion of patients who experience adverse events.

The number of patients required per regimen for a trial defined in terms of these characteristics will range anywhere from 125 to 164, depending upon whether one takes the point of view that the alternative hypothesis is one- or two-sided and also whether one adopts the worst case of the variance or adopts a position less conservative. It is important to note that a trial designed in the manner described above to detect a (δ) percent difference between two regimens will permit the statistical detection (at the 0.05 nominal significance level) of a difference as small as one-half (δ) percent at the analysis stage. However, a trial designed definitively in this manner is very unlikely to be able to furnish any information about an extremely rare event. For example, if the fraction of a population who would develop an adverse experience upon treatment with a drug at a given dose was 0.1%, one would require 4604 (Table 2.36) patients to be treated with the drug at the given dose in order to be 99% confident of observing at least 1 patient with a particular adverse experience. If one required a greater degree of certainty, say 99.99%, 9000–10,000 patients would require treatment. In fact, the definitively designed efficacy trial would not enable one to detect any adverse experiences with certainty that would occur less frequently than in 6% of the treated population.

Taking a trial with 150 patients per arm as representative of the definitively designed efficacy trial, one is not likely to observe in such a trial any patient experiencing a rare adverse event. For example, the probability of observing no patient with an adverse experience among 150 treated patients given that the true incidence in the population is 0.1% is 0.861. It is therefore highly likely that the outcome of such a trial will be 0 divided by 150: that is, an incidence of 0% among those patients treated. A corresponding exact 95% confidence interval based

TABLE 2.36 Number of patients required to be treated with a dose of a drug in order to be $100(1-\alpha)\%$ confident of observing at least one adverse experience (AE) given that the true fraction who would develop AEs in the population is P.

p	0.90	0.95	0.99	0.999	0.9999
0.001	2302	2995	4604	6906	9208
0.005	460	599	920	1380	1840
0.01	230	300	460	690	920
0.015	[153]	200	306	459	612
0.02	114	[149]	228	342	456
0.03	76	99	[152]	218	304
0.04	57	75	114	[171]	228
0.05	45	59	90	[135]	[180]
0.06	38	50	76	114	152
0.07	32	42	64	96	128
0.08	28	37	56	84	112
0.09	25	33	50	75	100
0.10	22	29	44	66	88
0.15	15	20	30	45	60
0.20	11	15	22	33	44
0.30	7	10	14	21	28
0.40	5	7	10	15	20
0.50	4	6	8	12	16

on this outcome ranges from 0 to 2.4%. If, in fact, what was known about the mechanism of action, the pharmacology, and/or the toxicology of the drug suggested certain untoward adverse events were possible and one monitored specifically for such events in a definitively designed efficacy trial, the fact that no such events were observed among 150 treated patients would probably be insufficient for regulatory approval in view of the upper limit of the 95% confidence interval being 2.4%.

For adverse events that would happen in 6% or greater of the population, the typical definitively designed trial for efficacy would permit discrimination between two arms of approximately a 20% difference in the incidences of adverse experiences with a power of 95% and a nominal false positive rate of 5%, or alternatively, discrimination between two arms of approximately a 10% difference with a power of 50% and a nominal false positive rate of 5%. The latter quantifies the smallest observed difference at the analysis stage that would be indicative of a real difference.

D. Monitoring for Safety

Since a trial designed to provide definitive efficacy information is not likely to provide much information about safety, it therefore becomes highly important to monitor all trials of new drugs for safety. Some reasons are (1) it is in the patient's best interest—that is, ideally one would want to know the earliest possible moment when anything untoward began to happen to the patient so that appropriate medical procedures could be initiated; (2) it is also in the primary investigator's best interest; and (3) it is certainly in the sponsor's best interest—in terms of credibility, in terms of prompt reporting to the regulatory agency, and also to minimize legal consequences.

However, there are logistical difficulties in monitoring trials for safety (or efficacy) information. These may depend on (1) the frequency of follow-up patient visits, (2) the rate of patient accession, (3) the data collection instrument, (4) the quality of the collection of data, (5) the staff of field monitors, (6) the ability to rapidly generate a quality assured database in an ongoing manner, (7) the ability to rapidly generate appropriate displays, summaries, or analyses, (8) the identification of who is going to review such displays or summaries, (9) the identification of who will make decisions based on such reviews, and (10) possibly other committees as well.

Kamm, Maloney, Cranston, Roe, and Haas (1984) provide an excellent reference on organizational structure reflecting the logistics of being able to rapidly monitor a trial (TASS) for safety. Briefly, the TASS trial was parallel, was stratified by sex, cardiovascular history, and previous stroke, and was quadruply blinded. Organizational structure consisted of an operations committee, a randomization center, a drug distribution center, clinical centers, a central lab, an end-point review committee, an interim statistical analysis group, a safety committee (which interacted with the FDA and IRB's), and a policy committee.

E. Statistical Methodology

Given that the logistics for monitoring a trial for safety can be put in place, what should be the appropriate analysis or summarization methodology for generating information to be reviewed? One first of all should distinguish between methodology that might be used for rare events versus methodology that might be used for common events. For rare events, each event is important especially if untoward. Procedures aimed at comparing treatment regimens may not be appropriate—particularly from individual trials designed for efficacy. Therefore a simple descriptor such as the number of patients experiencing the event compared to the number of patients exposed to treatment may be more appropriate. As more information accumulates, time-to-event methods may be applied, as well as some type of metaanalysis that would seek to dscriptively combine information across trials.

For common events, statistical methodology should be based on confidence intervals. Confidence intervals are statistically more appropriate than hypothesis testing in the absence of design considerations for safety. They also utilize both the observed incidence and the estimate of the variability of the observed incidence. Confidence intervals should also better facilitate a decision by an informed reviewer. For a two-sided confidence interval with a large confidence coefficient, the lower limit being greater than 0 might represent the drug not being safe whereas the upper limit, if small enough, might permit a conclusion of proof of safety. This would be particularly true if one were able to set an acceptable safety limit. If the upper limit of the confidence interval with a large confidence coefficient were, in fact, less than the acceptable safety limit, then proof of safety would be indicated, whereas the lower confidence limit exceeding the acceptable safety limit would be indicative of proof of being not safe.

In the utilization of confidence intervals, the confidence level (the complement of the Type I error) must be chosen. In addition, statistical rigor would require that the confidence level be preserved or adjusted if multiple or interim analyses are performed. However, it may not be as important to preserve the confidence level or the Type I error, particularly, if "absolute safety" of the sponsors compound alone is of interest. Presumably, one would want to know the first moment when the accumulated information on an untoward event was different from that of untreated patients at *some* level of confidence. If, however, it is important to preserve the Type I error, then there are procedures to do so. Most incorporate group sequential methods. Jennison and Turnbull (1984) provide an excellent reference.

1. Direct-Comparison Methodology

In using confidence intervals to display and to help monitor adverse experience information in clinical trials of new drugs, the more traditional approach would be to directly compare two regimens. The aim of the comparison would be to provide estimates of the *difference* between regimen incidences. To construct a two-sided $100(1-2\alpha)\%$ confidence interval on the true difference in incidences of adverse experiences between two regimens, one would proceed as follows: Let P_i and P_j denote the true incidences of some adverse experience in the populations to be treated with the i-th and j-th regimens, respectively; let $\hat{P}_i$ and $\hat{P}_j$ denote the corresponding observed incidences among N_i and N_j treated patients, respectively; then the difference, $\hat{\delta}_{ij} = \hat{P}_i - \hat{P}_j$, in observed incidences would represent the estimate of the difference in true incidences; and the estimate of the variance of the observed difference is given by $\hat{V}_i + \hat{V}_j$, where $\hat{V}_i$ is the estimate of the variance of the observed incidence in the i-th regimen given by $\hat{P}_i(1-\hat{P}_i)/N_i$.

The confidence interval can be represented as

$$L_{ij} \le P_i - P_j \le U_{ij} \tag{2.12}$$

where L_{ij} is the lower limit and U_{ij} is the upper limit. The limits may be specified as

$$L_{ij} = \hat{P}_i - \hat{P}_j - Z\alpha(\hat{V}_i + \hat{V}_j)^{1/2} \tag{2.13}$$

$$U_{ij} = \hat{P}_i - \hat{P}_j + Z\alpha(\hat{V}_i + \hat{V}_j)^{1/2} \tag{2.14}$$

where Z_α is the upper $(100(1-\alpha)$ percentile of the distribution of $\hat{P}_i - \hat{P}_j$ under the assumption of no difference in true incidences.

The direct comparison of two regimens via $100(1-2\alpha)\%$ confidence intervals also permits concluding that two regimens are different. If the lower limit L_{ij} were positive (presuming that the observed incidence in the i-th regimen exceeded the observed incidence in the j-th regimen), one would conclude that the two regimens were different at the nominal significance level α.

2. Indirect-Comparison Methodology

Another approach, which may be nonstandard, may be thought of as an indirect comparison of two regimens. The primary or initial aim of the approach is to provide estimates of the true incidences of each regimen. Let P_i, P_j, $\hat{P}_i$, $\hat{P}_j$, N_i, N_j, $\hat{V}_i$, and $\hat{V}_j$ be as identified before. A two-sided $100(1-2\alpha_1)\%$ confidence interval on the true incidence P_i in the i-th regimen is

$$L_i \leq P_i \leq U_i \tag{2.15}$$

where L_i is the lower limit and U_i is the upper limit. The limits are given by

$$L_i = \hat{P}_i - Z\alpha_1(\hat{V}_i)^{1/2} \tag{2.16}$$

$$U_i = \hat{P}_i + Z\alpha_1(\hat{V}_i)^{1/2} \tag{2.17}$$

where $Z\alpha_1$ is the $100(1-\alpha_1)$ percentile of the distribution of $\hat{P}_i - \hat{P}_j$ under the assumption that $P_i = P_j$.

In addition to such confidence intervals furnishing information on the true incidence in each regimen, they also permit two regimens to be indirectly compared. One would be able to say that regimens i and j were statistically different at the nominal significance level α_1 if the lower limit of the $100(1-2\alpha_1)\%$ confidence interval on the true incidence of regimen i was greater than the upper limit of regimen j, that is, if $L_i > U_j$, where again the observed incidence in the i-th regimen was greater than the observed incidence in the j-th regimen.

The direct-comparison and the indirect-comparison methods connect. To illustrate, think of the null hypothesis as no difference in true incidences (H_0: $P_i = P_j$) among the regimens, and the alternative hypothesis as, there is a difference (H_a: $P_i > P_j$). The rejection rule for the direct comparison method is that the incidence of regimen i statistically exceeds that of regimen j at the significance level α if $L_{ij} > 0$. The rejection rule for the indirect comparison method is that the incidence of regimen i statistically exceeds that of regimen j at the significance level α_1 if $L_i > U_j$, presuming that $P_i > P_j$.

The equivalence of the rejection rules is expressed as

$$Z\alpha_1 = \{[(\hat{V}_i)^{1/2} + (\hat{V}_j)^{1/2}]/(\hat{V}_i + \hat{V}_j)^{1/2}\}^{-1} Z\alpha \tag{2.18}$$

That is, they are equivalent if the relationship between the critical point for the indirect comparison is proportional to the critical point for the direct comparison where the proportionality constant is that ratio of the variances given in equation (2.18). As an example, under the null hypothesis of no difference and equal sample sizes, the critical point corresponding to the indirect comparison would be 1, divided by the square root of 2, times the critical point for the direct comparison. For the specific case where α equals 5%, α_1 would be 12.24%. That is, if one were using a nominal 90% two-sided confidence interval to directly compare two regimens and the lower limit of that confidence interval exceeded 0, one would say with a confidence level of 95% or a Type I error rate of 5% that the two regimens were in fact different. To reach the same decision using the indirect comparison, one would construct two-sided 75.53% confidence intervals on the true incidence in each regimen and require that the lower limit of one be greater than the upper limit of the other.

F. Summary and Suggestions

To summarize the points made thus far, it was recognized that it may be possible to design some trials to provide definitive safety information. Three occasions were presented where indeed that was the case. However, for most new drugs in clinical development it is not possible. Therefore, a rational approach is to design definitively for efficacy and to monitor and describe safety. This position is in fact consistent with the statutory requirement for approval to market new drugs in the United States. Statistical procedures involving confidence intervals were also suggested for monitoring trials for safety.

In addition, the following suggestion/observations are made. (1) Since open trials don't permit unbiased comparisons of groups and positive controlled trials may reflect an upward bias, the primary assessment of safety should come from double-blind, placebo-controlled trials. (2) Ideally, the clinical development plan for a new compound should address plans for assessing efficacy *and* safety as characteristics of the drug. This should include developing how the null hypotheses that the drug is not efficacious (HOE) and the drug is safe (HOS) would be contradicted. The ideal development plan would also include procedures for monitoring each trial for safety as well as the for monitoring the development plan as data accumulate across trials. (3) If rare adverse events are of interest, development plans should be designed to have a high probability of observing one or more events in each dose regimen—this may include postmarketing surveillance studies as well. (4) The preferred statistical methodology for monitoring and analyzing adverse experience data is per regimen confidence intervals with large coefficients. This approach allows one to provide interval estimates on the true incidence of each regimen; permits sequential procedures such as those of Jennison and Turnbull to be incorporated; also permits sequential procedures such as those of Schultz et al. (1973) or Fleming (1982) to be incorporated regarding a decision to terminate any arm independent of other arms; and would minimize breaking the blind of studies. (5) The impact on ideal clinical development plans if a Hauck and Anderson (1983) approach were taken to reverse the null and alternative hypotheses regarding safety should be investigated. That is, consider the null hypothesis to be "the drug is not safe," and the alternative hypothesis to be "the drug is safe." Such an approach would provide consistency between the regulatory risks for approval based on efficacy as well as based on safety. (6) The impact on ideal clinical development plans if we viewed efficacy and safety as compound hypotheses should be investigated. That is, view the null hypothesis as "the drug is not efficacious and the drug is not safe," and the alternative hypothesis as "the drug is efficacious and the drug is safe." Other alternative hypotheses less stringent may also be proposed. (7) If we continue to design only for efficacy, what the total sample size provides in the way of safety information per trial and across trials in a particular clinical development plan should be explored. If this is sufficiently uninformative, then larger sample sizes may be called for. (8) Perhaps a safety review committee of impartial observers should be formulated. (9) Finally, and ideally, each patient in each clinical trial conducted in the development of new drugs should be monitored for safety. When changes are noted that would give the physician concern, care for the patient and then assess whether such changes are different from those among untreated comparable patients. This in itself argues for accumulating large *experimental* data bases on placebo-treated patients from placebo-controlled trials.

APPENDIX: PROTOCOL OUTLINE

I. Background
II. Objective
III. Plan of study
    A. 1. Demography
        2. Criteria for patient inclusion
        3. Criteria for patient exclusion
    B. Study design
        1. Type of study
        2. Assignment of treatment

3. Blinding, dosage, and administration of study drugs
4. Concomitant medications
5. Procedures
   a. Treatment period
   b. Pretherapy
   c. During treatment period
   d. Posttherapy period
   e. Observers
   f. Data recording
   g. Dropouts

C. Problem management
   1. Adverse reactions
   2. Criteria for discontinuing study drug

IV. Data analysis
   A. Criteria for defining safety end points
   B. Statistical design considerations
   C. Early termination considerations, if any
   D. Statistical methods

V. Administration
   A. Review and consent requirements
   B. Record keeping
   C. Monitoring

VI. Bibliography

REFERENCES

Aalen, O. O. (1978). Nonparametric inference for a family of counting processes. *Annals of Statistics 6:* 701–726.

Agresti, A. (1983). A survey of strategies for modelling classifications having ordinal variables. *Journal of the American Statistical Association 78:* 184–197.

Amara, I. A. (1983). Strategies for multivariate randomization analyses and applications to health sciences data. Institute of Statistics Mimeo Series, No. 1446, University of North Carolina, Chapel Hill, NC.

Amara, I. A., and Koch, G. G. (1980). A macro for multivariate randomization analysis of stratified sample data. *Proceedings of the Fifth Annual SAS Users Group International Conference*. SAS Institute, Inc., Cary, NC.

Anderson, P. K., and Gill, R. D. (1982). Cox's regression model for counting processes: A large sample study. *Annals of Statistics 10:* 1100–1120.

Armitage, P. (1954). Sequential tests in prophylactic and therapeutic trials. *Quarterly Journal of Medicine 91:* 255–274.

Armitage, P. (1983). Exclusions, losses to follow-up, and withdrawals in clinical trials. In *Clinical Trials: Issues and Approaches*, edited by S. H. Shapiro and T. A. Louis. New York: Marcel Dekker, 99–113.

Atkinson, S. S. (1984). Poisson regression methods for the log-linear model. Master's paper submitted to the Biostatistics faculty of the University of North Carolina, Chapel Hill, NC.

Bartolucci, A. A., and Fraser, M. D. (1977). Comparative step-up and composite tests for selecting prognostic indicators associated with survival. *Biometrical Journal 19:* 437–448.

Beaumont, G. (1976). Antidepressant and anxiolytic trials. In *The Principles and Practice and Clinical Trials*, edited by C. S. Good. New York: Churchill Livingstone, 181–187.

Blum, A. L. (1982). Principles for selection and exclusion. In *The Randomized Clinical Trial and Therapeutic Decisions*, edited by N. Tygstrup, J. M. Lachin, and E. Juhl, New York: Marcel Dekker, 43–58.

Breslow, N. E. (1970). A generalized Kruskal–Wallis test for comparing K samples subject to unequal patterns of censorship. *Biometrika 57:* 579–594.

Breslow, N. E. (1974). Covariance analysis of censored survival data. *Biometrics 30:* 89–100.

Breslow, N. E. (1979). Statistical methods for censored survival data. *Environmental Health Perspectives 32:* 181–192.

Bristol, D. R., and Patel, H. I. (1985). A Markovian model for comparing incidences of side effects. Presentation at the Biometric Society meeting, Raleigh, NC.

Brown, B. W. (1980). The crossover experiment for clinical trials. *Biometrics 36:* 69–79.

Bulpitt, C. J. (1983). The evaluation of subjective well-being. In *Randomised Controlled Clinical Trials* by C. J. Bullpitt, Boston: Martinus Nijhoff Publishers, 194–209.

Buncher, C. R. (1972). Principles of experimental design for clinical drug studies. In *Perspectives in Clinical Pharmacy*, edited by D. E. Franke and H. A. K. Whitney, Jr. Hamilton IL: Drug Intelligence, 504–525.

Busfield, B. L., Schneller, P., and Capra, D. (1962). Depressive symptom or side effect? A comparative study of symptoms during pretreatment and treatment periods of patients of three antidepressant medications. *Journal of Nervous and Mental Disease 134:* 339–345.

Calimlim, J. F. and Weintraub, M. (1981). Selection of patients participating in a clinical trial. In *Statistics in the Pharmaceutical Industry*, edited by C. R. Buncher and J. Tsay. New York: Marcel Dekker.

Canner, P. L. (1979). Monitoring clinical trial data for evidence of adverse or beneficial treatment effects. Edited by J. P. Boissel and C. R. Klimt. In: *Multicenter Controlled Trials: Principles and Problems*. Paris: INSERM.

Canner, P. L. (1983). Monitoring of the data for evidence of adverse or beneficial treatment effects. *Controlled Clinical Trials 4:* 467–483.

Chalmers, T. C. (1982). Discussion following Chapter 5: Principles for selection and exclusion, by Andre L. Blum. In *The Randomized Clinical Trial and*

Therapeutic Decisions, edited by N. Tygstrup, J. M. Lachin, and E. Juhl. New York: Marcel Dekker, 43–58.

Cox, C. and Chuang, C. (1984). A comparison of chi-square partitioning and two logit analyses of ordinal pain data from a pharmaceutical study. *Statistics in Medicine 3:* 273–285.

Cox, D. R. (1970). *The Analysis of Binary Data*. London: Methuen.

Cox, D. R. (1972). Regression models and life tables. *Journal of the Royal Statistical Society, Series B, 34:* 187–220.

Cox, D. R. (1975). Partial likelihood. *Biometrika 62:* 269–276.

Davies, D. M. (1981). History and epidemiology. In *Textbook of Adverse Drug Reactions*, 2nd ed., edited by D. M. Davies. New York: Oxford University Press, 1–10.

DeMets, D., Friedman, L., and Furberg, C. D. (1980). Counting events in clinical trials. *New England Journal of Medicine 302:* 924.

Donner, A. (1984). Approaches to sample size estimation in the design of clinical trials—A review. *Statistics in Medicine 3:* 199–214.

Downing, R. N., Rickels, K., and Meyers, F. (1970). Side reactions in neurotics: 1. A comparison of two methods of assessment. *Journal of Clinical Pharmacology 10:* 289–297.

Eadie, M. J., Tyrer, J. H., and Bochner, F. (1981). Adverse drug reactions. In *Introduction to Clinical Pharmacology*. New York: ADIS Press, 117–124.

Elandt-Johnson, R. C. (1980). Time dependent logistic models in follow-up studies and clinical trials: I. Binary data. Institute of Statistics Mimeo Series, No. 1310, University of North Carolina, Chapel Hill, NC.

Elashoff, J. D. (1978). Combining results of clinical trials. *Gastroenterology 75:* 1170–1174.

Engleman, L. (1981). PLR: Stepwise logistic regression. In *BMDP Statistical Software*, edited by W. J. Dixon et al. Los Angeles: University of California Press, 330–344.

Fleming, T. R. (1982). Sample multiple testing procedure for phase II clinical trials. *Biometrics 38:* 193–151.

Food and Drug Administration. (1988). *Guidelines for the Format and Content of the Clinical and Statistical Sections of New Drug Applications*.

Friedman, L. M., Furberg, C. D., and DeMets, D. L. (1981). *Fundamentals of Clinical Trials*. Boston: John Wright PSG, 18–27.

Frome, E. L. (1983). The analysis of rates using Poisson regression models. *Biometrics 39:* 665–674.

Gart, J. J. (1969). An exact test for comparing matched proportions in crossover designs. *Biometrika 56:* 75–80.

Gehan, E. A. (1965). A generalized Wilcoxon test for comparing arbitrarily singly-censored samples. *Biometrika 52:* 203–223.

Glasser, M. (1967). Exponential survival with covariance. *Journal of the American Statistical Association 62:* 561–568.

Grady, F. (1976). Designing the report form. In *The Principles and Practice of Clinical Trials*, edited by C. S. Good. Edinburgh: Churchill Livingstone, 60–74.

Green, D. M. (1962). Side effects—Quantification. *Federation Proceedings 21:* 179.

Green, M. S., and Symons, M. J. (1983). A comparion of the logistic risk function and the proportional hazards model in prospective epidemiologic studies. *Journal of Chronic Disease 36:* 715–724.

Greenblatt, M. (1964). Controls in clinical research. *Clinical Pharmacology and Therapeutics 5:* 864.

Grizzle, J. E. (1965). The two period change-over design and its uses in clinical trials. *Biometrics 21:* 467–480.

Grizzle, J. E., Starmer, C. F., and Koch, G. G. (1969). The analysis of categorical data by linear models. *Biometrics 25:* 489–504.

Hadler, N. M., and Gillings, D. B. (1983). On the design of the Phase III drug trial: The example of rheumatoid arthritis. *Arthritis and Rheumatism 26:* 1354–1361.

Halperin, M., Rogot, E., Gurian, J., Ederer, F. (1968). Sample sizes for medical trials with special reference to long term therapy. *Journal of Chronic Disease 21:* 13–23.

Harrell, F. E., Jr. (1986a). The LOGIST Procedure. In *SUGI Supplemental Library User's Guide*, Version 5 Edition. SAS Institute, Cary, NC, 269–293.

Harrell, F. E., Jr. (1986b). The PHGLM Procedure. In *SUGI Supplemental Library User's Guide*, Version 5 Edition. SAS Institute, Cary, NC, 437–466.

Hassar, M., and Weintraub, M. (1976). "Uninformed" consent and the healthy volunteer: An analysis of patient volunteers in a clinical trial of a new anti-inflammatory drug. *Clinical Pharmacology and Therapeutics 20:* 379–386.

Hauck, W. W., and Anderson, S. (1983). A new procedure for testing equivalence in comparative bioavailability and other clinical trials. *Communications in Statistics: Theory and Methods 12:* 2663–2692.

Holford, T. R. (1980). The analysis of rates and survivorship using log-linear models. *Biometrics 36:* 299–305.

Hopkins, A. (1981). P2L: Regression with incomplete survival data. In *BMDP Statistical Software*, edited by W. J. Dixon et al. Los Angeles: University of California Press, 576–594.

Hsu, J. (1983). The assessment of statistical evidence from active control clinical trials. *American Statistical Association 1983 Proceedings of the Biopharmaceutical Section*, 12–16.

Huskisson, E. C., and Wojtulewski, J. A. (1974). Measurement of side effects of drugs. *British Medical Journal 2:* 698–699.

Idanpaan-Heikkila, J. (1983). A review of safety information obtained from Phases I–II and Phase III clinical investigations of sixteen selected drugs. Office of New Drug Evaluation, National Center for Drugs and Biologics, Food and Drug Administration, Rockville, MD.

Imrey, P. B., Koch, G. G., Stokes, M. E., et al. (1981). Categorical data analysis: Some reflections on the log linear model and logistic regression, Part I. *International Statistical Review 49:* 265–283.

Imrey, P. B., Koch, G. G., Stokes, M. E., et al. (1982). Categorical data analysis:

Some reflections on the log linear model and logistic regression, Part II. *International Statistical Review 50:* 35–64.

Jennison, C., and Turnbull, B. W. (1984). Repeated confidence intervals for group sequential trials. *Controlled Chemical Trials 5:* 33–45.

Jennrich, R. I. (1984). Some exact tests for comparing survival curves in the presence of unequal right censoring. *Biometrika 71:* 57–64.

Johnson, C., Amara, I. A., Edwards, S., and Koch, G. G. (1981). Some computational strategies for the analysis of longitudinal categorical data. *1981 Proceedings of the Statistical Computing Section of the American Statistical Association*, 293–298.

Jones, J. K. (1982a). Post-marketing surveillance, annual reports and long term follow-up. *Drug Information Journal 16:* 87–92.

Jones, J. K., session coordinator (1982b). Terms used in indicating causal relationship. In *Assessing Causes of Adverse Drug Reactions*, edited by J. Venulet. New York: Academic Press, 19–46.

Kalbfleisch, J. D., and Prentice, R. L. (1973). marginal likelihoods based on Cox's regression and life model. *Biometrika 60:* 267–278.

Kamm, B., Maloney, B., Cranston, B., Roe, R., and Hess, W. (1984). Ticlopidine aspirin stroke study organizational structure. Presented at the Society for Controlled Clinical Trials, May 13–16, Miami.

Karch, F. E., and Lasagna, L. (1977). Toward the operational identification of adverse drug reactions. *Clinical Pharmacology and Therapeutics 21:* 247–254.

Kellerer, A. M., and Chmelevsky, D. (1983). Small-sample properties of censored data rank tests. *Biometrics 39:* 675–682.

Kleinbaum, D. G., Kupper, L. L., and Morgenstern, H. (1982). *Epidemiologic Research Principles and Quantitative Methods*. London: Lifetime Learning Publications.

Koch, G. G. (1972). The use of nonparametric methods in the statistical analysis of the two period change-over design. *Biometrics 28:* 577–584.

Koch, G. G., Amara, I. A., and Atkinson, S. S. (1983). Mantel–Haenszel and related methods in analyzing ordinal categorical data with concomitant information. Presented at the 39th Annual Conference on Applied Statistics, Newark, NJ, November 30, 1983.

Koch, G. G., Amara, I. A., Davis, G. W., and Gillings, D. B. (1982). A review of some statistical methods for covariance analysis of categorical data. *Biometrics 38:* 563–595.

Koch, G. G., Amara, I. A., and Singer, J. M. (1985). A two-stage procedure for the analysis of ordinal categorical data. In *Biostatistics—Statistics in Biomedical, Public Health, and Environmental Science (The Bernard G. Greenberg Volume)*, edited by P. K. Sen. Amsterdam: Elsevier Science Publishers, 357–387.

Koch, G. G., Atkinson, S. S., and Stokes, M. E. (1986). Poisson regression. In *Encyclopedia of Statistical Sciences*, Vol. 7, edited by N. L. Johnson and S. Kotz. New York: John Wiley & Sons, 32–41.

Koch, G. G., and Bhapkar, V. P. (1982). Chi-square tests. In *Encyclopedia of*

Statistical Sciences, Vol. 1, edited by N. L. Johnson and S. Kotz. New York: John Wiley & Sons, 442–457.

Koch, G. G., Carr, G. J., Amara, I. A., Stokes, M. E., and Uryniak, T. J. (1989). Categorical data analysis. Chapter II in *Statistical Methodology in the Pharmaceutical Sciences*, edited by D. A. Berry. New York: Marcel Dekker, in press.

Koch, G. G., and Edwards, S. (1985). Logistic regression. In *Encyclopedia of Statistical Sciences*, Vol. 5, edited by N. L. Johnson and S. Kotz. New York: John Wiley & Sons, 128–133.

Koch, G. G., and Edwards, S. (1988). Clinical efficacy trials with categorical data. Chapter 9 in *Biopharmaceutical Statistics for Drug Development*, edited by Karl E. Peace. New York: Marcel Dekker, 403–457.

Koch, G. G. and Gillings, D. B. (1982). Statistical issues in comparative clinical trials: An academic perspective. Presented at the Drug Information Association Workshop on Comparative Advertising of Prescription Drugs, Dec. 5–7, 1982, New York.

Koch, G. G. and Gillings, D. B. (1983). Inference, design based vs. model based. In *Encyclopedia of Statistical Sciences*, Vol. 4, edited by N. L. Johnson and S. Kotz. New York: Wiley, 84–88.

Koch, G. G., Gillings, D. B., and Stokes, M. E. (1980). Biostatistical implications of design, sampling, and measurement to health science data analysis. *Annual Review of Public Health 1:* 161–225.

Koch, G. G., Imrey, P. B., Singer, J. M. Atkinson, S. S., and Stokes, M. E. (1985). *Analysis of Categorical Data*. Montreal: Les Presses de l'Universite de Montreal.

Koch, G. G., and Sollecito, W. A. (1984). Statistical considerations in the design, analysis, and interpretation of comparative clinical studies: An academic perspective. *Drug Information Journal 18:* 131–151.

Kramer, M. S. (1981). Difficulties in assessing the adverse effects of drugs. *British Journal of Clinical Pharmacology 11:* 105S–110S.

Kramer, M. S., Leventhal, J. M., Hutchinson, T. A., and Feinstein, A. R. (1979). An algorithm of the operational assessment of adverse drug reactions: I. Background, description, and instructions for use. *Journal of the American Medical Association 242:* 623–632.

Kuritz, S. J., Landis, J. R., and Koch, G. G. (1988). A general overview of Mantel–Haenszel methods; applications and recent developments. *Annual Review of Public Health 9:* 123–160.

Lachin, J. M. (1979). Sample size considerations for clinical trials of potentially hepatotoxic drugs. In *Guidelines for Detection of Hepatotoxicity Due to Drugs and Chemicals*, edited by C. S. Davidson, C. M. Levy, and E. C. Chamberlayne. Washington, DC: US Department of HEW, National Institutes of Health, NIH Publication No. 79–313, 119–130.

Lachin, J. M. (1981). Introduction to sample size determination and power analysis for clinical trials. *Controlled Clinical Trials 2:* 93–113.

Lachin, J. M. (1982a). Statistical inference in clinical trials. In *The Randomized*

Clinical Trial and Therapeutic Decisions, edited by N. Tygstrup, J. M. Lachin, and E. Juhl. New York: Marcel Dekker, 117–143.

Lachin, J. M. (1982b). Statistical analysis of the randomized clinical trial. In *The Randomized Clinical Trial and Therapeutic Decisions*, edited by N. Tygstrup, J. M. Lachin, and E. Juhl. New York: Marcel Dekker, 117–143.

Laird, N., and Olivier, D. (1981). Covariance analysis of censored survival data using log-linear analysis techniques. *Journal of the American Statistical Association 76:* 231–240.

Lal, H., Fielding, S., and Karkalas, J. (1975). Clinical evaluation of antidepressant drugs. In *Antidepressants*, edited by S. Fielding and H. Lal. Mount Kisco, NY: Futura Publishing, 301–317.

Landis, J. R., Cooper, M. M., Kennedy, T., and Koch, G. G. (1979). A computer program for testing average partial association in three-way contingency tables (PARCAT). *Computer Programs in Biomedicine 9:* 223–246.

Landis, J. R., Heyman, E. R., and Koch, G. G. (1978). Average partial association in three way contingency tables: A review and discussion of alternative tests. *International Statistical Review 42:* 237–254.

Lasagna, L. (1981). Bias in the elucidation of subjective side effects. *British Journal of Clinical Pharmacology 11:* 111S–113S.

Latta, R. B. (1981). A Monte Carlo study of some two-sample rank tests with censored data. *Journal of the American Statistical Association 76:* 713–719.

Leviton, A., Schulman, J., Kammerman, L., Porter, D., Slack, W., and Graham, J. R. (1980). A probability model of headache recurrence. *Journal of Chronic Disease 33:* 407–412.

Lewis, J. A. (1981). Post-marketing surveillance: How many patients? *Trends in Pharmacological Science 2:* 93–94.

Lininger, L., Gail, M. H., Green, S. B., and Byar, D. P. (1979). Comparison of four tests for equality of survival curves in the presence of stratification and censoring. *Biometrika 66:* 419–428.

Mantel, N. (1963). Chi-square tests with one degree of freedom: Extensions of the Mantel–Haenszel procedure. *Journal of the American Statistical Association 58:* 690–700.

Mantel, N. (1966). Evaluation of survival data and two new rank order statistics arising in its consideration. *Cancer Chemotherapy Reports 50:* 163–170.

Mantel, N., and Fleiss, J. (1980). Minimum expected cell size requirements for the Mantel–Haenszel one-degree-of-freedom chi-square test and a related rapid procedure. *American Journal of Epidemiology 112:* 129–134.

Mantel, N., and Haenszel, W. (1959). Statistical aspects of the analysis of data from retrospective studies of disease. *Journal of the National Cancer Institute 22:* 719–748.

McCullagh, P. (1980). Regression models for ordinal data (with discussion). *Journal of the Royal Statisical Society, Series B, 42:* 109–142.

McNemar, Q. (1947). Note on the sampling error of the difference between correlated proportions or percentages. *Psychometrika 12:* 153–157.

Mehta, C. R., Patel, N. R., and Gray, R. (1985). Computing an exact confidence interval for the common odds ratio in several 2×2 contingency tables. *Journal of the American Statistical Association, 80:* 969–973.

Mehta, C. R., and Patel, N. R. (1983). A network algorithm for performing Fisher's exact test in $r \times c$ contingency tables. *Journal of the American Statistical Association 78:* 427–434.

Metzler, C. M., and Schooley, G. L. (1981). Design and analysis of clinical trials of psychoactive drugs. In *Statistics in the Pharmaceutical Industry*, edited by C. R. Buncher and J. Tsay. New York: Marcel Dekker, 157–187.

Miettinen, O. S. (1976). Estimability and estimation in case-referent studies. *American Journal of Epidemiology 103:* 226–235.

Nagelkerke, N. J. D., Oosting, J., and Hart, A. A. M. (1984). A simple test for goodness of fit of Cox's proportional hazards model. *Biometrics 40:* 483–486.

O'Neill, R. T. (1988). Assessment of safety. Chapter 13 in *Biopharmaceutical Statistics for Drug Development*, edited by Karl E. Peace. New York: Marcel Dekker, 543–604.

Pagano, M., and Halvorsen, K. T. (1981). An algorithm for finding the exact significance levels of $r \times c$ tables. *Journal of the American Statistical Association 76:* 931–934.

Peace, K. E. (1987). Design, monitoring and analysis issues relative to adverse events. *Journal of Drug Information Association 21:* 21–28.

Peto, R., and Peto, J. (1972). Asymptotically efficient rank invariant procedures. *Journal of the Royal Statistical Society, Series A, 135:* 185–207.

Pogge, R. C., and Coats, E. A. (1962). The placebo as a source of side effects in normal people. *Nebraska Medical Journal 47:* 337–339.

Prentice, R. L. (1978). Linear rank tests with right censored data. *Biometrika 65:* 167–179.

Prentice, R. L., and Gloeckler, L. A. (1978). Regression analysis of grouped survival data with application to breast cancer data. *Biometrics 34:* 57–67.

Prescott, L. F. (1979). Factors predisposing to adverse drug reactions. *Adverse Drug Reaction Bulletin 78:* 280–283.

Puri, M. L., and Sen, P. K. (1971). *Non-parametric Methods in Multivariate Analysis*, New York: John Wiley & Sons.

Quade, D. (1967). Rank analysis of covariance. *Journal of the American Statistical Association 62:* 1187–1200.

Reidenberg, M. M., and Lowenthal, D. T. (1968). Adverse nondrug reactions. *New England Journal of Medicine 279:* 678–679.

Riis, P. R. (1982). How therapeutic decisions are motivated. In *The Randomized Clinical Trial and Therapeutic Decisions*, edited by N. Tygstrup, J. M. Lachin, and E. Juhl. New York: Marcel Dekker, 3–11.

Routledge, P. A. (1977). Adverse reactions to drug withdrawal. *Adverse Drug Reaction Bulletin 67:* 236–239.

Sackett, D. L., and Gent, M. (1979). Controversy in counting and attributing events in clinical trials. *New England Journal of Medicine 301:* 1410–1412.

Salzman, C., Kochansky, G. E., Porrino, L., and Shader, R. I. (1972). Emotional side effects of placebo. In *Psychiatric Complications of Medical Drugs*, edited by R. I. Shader. New York: Raven Press, 369–387.

SAS Institute, Inc. (1985). *SAS User's Guide: Statistics*, Version 5 Edition. SAS Institute, Cary, NC.

Savage, I. R. (1965). Contributions to the theory of rank order statistics—The two sample case. *Annals of Mathematical Statistics 27:* 590–615.

Schemper, M. (1984). A survey of permutation tests for censored survival data. *Communications in Statistics: Theory and Methods 13:* 1655–1665.

Schoenfeld, D. (1982). Partial residuals for the proportional hazards regression model. *Biometrika 69:* 239–241.

Schultz, J. R., Nichol, F. R., Elfring, G. L., and Weed, S. D. (1973). Multiple stage procedures for drug screening. *Biometrics 29:* 293–300.

Schultz, J. R., and Assenzo, J. R. (1982). Statistical involvement in the development of a new drug. *Drug Information Journal 16:* 70–82.

Shader, R. I., and DiMascio, A. (1970). *Psychotropic Drug Side Effects: Clinical and Theoretical Perspectives*. Baltimore: Williams and Wilkins.

Skegg, D. C. G., and Doll, R. (1977). The case for recording events in clinical trials. *British Medical Journal 2:* 1523–1524.

Stanish, W. M., Gillings, D. B., and Koch, G. G. (1978). An application of multivariate ratio methods for the analysis of a longitudinal clinical trial with missing data. *Biometrics 34:* 305–317.

Stanish, W. M., Koch, G. G., and Landis, J. R. (1978). A computer program for multivariate ratio analysis (MISCAT). *Computer Programs in Biomedicine 8:* 197–207.

Stokes, M. E., and Koch, G. G. (1983). A macro for maximum likelihood fitting of log-linear models to Poisson and multinomial counts with contrast matrix capability for hypothesis testing. *Proceedings of the Eighth Annual SAS Users Group International Conference*. SAS Institute, Cary, NC, 795–800.

Streichenwein, S. M., and Blomer, R. (1982). Computer documentation of adverse drug reactions with a multinational pharmaceutical company. *Drug Information Journal 16:* 109–111.

Tarone, R. E., and Ware, J. (1977). On distribution-free tests for equality of survival distributions. *Biometrika 64:* 156–160.

Temple, R. (1982). Government viewpoint of clinical trials. *Drug Information Journal 16:* 10–17.

Temple, R. (1983). Difficulties in evaluating positive control trials. *American Statistical Association 1983 Proceedings of the Biopharmaceutical Section*, 1–7.

Thomas, D. G. (1975). Exact and asymptotic methods for the combination of 2×2 tables. *Computers and Biomedical Research 8:* 423–446.

Trouton, D. S. (1957). Placebos and their physiological effects. *Journal of Mental Science 103:* 344–354.

Vere, D. W. (1976). Drug adverse reactions as masqueraders. *Adverse Drug Reaction Bulletin 60:* 208–211.

Wade, O. L. (1970). *Adverse Reactions to Drugs*. London: William Heinemann Medical Books, 11–24.

Walker, S. H., and Duncan, D. B. (1967). Estimation of the probability of an event as a function of several independent variables. *Biometrika 54:* 167–179.

Wallin, J., and Sjovall, J. (1981). Detection of adverse drug reactions in clinical trials using two types of questioning. *Clinical Therapeutics 3:* 450–452.

Westland, M. M. (1982). Frequency distribution of adverse drug reaction terms. *Drug Information Journal 16:* 145–147.

Wilcoxon, F. (1945). Individual comparisons by ranking methods. *Biometrics 1:* 80–83.

Wilcoxon, F. (1949). *Some Rapid Approximate Statistical Procedures*. Stamford, CT: American Cyanimid.

3
Two Treatment Crossover Designs

Sylvan Wallenstein* *Columbia University, New York, New York*

Harji I. Patel *Hoechst-Roussel Pharmaceuticals, Inc., Somerville, New Jersey*

Gerald M. Fava *Knoll Pharmaceuticals, a Unit of BASF K & F Corporation, Whippany, New Jersey*

Marcia Polansky *Hahnemann University, Philadelphia, Pennsylvania*

Karl E. Peace† *Biopharmaceutical Research Consultants, Inc., Ann Arbor, Michigan*

Satya D. Dubey *Food and Drug Administration, Rockville, Maryland*

Ronald P. Kershner *Sterling-Winthrop Research Institute, Rensselaer, New York*

George Lynch *Ancaster, Ontario, Canada*

Matthew Koch *University of North Carolina, Chapel Hill, North Carolina*

**Present affiliation:* Mount Sinai Medical Center, New York, New York
†*Previous affiliation:* Warner-Lambert Company, Ann Arbor, Michigan.

I. INTRODUCTION

Sylvan Wallenstein

At the inception of the crossover designs work group in 1984, there was a feeling that problems in the crossover design have not been fully explored, particularly with respect to the ideas of using baseline values and multiple periods, and considerations of costs and efficiency. Also, nonparametric analysis and more complex designs had not received adequate attention. Presumably, one anticipated outcome from this work group could have been a definitive discussion of all these issues, particularly, since so few papers had appeared in 1982–1984. However, as can be seen by the references, numerous papers have recently appeared on the topics noted above. Some papers have encouraged the use of the design in clinical trials, and others have discouraged its use. Thus there is now less need for a comprehensive document detailing all aspects of analysis for crossover trials.

The format of this final report allows readers to become familiar with the controversies concerning the design, some resolution of issues, and some personal viewpoints. The document begins with a brief historical review of the issue, with perhaps a slight overemphasis describing the work that will not be detailed here. A general consensus statement is given that has been reviewed by all members on the committee on use of the crossover. Members of the committee with expertise on certain areas give their own viewpoint on several issues much as they would in a contributed paper session. Attempts have been made to keep these noncontradictory and cohesive, although the perspective can vary and differ from the consensus statement.

II. CONSENSUS STATEMENT

Sylvan Wallenstein, Harji I. Patel, Ronald P. Kershner, Gerald M. Fava, George Lynch and Matthew Koch

The 2×2 crossover design and its variants are not the design of choice if demonstration of unequivocal efficacy is required, and carryover effects may exist. When one has to live with less than unequivocal demonstrations, the design has merit based on ethical issues, acceptability on clinical grounds, and the relatively shorter time required to recruit subjects. Crossover studies can be performed quickly based on both a smaller number of required subjects and a perceived greater willingness of physicians and patients to participate in crossover trials. Three-period designs are to be preferred to two-period designs on statistical grounds. Good research practice requires baseline values when possible, but their help in demonstrating unequivocal efficacy is subject to controversy. A crossover design can play an important role in early phase studies and in exploratory research, and is the preferred analysis in comparative bioavailability trials. It is not recommended for safety trials.

The principal argument against using the 2×2 crossover is that the estimate of treatment difference is biased if unequal carryover effects are present. In the two-period, two-treatment crossover, the tests of unequal carryover effects, period-by-treatment interaction, and sequence effects are completely confounded. Differentiating which is the cause of a significant effect is difficult to impossible. The test of assumptions has generally poor power.

The second baseline value is of use for testing for direct treatment effects in two-period designs that have long washout periods; their use in designs with short washouts is doubtful. When recruitment costs are not prohibitively high or when there is a sufficient pool of subjects, the cost savings of a crossover design may be minimal. Three-period designs offer the combination of efficient within-patient estimation of a variety of treatment effects under several different modeling assumptions on the length of the carryover effects. These designs do, however, require some assumptions regarding the duration of carryover effects and interactions between carryover and direct effects.

III. OVERVIEW

Sylvan Wallenstein, Harji I. Patel, Ronald P. Kershner, Gerald M. Fava and Matthew Koch

A. Introduction

To compare the efficacy of two or more noncurative treatments, many researchers have found it appealing to utilize the subject as his own control by giving some or all treatments to each subject at different times in random order. This type of design is called a crossover or changeover design.

In the simplest crossover design, subjects are allocated randomly to two groups with the first group receiving the treatment in order AB (with a suitable "washout" period separating the treatments) and the second group receiving the treatments in the reverse order, BA. This design is called a 2×2 crossover design.

The simple 2×2 crossover design is appealing because of its simplicity in using subjects as their own controls, its use of within-subjects variance, possible economy of costs, and possible ease in recruiting patients. Recruitment is facilitated both by statistical considerations (only half the subjects required even if observations are uncorrelated) and for possible administrative/ethical reasons (e.g., each patient will be exposed to the "better" treatment).

This report will consider two-treatment design. The considerations for comparing more than two treatments are similar to those for two treatments and will not be explicitly discussed here.

B. Literature Review up to the BEMAC Report

Cox (1958) emphasized that the 2×2 crossover design is a special case of the split-plot design and, along with Cochran and Cox (1957), described use of the crossover design for the situation when there is no residual treatment effects. Cochran and Cox (1957) and other authors proposed methods for estimating the carryover effect. These designs included additional combinations of orders of treatments (e.g., AA, AB, BA, BB). Probably because of the loss of simplicity and the increased costs associated with these more complex designs, there was not an overwhelming support for them.

For the 2×2 crossover design, Grizzle (1965) estimated the direct treatment effect and the residual effect of the previous treatment, and constructed the proper error term for testing the equality of treatment means effects given no carryover. A preliminary test for carryover effects was also described, and the efficiency of the crossover design (assuming no carryover) relative to the completely randomized design was given for different correlations.

Chassan (1970) computed the efficiency of the crossover design relative to the completely randomized design (CRD), showed that this efficiency bears a simple relationship to the correlation between pairs of measurements in Periods 1 and 2, and discussed some implications of baseline measurements.

One of the manifestations of the support for Grizzle's (1965) work was in the form of many presentations to the Bureau of Drugs of the Food and Drug Administration (FDA)—despite the fact that Grizzle (1965) advised, as did Cox (1958), that the 2×2 crossover design be used only when it could be safely assumed that there are no residual effects.

C. The BEMAC Report (1977) Hill and Armitage (1980), and Brown (1980a)

Following the presentation to the FDA of many 2×2 crossover trials supporting claims of efficacy of new drugs, there was renewed interest in the evaluation of the criteria for judging the validity of these trials. One early result of this renewed interest was the report of the Biometrics and Epidemiology Methodology Advisory Committee (BEMAC) in 1977.

This report concluded that "the two-period crossover design, except in some circumstances is not the design of choice in clinical trials where unequivocal evidence of treatment effect is required." These points were discussed in more detail by Brown (1980a) and Hills and Armitage (1980).

The main points of these studies can be summarized as follows:

1. The usual analysis for direct treatment effect assumes no "period × treatment" interaction, and such an interaction could be due to (see Hills and Armitage):
   a. Inadequate washout period.
   b. Physiological or psychological state induced by first treatment.
   c. Treatment level may vary with general level of response. A period effect could change nature of response (may be resolved by a transformation).
2. The number of subjects needed to test the validity of the model exceeds the number required for a completely randomized design, negating use of design (Brown, 1980).
3. Assumption of no period × treatment interaction not justified if there is (a) cure, (b) slow excretion, (c) delayed effects beyond end of washout period, or (d) natural history of rapid change in disease.
4. Justification for the model could be better based on data collected outside of study.
5. Adding a baseline value to (a placebo-controlled) CRD design allows the investigator to make use of intrasubject variability.
6. Cost savings may not be as great as one might believe (Brown, 1980).

D. Post BEMAC

Baseline values have two primary uses in the analysis of crossover designs: (1) to permit more powerful test(s) of assumption of no carryover effects, and (2) to permit a more powerful test of direct effects assuming no carryover effects are present. Such uses are implicit in the BEMAC report, in Wallenstein (1979), and in several tests cited in the papers referred to below. Patel (1983) presented a series of preliminary tests involving the baseline values, and suggested use of the analysis of covariance with the baseline of period j as covariate for the posttreatment value in period J. Fleiss, Wallenstein and Rosenfeld (1985) cautioned about possible misleading results that could be obtained by use of this test. Wallenstein (1986) and Wallenstein and Fleiss (1988) examined under what assumptions use of the second baseline actually improves power for detection of direct and carryover effects. Fleiss (1989) concluded that the analysis of change from baseline is best avoided. Section IV gives the viewpoint of Harji Patel on this issue.

Willan and Pater (1986a) argued that existence of a carryover effect does not necessarily invalidate the test for direct treatment effects, since the bias will usually be in the direction of making differences in main effects difficult to detect. This (biased) test is often more powerful than that based on first-period effects. Possible problems with routine use of biased tests have been noted by Fleiss (1989).

In many trials, patients are only crossed over if they do not succeed on the first treatment. K. Peace in Section V and G. Fava in Section VI discuss analyses of such trials. Section V was included by the editor because of its relevance to Section VI.

The issues of cost savings relative to the completely randomized design, and whether data from the crossover can validate the no-interaction model, are discussed by Brown (1980). Koch (1986) has applied similar approaches to compare the baseline-adjusted crossover with the baseline-adjusted completely randomized design, assuming costless baseline measurements and a variance–covariance matrix with independent subject effects and either independent or autocorrelated within subject errors. Cost savings were less than those in the no-baseline case for the correlation patterns studied. In addition, although baseline adjustments improved precision in estimating the carryover effects, the improvement was not sufficient to alter Brown's conclusions regarding the requirement for a priori justification of carryover assumptions.

It has been clearly established that the two-period two-sequence crossover design is not the design of choice for comparing two treatments. Extra-period designs offer the combination of efficient within-patient estimation.

Kershner and Federer (1981) considered several two-treatment designs incorporating extra periods and/or sequences under a number of different models both with and without baseline observations. Among the designs that they considered, the extra-period design (EPD) of Lucas (1950) provided the most efficient estimators of contrasts between direct treatment effects when one-period carryover effects were present. This design is constructed by repeating the last period of the two-period two-sequence design. Laska, Meisner, and Kushner (1983) describe optimality properties of this test among the class of two- and three-period designs.

Based on the calculations of Laska et al. (1983), the conventional design requires 1.3 to 2 times as many patients than the extra-period design in order to obtain the same precision on the contrast between direct effects. The additional increase in efficiency from adding more treatment periods diminishes rapidly after three periods.

Fleiss (1986a, 1989) critiqued these designs by arguing that they in turn depended on other (more benign) assumptions, mainly the assumption of additivity among the direct and carryover effects and the assumption of no two-period carryover. Whether or not the assumptions of the multiperiod design are reasonable depends on the design of the trial and type of treatment. In many trials the assumptions required, that treatment effects persist into the following treatment period even after a washout and that they be small relative to the direct effects, are reasonable, and use of the design could be encouraged.

In designs with more than two periods, or multiple observations within periods, the correlation between errors should be considered when planning an analysis. Marcia Polansky discusses this issue in Section VII.

Section VIII reports the result of a survey undertaken by Fava and Patel on the use of the crossover design in the pharmaceutical industry. In general, the respondent companies indicated that efficiency and clinical insistence/preference were the major reasons for using crossover designs and that the 2×2 crossover design was employed most frequently. Finally, Satya Dubey, who is not a member of the workgroup, but who has some thoughts on crossover designs, was given the opportunity by the editor to contribute to the chapter. His thoughts appear in Section IX.

IV. BASELINE MEASUREMENTS IN A 2×2 CROSSOVER TRIAL

Harji I. Patel

A. Introduction

While designing and analyzing clinical trials, one seeks devices that reduce bias and noise due to extraneous sources of variation. These devices are based on principles of randomization and local control. The local control can be either in the form of blocking or in the form of covariate adjustments with respect to important prognostic factors. For example, if patient's sex is a good predictor of the response at the end of the treatment period, it is advantageous to randomly assign the treatments to males and females separately and compare the treatment effects after removing the sex effect. When prognostic factors are continuous variables and not usable for blocking, the treatment differences can be adjusted for the prognostic factors using an analysis of covariance model.

Several factors can be used for blocking, and in an extreme situation blocking reduces to a matched-group design. In a matched-group design with k treatments, groups (blocks) of k patients each are formed in such a way that a patient within a group is more similar to the remaining $(k-1)$ units of the group than to any other units. A matched-group design is referred to as a matched-pair design when $k = 2$. Because of practical difficulties in matching, matched-group designs have limited scope in clinical trials. An alternative to a matched-group design is within-patient design where each patient receives t_i of k treatments during m treatment periods in a randomly assigned order. For example, in an AA, BB, AB, BA design some patients would take the same treatment during both periods, so for those patients $t_i = 1$ and for the remaining patients $t_i = 2$. In a matched-group design similar but different patients form a block, whereas in a within-patient design each patient itself is a block.

In a within-patient design, a patient is a physical unit for the treatments administered at successive time points. However, in contrast to a matched-group design, the time (environmental) effects and residual or carryover effects interfere with the treatment effects, and this causes serious concern regarding bias. If a within-patient design is conducted in a proper setting and analyzed validly, this bias can be reduced.

This note briefly reviews the work done on a 2×2 (two-treatment, two-period) crossover design with baseline measurements. It also points out practical problems in meeting the underlying model assumptions, outlines an analysis strategy, and gives some guidelines for designing a 2×2 crossover trial.

B. Why Baseline Measurements?

When baseline measurements are not obtained in a 2×2 crossover design, a test for the treatment $\times$ period interaction is regarded as a preliminary test for examining the validity of the test for the treatment difference. However, as discussed by Brown (1980) and others, this preliminary test does not have adequate power, especially when the sample size is small. Consequently, the interpretation of the results of the inference about the treatment difference may remain clouded.

Another problem with this preliminary test in the absence of baseline measurements is that the treatment $\times$ period interaction is a consequence of several factors. These factors are (1) differences in prognostic factors of the patients in the two sequences, (2) difference in the carryover effects, (3) physiological or psychological state induced by the first period, and (4) the influence of differential period effects when the treatment difference depends on the general level of response. Simultaneous occurrence of two or more of these causes might result in acceptance of the hypothesis of no treatment $\times$ period interaction, and this might lead to a false validation of a treatment comparison test.

The use of baseline measurements in the analysis tries to correct these problems. Therefore, we propose a 2×2 design with run-in and washout periods of adequate lengths and baseline measurements before the start of each treatment period. Numerous researchers have proposed methods of analyzing a 2×2 design with baseline measurements under different models and assumptions.

Now we discuss what improvement the use of baseline measurements offers over the analysis that does not use the baseline measurements. Let x_{ijk} and y_{ijk} $(k = 1, \ldots, n_i;\ i = 1, 2;\ j = 1, 2)$ be the baseline and treatment measurements, respectively, for the kth patient and the jth period of the ith sequence.

Now $\theta_i = E(x_{i1k} - x_{i2k})$ measures the expected change in the state of disease from the first baseline to the second baseline for the patients in sequence i. Hence the carryover effects can best be measured by θ_i in sequence i. Considering the principle of matching discussed in Section IV.A, an ideal experimental situation would be provided if $\theta_1 = \theta_2 = 0$. However, this is too much to expect in reality and therefore, contrary to Patel's (1983) suggestion, such a stringent requirement is perhaps not necessary. On the other hand, one should not ignore large values of θ_1 and θ_2, because large θ values would mean drastic changes in the disease conditions between the two periods. This is why crossover designs are not recommended in diseases with acute conditions.

The difference $\theta_1 - \theta_2$ measures the difference in carryover effects. The test for H_0: $\theta_1 - \theta_2 = 0$ is obtained after removing the between-patient variability and therefore is associated with a high power. Hence, this test should be considered a primary preliminary test. If H_0: $\theta_1 - \theta_2 = 0$ is not rejected at some prespecified level of significance (generally greater than 0.05 level), we proceed further to test the hypothesis of no period $\times$ treatment interaction. This again is a preliminary test for the test for comparing the treatment effects. These last two tests can be performed after adjusting for the baseline measurements. The test for the period $\times$ treatment interaction after making use of baseline measurements is more valid and is generally associated with a higher power than the test without the use of baseline measurements. For the test for the treatment comparison, however, the literature suggests that the adjustment due to baseline measurements improves the validity but does not necessarily increase the power. The efficiencies of these tests depend on the underlying dispersion matrix of the vector $(x_{i1k}, y_{i1k}, x_{i2k}, y_{i2k})$.

In summary, the use of baseline measurements

1. Allows us to interpret the difference between the carryover effects separately from the treatment $\times$ period interaction;
2. Makes the first preliminary test (test for the hypothesis of equal carryover effects) reasonably powerful;
3. Offers a better screening procedure for checking the validity of a test for the treatment comparison by allowing two preliminary

tests; and

4. Allows adjustment for the baseline measurements in estimating and testing the treatment difference and testing the treatment × period interaction.

C. Importance of Adequate Run-In and Washout Periods

Baseline is a very important prognostic variable, since it represents the disease severity before the start of the treatment. The importance of run-in and washout periods, therefore, should not be underestimated. Their lengths should be adequate to remove the effects of the previous therapies. Especially when the washout period is not of adequate length, the second baseline measurements x_{i2k} might not be independent of the sequences or the treatments received during the first period. Because the patients are randomly assigned to the treatment sequences, the baseline measurements for the first period can be assumed to be a random sample from a single population. Therefore, the rejection of H_0: $\theta_1 - \theta_2 = 0$ implies that the second-baseline measurements are not independent of the treatments the patients received during the first period. In this situation, of course, no valid test for the treatment × period interaction is possible, and a test for the treatment comparison should therefore be performed from the first-period data only. One can of course consider the latter test after making adjustment for the first-baseline values to increase the validity and efficiency of the test.

If for ethical reasons it is not possible to plan a washout period sufficiently long to achieve the independence of the second baseline from the treatments received during the first treatment period, then a parallel group design should be preferred to a 2 × 2 crossover design.

D. How Many Baselines for Analyzing Treatment Responses?

When H_0: $\theta_1 = \theta_2$ holds, x_1 and x_2, the first and second baselines, are valid baselines for the treatment responses y_1 and y_2, respectively. Although treatments are not randomly assigned to the patients at the start of Period 2, x_2 is a valid baseline for y_2, because in this case the x_2 values are independent of the treatments received during the first period. Alternatively, it is also appropriate to ignore x_2 and use x_1 as a common baseline for both y_1 and y_2, because x_1 and x_2 are expected to be highly correlated under H_0: $\theta_1 = \theta_2$.

If there exist different carryover effects (i.e., when $\theta_1 \neq \theta_2$), the second-baseline measurements are not independent of the treatments received during the first period and therefore neither baseline can validly be used for adjusting the tests involving the treatments. When H_0: $\theta_1 = \theta_2$ does not hold and when a design does not include a washout period, some researchers still recommend the use of x_1 as a common baseline for adjusting the treatment × period interaction and the treatment difference. But in this case the use of the first baseline as covariate for the treatment response of Period 2 does not seem to be appropriate. In a repeated measures, parallel-group design where each patient receives a randomly assigned treatment throughout the trial without any interruption, the first baseline would be appropriate for adjusting the treatment difference at any visit. In a crossover design the situation is different, however. For example, in sequence AB the first baseline cannot represent the state of the disease at the start of Treatment B. Hence, when $\theta_1 \neq \theta_2$, it is not appropriate to use any baseline for adjusting either a test for the treatment × period interaction or a test for the treatment comparison. In fact, when $\theta_1 \neq \theta_2$, the use of data from both periods should be considered inappropriate for further inferences. In this case, analysis of covariance of y_1 using x_1 as a covariate is recommended.

E. Adjustment: Change or Covariance?

If x is an initial measurement and y is the treatment response in a comparative trial, we make an adjustment in the analysis of the y values by removing the influence of the x values. The purpose of adjustment is to increase the validity and precision of the inference on the treatment difference(s). The simplest adjustment is the analysis of the change $y - x$. A better method of adjustment is the analysis of covariance where the influence of the x values is removed from the y values through a linear regression model or a covariance adjustment.

For ease of interpretation, some researchers have analyzed a 2×2 crossover design using the change from baseline. It should be noted, however, that the inference based on the covariance adjustment is generally more precise than that based on the change adjustment. The readers are referred to Patel (1983, 1986) and Kenward and Jones (1987b) for covariance-adjusted methods.

F. Structure of the Dispersion Matrix

In an analysis based on changes from baseline measurements, one needs to estimate the elements of the dispersion matrix Σ of (x_1, y_1, x_2, y_2). In a given situation one can assume a specific structure on Σ, so that it would require estimation of fewer parameters, which makes an estimate of Σ more precise. But in reality it is difficult to verify a given structure on Σ, especially when the sample size is small.

Kenward and Jones (1987b) have examined a few data-sets to see how well three structures—(1) compound symmetry, (2) structure based on a simple autoregression model, and (3) structure 2 modified to include a relative length of a washout period—fit to the data. Their experience showed that in reality no specific structure can be recommended for future use. Structure 3 is studied by Wallenstein (1986) and Koch (1986).

Until we gain more knowledge about some specific structures that would commonly hold in a 2×2 crossover trial with baseline measurements, we should continue using Σ without assuming any specific structure.

G. Analytical Procedures

Under the assumption of normality, various change-adjusted procedures for analyzing a 2×2 crossover design with baseline measurements have been proposed by several researchers, including Zimmerman and Rahlfs (1980), Armitage and Hills (1982), Fleiss et al. (1985). Wallenstein (1979, 1986), Koch (1986), Willan and Pater (1986b), and Wallenstein and Fleiss (1988). These procedures make use of either one or both baseline measurements, and some of them assume a specific structure on Σ, the dispersion matrix of (x_1, y_1, x_2, y_2). For covariance-adjusted procedures the readers are referred to Patel (1983, 1986) and Kenward and Jones (1987b), where no specific structure on Σ is assumed.

In all these procedures, one or more preliminary tests have been recommended for checking the validity of a test for the treatment comparison. Patel (1983) has proposed an ad hoc procedure for the covariance-adjustment. His first preliminary test is more stringent, as it tests the hypothesis of equal carryover effects and equal baselines. Although it is desirable to have equal baseline distributions, this desirability may not warrant a statistical test for verifying it. Patel (1986) has given likelihood ratio tests (under the normality assumption) for testing the hypotheses of no period $\times$ treatment interaction and no treatment difference.

Kenward and Jones (1987b) have tested various hypotheses in a stepwise manner through a generalized least-squares method that is equivalent to the analysis of covariance after making adjustment with respect to the baseline measurements and/or transformed response variable(s) involved in the previously tested effects. Both Patel (1983, 1986) and Kenward and Jones (1987b) have used the same numerical data for the analysis, and their results are similar even though they have used different approaches. This does not mean, however, that these approaches will yield similar results all the time. Future research should examine these two approaches closely.

Castellana and Patel (1985) have studied a problem in a multicenter framework under the assumption of normality of $(y_1 \mid x_1, y_2 \mid x_1)$. They have used x_1 alone as a covariate, which is justifiable because this analysis is done after knowing that H_0: $\theta_1 = \theta_2$ holds. Recently, Tsai and

Patel (1987) have studied robust procedures for analyzing the data from a 2×2 crossover trial.

H. Discussion

A 2×2 crossover design with baseline measurements allows us to model the experimental situation more closely than that without baseline measurements. Hence the use of baselines leads to a better screening procedure for checking the validity of a test for the treatment effects.

There are various approaches of making use of baseline measurements under different model assumptions. One should use an approach that is clinically meaningful and statistically valid and efficient. Assumptions of normality and a structure on the dispersion matrix of the baselines and response measurements are difficult to verify, especially when the sample size is small. One may rely on historical data for these assumptions, but in a doubtful situation robust procedures would be more appropriate to use.

If a crossover design with baseline measurements is used in a proper setting, it can turn out to be a very valuable design in clinical trials.

While designing a crossover trial experimenters generally express a fear about the outcomes of preliminary tests. A biostatistician should raise certain questions that would help decide whether to consider a crossover design in a given situation. These questions are:

1. Can we allow sufficiently long run-in and washout periods?
2. Is the underlying disease such that after a washout period the state of the disease would return approximately to the level observed at the start of Period 1?
3. Is there any historical evidence of preliminary test results implying the treatment comparison invalid in situations similar to those of the current trial?
4. Is the comparative treatment a negative control or a positive control? (In a crossover trial with a positive control, the assumptions of equal carryover and psychological effects are more likely to be satisfied than in a trial with a placebo treatment.)
5. What is the likelihood of patient withdrawals during the trial? [If a relatively large number of patients drop out before the completion of the trial, there may be a substantial loss in efficiency. Patel (1985) has analyzed incomplete data in a 2×2 crossover without baseline measurements. Future research should focus on incomplete data when baseline measurements are obtained.]

Ultimately, the decision for planning a crossover trial depends on whether one is willing to compromise between the validity and efficiency of a test for the treatment comparison. If the validity is given a higher priority, as it should be, and if the confidence of getting favorable outcomes from preliminary tests is low, then a parallel group design is a better choice.

ACKNOWLEDGMENT

The author would like to thank Dr. Byron Jones and Dr. Michael Kenward, University of Kent at Canterbury, Kent, UK, for their useful comments.

V. THE TWO-TREATMENT, TWO-PERIOD, FOUR-SEQUENCE DESIGN*

Karl E. Peace

A. Introduction

Grizzle (1965) proposed a two-treatment, two-period, two-sequence crossover design that permits assessment of carryover effects and direct effects in a stepwise manner. That is, the carryover effect is first assessed. If it is found not significant, then the direct effect of treatment is then assessed. The assessment in this case utilizes information from both periods. If the carryover effect is found significant, then the direct effect of treatment is assessed utilizing only the first-period information. This is true (Shah, 1980) whether or not one makes the assumption, as did Grizzle, of stochasticity of subjects within sequences.

Thus, a significant carryover effect imposes a severe penalty for having conducted the experiment in a crossover rather than in a parallel fashion. Other criticisms of the Grizzle model have appeared (Brown, 1980a). The Food and Drug Administration, due largely to meetings (June 23, 1976; December 20, 1976) of the Biometric and Epidemiological Methodology Advisory Committee (BEMAC), has taken the position (O'Neill 1977) that the crossover design should be avoided in studies requiring demonstration of efficacy.

Balaam (1965) proposed a design that is an augmentation of the Grizzle model. Two additional sequences in which patients are not crossed over are added. This design is one of a class of designs, proposed by Laska, Meisner, and Kushner (1981), that permit investigation of carryover effects. In this section, the Balaam design is reviewed. It is noted that the design permits assessment of direct effects regardless of

*A version of this section was originally presented at a regional meeting of A. H. Robins Company and Burroughs Wellcome Corporation statisticians in May 1981.

the outcome of the assessment of carryover effects. The model, methodology and hypotheses of interest are reviewed in Sections B–D. Illustrative examples are given in Section E.

B. The Model

The proposed model is given by

$$Y_{ijk} = \mu + \pi_i + S_{k(j)} + \phi_l + C_l + \eta_{ijk} \tag{3.1}$$

Notationally, Y_{ijk} is the response observed on the jth subject in the kth sequence in the ith period; μ is the effect common to all responses; π_i is the effect of the ith period; $S_{k(j)}$ is the effect of the jth subject in the kth sequence; ϕ_l is the direct effect of the lth treatment; C_l is the carryover effect of the lth treatment; and η_{ijk} is the random component reflecting observation error.

The assumptions that are made on the model are

$$\sum_i \pi_i = \sum_j S_{k(j)} = \sum_l \phi_l = \sum_l C_l = 0 \tag{3.2}$$

and

$$\eta_{ijk} \approx NiD(0, \sigma_e^2) \tag{3.3}$$

where $i = 1, 2$; $j = 1, 2, \ldots, n$; $k = 1, 2, 3, 4$; $l = 1$ (treatment A), 2 (treatment B).

To contrast, in the Grizzle model, C_l (which would be indexed by k instead of l) respresents the sequence, treatment-by-period interaction, or carryover effect and $S_{k(j)}$ is assumed to follow an $N(0, \sigma_s^2)$ distribution, independently of η_{ijk}. In model (3.1), the sequence effect is partitioned into two components; one representing carryover effect (C_l), and another that is lumped into error, and $S_{k(j)}$ is a fixed effect.

C. Data Layout and Estimators

The data that model (3.1) explains may be displayed as in Table 3.1.

Using linear models theory, the maximum likelihood estimators of the effects in model (3.1) may be obtained. These are given in Table 3.2.

TABLE 3.1 Data layout for model (3.1)

Period	AA(1)	AB(2)	BA(3)	BB(4)	Total
π_1	y_{1j1}	y_{1j2}	y_{1j3}	y_{1j4}	
Total	$y_{1.1}$	$y_{1.2}$	$y_{1.3}$	y_{1j4}	$y_{1..}$
π_2	y_{2j1}	y_{2j2}	y_{2j3}	y_{2j4}	
Total	$y_{2.1}$	$y_{2.2}$	$y_{2.3}$	$y_{2.4}$	$y_{2..}$
Grand total	$y_{..1}$	$y_{..2}$	$y_{..3}$	$y_{..4}$	$y_{..}$

TABLE 3.2 Estimators of the effects of model (3.1)

Source	Estimator[a]
π_i	$\bar{\bar{y}}_{i..} - \bar{\bar{\bar{y}}}_{...}$
$S_{k(j)}$	$\bar{y}_{.jk} - \bar{\bar{y}}_{..k}$
ϕ_l	$\bar{\bar{\bar{y}}}_{...}{}^{l} - \bar{\bar{\bar{y}}}_{...}{}^{a}$
C_l	$\bar{\bar{y}}_{2..}{}^{l} - \bar{\bar{y}}_{2..}{}^{b}$

[a] $\bar{\bar{\bar{y}}}_{...}{}^{l}$ is the mean of all observations on treatment l, and [b] $\bar{\bar{y}}_{2..}{}^{l}$ is the mean of all observations in the second period that correspond to treatment l in the first period.

D. Hypothesis, Contrasts, and ANOVA

Hypotheses of interest are H_{01}: $\phi_A = \phi_B$, $C_A = C_B$, H_{02}: $\phi_A = \phi_B$, and H_{03}: $C_A = C_B$. The hypothesis H_{01} may be addressed by applying the two degrees of freedom contrast matrix , given in Table 3.3, to the cell means of Table 3.1.

The rows of C are orthogonal contrast constants that may be applied to the cell means of Table 3.1 to test the hypotheses H_{02} (row 1) and H_{03} (row 2) individually. It is noted that the rows of C when applied to the cell means of Table 3.1 yield unbiased estimators of the difference in direct effects and in carryover effects, respectively.

The analysis of variance (ANOVA) reflecting the null hypotheses and other effects appears in Table 3.4.

TABLE 3.3 Contrast matrix for hypothesis H_{01}

	Sequence within Period 1				Sequence within Period 2			
Row 1	$\frac{1}{4}$	$\frac{1}{4}$	$-\frac{1}{4}$	$-\frac{1}{4}$	$\frac{1}{4}$	$-\frac{1}{4}$	$\frac{1}{4}$	$-\frac{1}{4}$
Row 2	0	0	0	0	$\frac{1}{2}$	$\frac{1}{2}$	$-\frac{1}{2}$	$-\frac{1}{2}$

The formulas for the sums of squares referenced in Table 3.3 appear below.

$$\mathrm{SS}\,H_{02} = (y_{..1} + y_{1.2} + y_{2.3})^2/4n + (y_{2.2} + y_{1.3} + y_{..4})^2/4n - (y_{...})^2/8n \tag{3.4}$$

$$\mathrm{SS}\,H_{03} = (y_{2.1} + y_{2.2})^2/2n + (y_{2.3} + y_{2.4})^2/2n - (y_{2..})^2/2n \tag{3.5}$$

$$\mathrm{SS}\,H_{01} = \mathrm{SS}\,H_{02} + \mathrm{SS}\,H_{03} \tag{3.6}$$

$$\mathrm{SS}\,\pi = (y_{1..})^2/4n + (y_{2..})^2/4n - (y_{...})^2/8n \tag{3.7}$$

$$\begin{aligned} \mathrm{SSS}(S) = {} & (y_{.11})^2/2 + \cdots + (y_{.n1})^2/2 + (y_{.12})^2/2 + \cdots \\ & + (y_{.n2})^2/2 + (y_{.13})^2/2 + \cdots + (y_{.n3})^2/2 \\ & + (y_{.14})^2/2 + \cdots + (y_{.n4})^2/2 - (y_{..1})^2/2n \\ & - (y_{..2})^2/2n - (y_{..3})^2/2n - (y_{..4})^2/2n \end{aligned} \tag{3.8}$$

$$\mathrm{SSTOT} = \sum_i \sum_j \sum_k y_{ijk}^2 - (y_{...})^2/8n \tag{3.9}$$

TABLE 3.4 ANOVA for model (3.1)

Source	df	SS	MS	F
H_{01}	2	$\mathrm{SS}\,H_{01}$	$\mathrm{SS}\,H_{01}/2$	$\mathrm{MS}\,H_{01}/\mathrm{MSE}$
H_{02}	1	$\mathrm{SS}\,H_{02}$	$\mathrm{SS}\,H_{02}$	$\mathrm{MS}\,H_{02}/\mathrm{MSE}$
H_{03}	1	$\mathrm{SS}\,H_{03}$	$\mathrm{SS}\,H_{03}$	$\mathrm{MS}\,H_{03}/\mathrm{MSE}$
Period	1	$\mathrm{SS}\,\pi$	$\mathrm{SS}\,\pi$	$\mathrm{MS}\,\pi/\mathrm{MSE}$
Sub(seq)	$4(n-1)$	$\mathrm{SSS}(S)$	$\mathrm{SSS}(S)/4(n-1)$	$\mathrm{MSS}(S)/\mathrm{MSE}$
Error	$4n$	SSE	$\mathrm{SSE}/4n$	
Total	$8n-1$	SSTOT		

and

$$\text{SSE} = \text{SSTOT} - \text{SS}H_{01} - \text{SS}\pi - \text{SSS}(S) \tag{3.10}$$

Alternatively, $\text{SS}H_{02}$ and $\text{SS}H_{03}$ may be expressed as

$$\text{SS}H_{02} = 2n(C_1)^2 \tag{3.11}$$

and

$$\text{SS}H_{03} = n(C_2)^2 \tag{3.12}$$

where C_i is the contrast obtained by applying row i of C to the cell means of Table 3.1, $i = 1, 2$.

E. Examples

Two examples illustrating the hypotheses of interest and the ANOVA necessary to address these hypotheses are presented. The data for the first example appear in Table 3.5. The data for the second example appear in Table 3.6. The ANOVA (Table 3.7) of the data in the first example illustrates a significant (at the 0.05 level) direct effect but a nonsignificant carryover effect. The ANOVA (Table 3.8) of the data in the second example illustrates significant direct and carry-over effects.

The ANOVA in Table 3.7 illustrates that the joint hypothesis of equality of direct effects and of carryover effects is rejected. Further inspection indicates that only direct effects are significantly different. The ANOVA in Table 3.8 also illustrates that the joint hypothesis of equality of direct effects and of equality of carryover effects is rejected. However, further inspection indicates that direct effects are significantly different and carryover effects are significantly different.

F. Discussion

The design of Balaam has been reviewed. Data generated using the normal random number generator of SAS have been presented. These data illustrate the ANOVA appropriate for the design. Further, one set of data illustrates that the rejection of the joint hypothesis of equality of direct effects and of carryover effects is due only to the significance of direct effects. The other set of data illustrates that the rejection of the joint hypothesis of equality of direct effects and of carryover effects is due to both the significance of direct effects and the significance of carryover effects.

The design presented should overcome the major criticism leveled at

TABLE 3.5 Data exhibiting significant direct effect but nonsignificant carryover effect

(a) Raw data

Period	Sequence	Patient	Drug	Y
1	1	1	1	11.10
1	1	2	1	8.25
1	1	3	1	11.12
1	1	4	1	9.69
1	2	5	1	9.33
1	2	6	1	7.03
1	2	7	1	11.92
1	2	8	1	5.79
1	3	9	2	3.54
1	3	10	2	11.74
1	3	11	2	7.08
1	3	12	2	8.90
1	4	13	2	7.68
1	4	14	2	7.54
1	4	15	2	4.74
1	4	16	2	6.18
2	1	1	1	9.90
2	1	2	1	11.59
2	1	3	1	11.06
2	1	4	1	10.78
2	2	5	2	5.36
2	2	6	2	2.04
2	2	7	2	7.20
2	2	8	2	2.87
2	3	9	1	13.22
2	3	10	1	9.05
2	3	11	1	12.31
2	3	12	1	8.59
2	4	13	2	9.62
2	4	14	2	7.77
2	4	15	2	8 55
2	4	16	2	9.10

(b) Summary (means) Sequence

Period	AA(1)	AB(2)	BA(3)	BB(4)	Combined
π_1	10.04	8.51	7.82	6.53	8.2
π_2	10.83	4.37	10.79	8.76	8.68
Combined	10.44	6.44	9.30	7.64	8.45
Drug effects	10.04(ϕ_1)	6.86(ϕ_2)	7.60(C_1)	9.77(C_2)	

TABLE 3.6 Data exhibiting significant direct effect and significant carryover effect

(a) Raw data

Period	Sequence	Patient	Drug	Y
1	1	1	1	11.10
1	1	2	1	8.25
1	1	3	1	11.11
1	1	4	1	9.69
1	2	5	1	9.33
1	2	6	1	7.03
1	2	7	1	11.92
1	2	8	1	5.79
1	3	9	2	3.54
1	3	10	2	11.74
1	3	11	2	7.08
1	3	12	2	8.90
1	4	13	2	7.68
1	4	14	2	7.54
1	4	15	2	4.74
1	4	16	2	6.18
2	1	1	1	13.90
2	1	2	1	15.58
2	1	3	1	15.06
2	1	4	1	14.78
2	2	5	2	11.36
2	2	6	2	8.03
2	2	7	2	13.19
2	2	8	2	8.86
2	3	9	1	7.21
2	3	10	1	3.04
2	3	11	1	6.30
2	3	12	1	2.58
2	4	13	2	3.61
2	4	14	2	1.76
2	4	15	2	2.54
2	4	16	2	3.10

(b) Summary (means) Sequence

Period	AA(1)	AB(2)	BA(3)	BB(4)	Combined
π_1	10.04	8.51	7.81	6.53	8.22
π_2	14.83	10.36	4.78	2.75	8.18
Combined	12.43	9.44	6.30	7.64	8.20
Drug effects	9.54(ϕ_1)	6.86(ϕ_2)	12.59(C_1)	3.77(C_2)	

TABLE 3.7 ANOVA of data given in table 3.5

Source	df	SS	MS	F value	p Value
H_{01}	2	99.62	49.81	8.60	0.0029
H_{02}	1	80.71	80.71	13.93	0.0018
H_{03}	1	18.91	18.91	3.26	0.0896
Period	1	1.68	1.68	<1	
Sub(seq)	12	47.81	3.98	<1	
Error	16	92.68	5.79		
Total	31	241.81			

TABLE 3.8 ANOVA of data given in table 3.6

Source	df	SS	MS	F Value	p Value
H_{01}	2	368.84	184.42	40.22	1×10^{-6}
H_{02}	1	57.30	57.30	12.49	0.0028
$H_{0}3$	1	311.54	311.54	67.95	1×10^{-6}
Period	1	0.01	0.01	<1	
Sub(seq)	12	47.81	3.98	<1	
Error	16	73.35	4.58		
Total	31	490.03			

the Grizzle two-treatment, two-period, two-sequence crossover design, since significant carryover effect imposes no penalty in the sense of data reduction. Essentially, this design provides an alternative for those trials where a crossover design is of interest. Instead of randomizing patients to two treatment sequences, randomize patients to four treatment sequences.

VI. CONDITIONAL 2×2 CROSSOVER DESIGNS IN CLINICAL TRIALS

Gerald M. Fava

A. Introduction

The classical two-treatment, two-period crossover is generally more efficient than the parallel-group design and has much more ethical appeal. It cannot be used, however, in a variety of clinical settings. It cannot be used, for example, when one of the treatments produces a cure; nor can it be used when it would be unethical to subject a patient to treatment in the second period when the patient has shown improvement to the first treatment.

The conditional (or incomplete) crossover design can be used in these situations. This design is similar to the classical crossover with the exception that only patients who fail to respond to their first-period treatment go on to receive the alternate treatment in the second period. Patients who respond to their first treatment do not enter the second period, but are terminated from the study as completers. A variation of this design has responders in Period 1 continue on the same treatment in Period 2. This design bridges the gap between the parallel-group design and the full crossover; it retains the ethical appeal of the latter while having utility in situations where the full crossover cannot be used. It also mimics clinical practice better than the other designs.

The efficiency of classical crossover designs stems from the estimation of treatment differences with each patient serving as his/her own control. Models by Grizzle (1965), Wallenstein and Fisher (1977), Hills and Armitage (1979), Gart (1969), McNemar (1947), and others all presuppose patients will receive both treatments. In the conditional crossover design, this is not the case. In fact, some of the strongest evidence of treatment effect is derived from patients who receive only one treatment. Since traditional models tend to give zero weight to patients who have received only one treatment, they are not appropriate for analyzing conditional crossovers.

B. Methods of Analysis

The basic difficulty then with analyzing conditional crossover designs is finding ways to give full weight to patients who respond during the first period. Methods have been proposed by Fava and Buhite (1981) and White (1979) specifically to handle this class of design. Both methods deal with analyzing responders. Fava and Buhite also define an ordered categorical response variable. Boadi-Boateng (1983) assumes a bivariate normal distribution in his proposed method to analyze the variant design of observing Period 1 responders on the same treatment in Period 2.

White's methodology is based on finding maximum likelihood estimators (MLE) and their variance–covariance matrix under a multinomial model for four mutually exclusive subgroups. These are patients who respond to:

- neither treatment

- both treatments
- Treatment A but not B
- Treatment B but not A

From this he derives the MLEs and variance for a test of treatment difference. Treatment difference is defined as the difference between the proportion of patients who respond to A minus the proportion of patients who respond to B. The proportion of patients who respond to A is the sum of the estimators for patients who respond to both treatments plus those who respond to A but not B, and similarly for those who respond to B. White (1979) assumes that washout periods eliminate any sequence effects. This methodology does not make specific allowance for period effects.

White (1979) finds the estimators for the four subgroups defined above from an iterative computational procedure. There is no closed-form solution. There is a closed-form solution for initial values. As one might expect, in dealing with proportions, the variance of the estimated treatment difference is also a function of the unknown population parameters. Estimates of the parameters are used to estimate the variance.

An example of an analysis with this procedure is given in Sato (1982), with more complete details given in White (1979).

Fava and Buhite test the null hypothesis of no treatment difference by using a modified version of the sign test to test that the proportion of responders is the same for each treatment. They proceed by letting

x = number of responders to Treatment A over both periods
y = number of responders to Treatment B over both periods
$n = x + y$

Then the Fava and Buhite test computes the binomial probability of observing x or a more extreme value of successes in n trials with $p = 0.5$. The test accepts or rejects the null hypothesis against a one-sided alternative depending on whether or not this probability is less than or equal to alpha. Tests against a two-sided alternative are also easily carried out.

This methodology is valid in the presence of period effects, but assumes the absence of carryover effects.

Fava and Buhite also define an ordered categorical response variable in the way described below. They consider patients randomized to the sequence AB and the sequence BA as two independent groups. They argue that for a patient in either sequence, the possible ordered outcomes of the trial are:

- full response to the Period 1 drug, no further treatment required
- better (but not full) response to Period 1 drug than Period 2 drug
- equivalent response to both drugs
- better (but not full) response to Period 2 drug than Period 1 drug
- full response to Period 2 drug

Patients in the two sequences are compared via an appropriate test for ordered categories (e.g., Klotz, 1966). This test has similarities to Koch's (1972) test for direct (treatment) effect in the absence of residual effects. The proposed procedure categorizes the results with the best scores being assigned to patients who are missing Period 2 due to a response in Period 1.

When responders in Period 1 remain on the same treatment in period 2, Boadi-Boateng (1983) has worked out MLEs of treatment difference and its variance for continuous variables under the assumption of a bivariate normal distribution. The methodology is an application of the selection problem. This situation arises when a selection procedure based on certain variables eliminate some subjects from further observation with respect to other variables. The model includes period and residual effects. However, it assumes that the variances and covariances are known.

C. Discussion

1. Design Efficiency

Comparisons of competing crossover designs have been carried out by Kershner and Federer (1981), Laska et al. (1983), and Ebbutt (1984). A design described by Balaam (1965) randomizes patients to four sequences: AB, BA, AA, and BB. The main advantage to this design is that treatment differences can be tested whether or not carryover effects are present. Laska et al. (1983) have shown that among all two-period, two-treatment designs, this design minimizes the variance of the unbiased estimator of treatment difference in the presence of carryover. However, if carryover effects are not present, the usual crossover is optimal.

Peace (1983) has shown that the efficiencies of the complete crossover and Balaam's design are greater than that of either variant of the incomplete crossover.

For estimating proportions, White (1979) has shown in simulations with $N = 50$ and $N = 100$ that the efficiency of the incomplete crossover design is substantially greater than that of the parallel group design. Boadi-Boateng (1983) derived the similar conclusion for his model for the variant design.

Since the efficiency of a design (for a fixed sample size) should be related to the number of observations and the efficiency of a crossover design should be related to the number of patients receiving both treatments, these are the expected results. For the same reason, the variant design should be more efficient than the basic design.

White (1979) also compared two forms of the conditional crossover design: one assigns patients to treatment sequence at random, and the other assigns them based on the outcome of a prognostic test at baseline (or profile assessment). Under the simulation conditions with $N = 50$ and $N = 100$, White (1979) found that the design with random allocation of patients to treatment sequence had uniformly more precise estimates. In addition, the assignment by profile assessment does not yield an unbiased estimate of treatment difference in the presence of period by treatment interaction even if only the first-period data are used (White, 1979).

2. Efficiency and Validity of Methods

The methods proposed for the basic design reduce all measurements to a nominal or ordinal scale. Only under the variant design that requires additional observations on first-period responders can the proposed methods take advantage of higher scales. None of the methods directly include baseline values. While the merit of using baselines in the full crossover can be argued, their use in the conditional crossover has not been explored.

The Boadi-Boateng estimate of treatment difference reduces to using only Period 1 data in the presence of unequal residual effects (unless exactly one-half of the patients in each treatment sequence cross over). Each of the other methods was developed under the assumption that the completely confounded effects of sequence, carryover, and period by treatment interaction are absent. The term "order effect" is more appropriate and will be used in the remainder of this discussion.

Given the generally high efficiency of the sign test (e.g., Lehmann, 1975; Dixon, 1953), we would expect it to be a relatively powerful test in the analysis of incomplete crossover designs, particularly when sample sizes are small. Fava and Buhite (1981) have shown that the power of this method is diminished when order effects are present. This implies that the resultant level of the test is larger than it should be. This corresponds to the result of Nam (1971), who showed that the true level of the two-sided McNemar test is always greater than the stated level in the presence of order effects. The bias is a function of the magnitude of the order effect and the difference in the number of patients randomized to the two treatment sequences.

It seems intuitive that the distortion of the true level of the test in the presence of order effects would also hold for the ordered categorical response parameter as well as for White's procedure. It also seems intuitive that the results of Willan and Pater (1986a) would apply as well. Under the assumption that the order effect is caused by the residual effect of treatment, they showed that unless the carryover effects are very large, the usual analysis of the full crossover is more powerful than that of using the first period data alone.

It is easily shown that the sign test approach by Fava and Buhite has the correct distribution under the null hypothesis only if the probability of a patient's being assigned to each treatment sequence is 0.5. Any other weighting scheme (with positive probability of response) results in a biased test—even in the absence of order effects. We infer that the test is biased if we condition on the (unequal) number of patients in each sequence, despite an equiprobable randomization. Small imbalances probably have a negligible effect, however, with medium to large sample sizes. With small sample sizes, when the sign test approach is expected to have the greatest utility, the influence of even small imbalances is unknown.

Since White's (1979) procedure was developed using equal numbers of patients in each treatment sequence, it is not clear that it applies as is to the unbalanced case. The difficulty may be with the variance of the estimates rather than with the estimates themselves.

The ordered categorical response parameter employs a two-sample test. The number of patients in each treatment sequence is taken into account in the test statistic. It should provide a true alpha-level test in the absence of order effects.

For the variant design, formal tests of hypothesis need to be proposed, and the requirement of known (co)variances removed. The performances of the tests would need to be studied under departures from the model assumptions. The power of the test of equal residual effects needs to be addressed.

D. Conclusion

The conditional crossover design has even more restricted use than the complete crossover. Its strongest features are that it can be used when one of the treatments produces a cure, and that it mimics the actual clinical treatment of patients. From this standpoint it has ethical appeal. The robustness of the proposed analytical methods has not been adequately studied even in the common case of sequence imbalance or unknown covariance structure. At this time, its best use may be as a follow-up to a parallel study. The cost of the extra period may be relatively little, and some important information on the practical performance of this design and methods can be gained.

VII. ANALYSIS OF CROSSOVER DESIGNS WHEN THE ERRORS ARE NOT INDEPENDENT

Marcia Polansky

In the case of the most basic type of crossover design response is measured only twice for each subject, once during the first treatment period and once during the second treatment period, but more commonly there will be multiple measurements of response for each subject. There may be more than two treatment periods, response may be measured more than once in each treatment period, or there may be a washout period and/or baseline measurements. When there are more than two measurements of response for each subject it is necessary to consider whether the correlations between all pairs of responses from the same individual are the same, since it is only in this case that a random subject effect can be used to model the correlation between observations. However, in practice, measurements of clinical response closer in time may be more highly correlated than those farther apart. Consequently, repeated-measures analysis of variance, which assumes constant covariance between responses, would not be an appropriate method of analysis. As will be discussed in more detail, when there is only one crossover this problem can be avoided by averaging the responses during each period of treatment administration, which reduces the number of measurements to two. Then these means can be treated as the unit of observation and analyzed using a paired *t*-test or the standard repeated-measures model with treatment, period, and order effects. This kind of approach is often used but is not always the most efficient approach and does not permit comparisons between time periods.

An alternative approach that can be used for repeated-measures data including data from crossover studies is a multivariate approach in which the only assumption made is that the covariance matrix is the same for all subjects. However, when there is a limited number of subjects, as is often the case in crossover studies, this approach results in a highly parameterized model and in some cases an overparameterized model. Another general method of analysis for designs in which response is measured repeatedly over time is to model the errors as a first-order autoregressive process. When the autocorrelation is positive, the correlation between observations decreases exponentially as the distance between the observations increases. Generally, a random subject effect is also included in the model. Albohali and Milliken (1984), Azzalini (1984), Lee (1988), Pantula and Pollock (1985), and Polansky (1988), among others, give methods for estimating and testing hypotheses when the errors are assumed to follow a first-order autoregressive process for various linear models. Jennrich and Schlucter (1986) and Laird and Ware (1982), among others, give general methods for fitting linear models with structured covariance matrices. Before describing these alternative approaches in more detail, we will first consider the magnitude of the error that can result from the use of a standard repeated-measures ANOVA when the errors are positively correlated.

Polansky (1988) evaluated the bias of the E(MSE) (within subject variance) and the variance of various contrasts for crossover designs with one crossover and no washout periods when a saturated model was fitted to the data (i.e., the time treatment interaction was included) and response was measured multiple times at equally spaced intervals during each treatment period. Although the variance of contrasts depends on the number of crossovers and whether there was a washout period, the bias of E(MSE) depends only on the total number of periods, so that the results that follow concerning the bias of the MSE can be directly applied to more complicated crossover designs.

Small and moderate positive autocorrelations were found to cause substantial downward biases in the estimates of the E(MSE) except when the number of measurements per subject was quite large. For example, when response was measured three times during each treatment period and the autocorrelation was greater than or equal to 0.4, the bias was greater than 20%. With 5 measurements of response, an autocorrelation of 0.5 or greater caused biases in excess of 20%. When there were 7 periods, the bias did not exceed 20% until the autocorrelation reached 0.6.

Of more practical importance are the biases of the estimates of the variances of important contrasts and F-tests based on the standard repeated-measures ANOVA. The biases of the variances of within-subject contrasts depend indirectly on the autocorrelation in that these estimates are a function of the MSE, but also directly in that the true variance of a contrast depends on the autocorrelation and the distances between the observations used in the contrast. When there is no missing data, between-subject contrasts will not be affected by the autocorrelation.

A type of contrast that is often of interest is the difference in the mean responses at different points in time, since this type of contrast can be used to determine the changes in response over time during the administration of a treatment or to compare the responses at the same point in time for different treatments. The variance of the difference in mean responses between two time periods is $(2/n)(1-r^k)\hat{\sigma}_e^2$ where n is the number of subjects and k is the distance between the periods. However, the estimate of the variance based on a standard repeated-measures analysis is $(2/n)\hat{\sigma}_e^2$ where $\hat{\sigma}_e^2$ is the MSE. The downward bias of the MSE causes a downward bias in the estimate of the variance, but excluding the autocorrelation coefficient causes an upward bias. The net result is that variance of differences between adjacent means is either only slightly underestimated when the number of time periods is small and overestimated when it is large. However, as the distance between the time periods increases, the variance of the mean difference increases, so there is a net downward bias. The bias is greatest when the number of periods is limited.

For example, it is often of interest to compare responses at the same point in time during each of the treatment regimes. If response is measured 3 times in each of the treatment periods, even for moderate autocorrelations (0.5 or greater) the bias of the standard estimate of the variance is greater than 20%. When the number of periods is 4, the bias exceeds 20% when the autocorrelation reaches 0.6. When the number of periods is between 5 and 7, the bias does not exceed 20% until the autocorrelation reaches 0.7. If there is a washout period and the response is measured at the same time intervals during this period, the biases would be the same except that the number of periods would be the total number of periods (including the washout periods) divided by 2.

However, the most important comparison in a two-period crossover study is the difference in the mean responses of the two treatment periods. The computationally simpliest approach and a commonly used approach to estimating the variance of the mean treatment difference would be to estimate it directly. That is, treat the averages of the observations during each of the treatment periods as the unit of observation and then compute the standard deviation of the differences of these means (multiply by 2 and divide by the number of subjects). Since there would be only two responses per subject, this estimate of the variance of the treatment difference would not be biased by the autocorrelation. However, there would be a loss in efficiency due to averaging. We will refer to this estimate of the variance of the difference between the difference in the treatment means as the direct estimate, since it can be viewed as the "observed" variance (as compared to an approach in which the autocorrelation is estimated).

An alternative approach that might be expected to be more efficient that averaging responses in each treatment period would be to model the errors as a first-order autoregressive process and use the actual measurements of response as the unit of observation. Pantula and Pollock (1985) proposes consistent estimators for the parameters of the autoregressive process and the other parameters of the model (the between-subject variance and the fixed effects). Their estimates have closed-form solutions and can be used for any repeated-measures model. However, simulations done by Polansky (1987) have shown that when the number of time periods is limited, the Pantula et al. estimates of the autocorrelation and variance have large variances. Polansky gives a method of moment estimates that can be used when the model is saturated with respect to time (includes all interactions with time) and there is no missing data. The latter have considerably smaller variances and are much less biased than Pantula's estimates, particularly when the number of measurements of responses for each subject is limited. In a standard crossover design a saturated model would include the time by treatment interactions and time effects as well as the treatment effect.

It is of interest to compare the direct estimates of the variance of the difference between the mean response in the two treatment periods with the method of moment estimates, because the former are much easier to compute and involve no assumptions about the structure of the covariance matrix. Simulations showed that when the number of measurements of response in each period was less than 5, the variance of the method of moment estimates was less than the variance of the direct estimates but generally by only a modest amount. However when the number of responses in each treatment period was 5 to 7, the variance of the method of moments estimates range was typically less by more than 50%. The method of moment estimates becomes relatively even more efficient as the number of periods increases.

In summary, when the number of measurements of response in each treatment period is limited, or when there are more than two treatment periods, standard repeated-measures analysis of variance may give misleading results. Specifically, estimates of the variances of the treatment means and comparisons between time periods within the same or in different treatment periods and other contrasts obtained using a standard repeated-measures analysis of variance without taking into account the dependence of the correlation on time can be considerably biased. Furthermore, it is difficult to determine when the errors are not independent because the observed correlation of the errors from the repeated measures analysis is also biased downward. An unbiased estimate of the variance of the treatment difference can be obtained by averaging responses in each treatment period so that there are only two measurements of response for each subject. However, this approach is highly inefficient when the number of periods exceeds 5. "Direct" estimates of the variance are not efficient for contrasts that do not include all the data, since only the data included in the contrast are used in estimating its variance. For example, in the case of contrasts between time periods or between the same time period in the different treatment periods, the only observations that would be used would be the observations in that period. A better approach is to model the autocorrelation using a first-order autoregressive process and estimate the parameters using the method of moment estimators if there is no missing data or Pantula's estimates when there is missing data.

VIII. A SURVEY OF CROSSOVER DESIGNS USED IN INDUSTRY

Gerald M. Fava and Harji I. Patel

A. Introduction and Methods

The crossover group planned to conduct a survey of the use of crossover designs in the pharmaceutical industry. The objective of the survey was to summarize the information for the benefit of the statistical community in industry. A list of pharmaceutical companies who sent representatives to the Biostatistics Subsection meeting of the Pharmaceutical Manufacturers Association (PMA) in the fall of 1985 was reviewed. Relatively large companies were then targeted for receipt of a questionnaire. The survey was restricted to large companies, as it was felt they would have both the largest cross section of indications and also more experience with the most disease types. Obviously, the companies selected do not constitute a random sample of the population of companies.

The questionnaire itself (Appendix 1) asked only eight questions: the design type (basically the number of periods and treatments), the therapeutic indication, clinical phase of development, whether or not washout periods were used, whether or not baseline values were used in the analysis, the primary reason for using this design, the year used, and comments/suggestions. Many of the critical questions were open-ended in nature, resulting in nonstandard completion of the form. This made combining answers across companies very difficult. It also made combining answers within the same company only somewhat less difficult.

About 25 companies were contacted. A cover letter explaining the objective of the survey and emphasizing confidentiality was sent to these companies. The questionnaires were filled out anonymously and returned to a central point by 12 of the companies. These responses were received before the end of June 1986. The responses were then collated and forwarded to another place for tallying. In the tally, any entries that fell outside the preceding 5 years were excluded, as the instructions indicated only clinical trials within the last 5 years were to be included. Also, any studies indicated as being bioequivalence, bioavailability, or pharmacokinetic in nature were also exluded. Crossover designs are well recognized as being the design of choice in these areas. Therapeutic indications were combined where possible, as were the primary reasons for use of the design.

B. Results

As used in this report, the term relative frequency means the number of times the specific item was listed as an answer to the question. It cannot be interpreted as being the number of studies that have that specific attribute. In many instances, the comments state that a particular design was used more than once. Since it was not generally possible to determine the number of times a design was used, no attempt was made to weigh an answer by the number of protocols or studies it may have represented.

A complete list of indications (after combining) is reported in Table 3.9, with the number of companies reporting crossover studies for the indication. As can seen, crossover designs were used in studying many diverse diseases. The area most studied via the crossover were acid secretion, analgesics, angina, and bronchoconstriction, each reported as being studied by three companies. Table 3.10 provides the relative frequency of each of the indications. Antiarrhythmic studies were performed most frequently, followed closely by asthma. Analgesia studies, antianginal, antiinflammatory, and bronchoconstriction were next most frequently mentioned.

The overwhelming reason for using a crossover design is what was classified as efficiency. The next most prevalent reason reported was clinical insistence or preference. Scarcity of patients was the third most prevalent reason listed. These results are given in Table 3.11.

Tables 3.12 and 3.13 present the number of treatments and periods in each design. The 2×2 design was by far the most widely used. The next most popular design was the 4×4. This was particularly surprising since the format of the questionnaire tended to group 3×3 and all higher-order designs. It is an aspect that shows that the answers were provided to a degree of exactness largely dependent on the respondent. When comments were provided for these 4×4 designs, it generally was that the design was balanced for residual effects.

There were few studies carried out where the number of periods did not equal the number of treatments. The most prevalent of these was the two-treatment, four-period design, which was mentioned only three

TABLE 3.9 Counts of companies doing studies in specified indication

Indication	No. of companies[a]
Acid secretion	3
Analgesia	3
Angina	3
Antiarrhythmic	2
Antiinflammatory	1
Antiviral	1
Appetite suppression	1
Arthritis	1
Asthma	2
Bronchoconstriction	3
Cardio: metabolic balance	1
Cardiovascular reflexes	1
Cardio hemodynamics	1
CHF	1
Cough/cold	1
Diuretic: metabolic balance	1
Epilepsy	1
Gastric emptying	1
Hypertension	1
Hypertension dose response	1
Juvenile larygeal papillomatoses	1
Menstrual disorders	1
Migraine	1
Panic disorder	1
Parkinson's	1
Partial seizure	1
Preference	1
Reduce chemotherapy side effects	1
Renal function	1
Safety	1
Uterine contractions	1

[a] A given company may have done trials in more than one indication. Number of companies responding = 12.

times. No comments were entered on the form by the respondents reporting the use of this design.

About 75% of the trials used baseline values in their analysis (Table 3.14). This value was consistent regardless of the number of treatments in the design. An even greater number (nearly 90%) of studies used

TABLE 3.10 Relative frequency of indications for using crossover designs[a]

Indication	Relative frequency
Acid secretion	3
Analgesia	6
Angina	5
Antiarrhythmic	12
Antiinflammatory	4
Antiviral	1
Appetite suppression	1
Arthritis	1
Asthma	10
Bronchoconstriction	4
Cardio: metabolic balance	3
Cardiovascular reflexes	1
Cardio hemodynamics	2
CHF	1
Cough/cold	1
Diuretic: metabolic balance	1
Epilepsy	1
Gastric emptying	1
Hypertension	1
Hypertension dose response	1
Juvenile larygeal papillomatoses	1
Menstrual disorders	2
Migraine	1
Panic disorder	1
Parkinson's	1
Partial seizure	1
Preference	1
Reduce chemotherapy side effects	1
Renal function	1
Safety	1
Uterine contractions	1
Total	72

Number of companies responding = 12.

washout periods. This percentage was also consistent regardless of the number of treatments in the design (Table 3.15). In 45 of 61 trials where a washout period was used, the analysis incorporated baseline values (Table 3.16).

Table 3.17 displays the relative frequency of crossover trials by the

TABLE 3.11 Reason for using crossover designs

Reason	Percentage
Efficiency	56.1
Clinical insistence/preference	12.3
Scarcity of patients	7.0
Investigator insisted/designed	3.5
Many dose levels	1.8
Pilot efficacy	3.5
Safety study	1.8
Ethics	1.8
FDA guidelines/requested	3.5
Indication	3.5
Therapy equivalence	3.5
Treatment effect not conditional upon test for carryover (Balaam design)	1.8
Total	100%

year when the trials were conducted. In some instances, a range of years was given in answer to this question. Table 3.18 displays the relative frequency by the phase of clinical trial. The number of trials is relatively constant between 1982 and 1985. The trials were also employed about equally in each of the major phases of clinical research (Phases I, II, and III).

TABLE 3.12 Number of treatments and periods in design

Number of treatments	Percentage	Number of periods	Percentage
2	61.1	2	59.2
3	11.1	3	9.9
4	11.1	4	15.5
5	8.5	5	7.0
>3	5.6	>3	5.6
3–4	1.4	3–4	1.4
BIB	1.4	BIB	1.4
	100%		100%

TABLE 3.13 Cross counts of design by number of treatments and periods

Number of treatments	Number of periods								
	2	3	4	5	6	3–4	>3	BIB	Total
2	40	1	3	0	0	0	0	0	44
3	1	6	0	0	1	0	0	0	8
4	0	0	8	0	0	0	0	0	8
5	1	0	0	5	0	0	0	0	6
3–4	0	0	0	0	0	1	0	0	1
>3	0	0	0	0	0	0	4	0	4
BIB	0	0	0	0	0	0	0	1	1
Total	42	7	11	5	1	1	4	1	72

C. Discussion

The objective of the survey was to collect the 5-year history of the use of crossover designs. The results should be interpreted within the limitations of this survey and the regulatory atmosphere in which pharmaceutical companies operate.

TABLE 3.14 Cross counts of designs by number of treatments in design and whether baseline values were used in analysis

Number of treatments	Baseline used in analysis?		
	No	Yes	Total
2	10	32	42
3	2	5	7
4	2	5	7
5	0	5	5
3–4	1	0	1
>3	1	3	4
BIB	1	0	1
Total	17	50	67[a]

[a] Baseline question was not answered 5 times, and these counts are omitted from the table.

TABLE 3.15 Cross counts of designs by number of treatments in design and whether washout periods were used

Number of treatments	Washout periods? No	Yes	Total
2	6	38	44
3	1	7	8
4	0	8	8
5	1	5	6
3–4	0	1	1
>3	0	4	4
BIB	0	1	1
Total	8	64	72

The results of the survey are limited in scope due to incomplete coverage of the population of institutions conducting clinical trials. For example, medical colleges, hospitals, government health agencies, and small pharmaceutical companies were excluded from the survey. A slightly different type of survey was conducted by Louis et al. (1981). They investigated 13 crossover studies that had been published in 1978 and 1979 (Volumes 298–301) of the *New England Journal of Medicine* and highlighted relevant design and analysis issues. The frame available

TABLE 3.16 Cross counts of designs by the use of washout periods and baseline values

Washout periods?	Baseline values used in analysis? No	Yes	Total
No	1	5	6
Yes	16	45	61
Total	17	50	67[a]

[a] Baseline question was not answered 5 times, and these counts are omitted from the table.

TABLE 3.17 Distribution of crossover trials by year of study

Year	Relative frequency
1980–1984	1
1981	2
1981–1982	1
1981–1983	1
1982	15
1982–1983	2
1983	16
1983–1984	2
1983–1986	1
1984	14
1984–1985	1
1984–1986	1
1985	12
1986[a]	3
Total	72

[a]Partial year.

for this survey included only those PMA member companies whose employees attended the 1985 PMA meeting. Furthermore, as mentioned in the survey method section, the companies selected for the survey did not constitute a random sample from the available frame.

No attempt was made to recontact nonrespondents. Also to be

TABLE 3.18 Distribution of crossover trials by clinical phase

Phase	Relative Frequency
I	26
II	21
III	20
IV	3
V	2
Total	72

considered is that returned questionnaires may have incomplete information. No attempt was made to collect company viewpoints or their analytical methods.

The second most prevalent reason for using the survey was clinical preference. Taken with studies designed by the investigator and those performed because of the FDA guidelines, about 20% of the crossover studies were initiated strictly from the clinical viewpoint.

We hope that in the future such surveys will be conducted to collect mutually beneficial information on various important topics in applied statistics. We also hope that the future surveys will have a broader coverage of the population of interest, include a better survey design, and have a higher response rate.

IX. CURRENT THOUGHTS ON CROSSOVER DESIGNS*

Satya D. Dubey

A. Historical Perspective

During the early years of the 1970s while reviewing statistical reviews of IND/NDA submissions the Division of Biometrics concluded that in some situations the use of the two-period crossover design in clinical trials presented many difficulties in drawing valid statistical inferences. Our statistical reviews pointed out a variety of problems, including inappropriate use of crossover design, lack of baseline data for each period, lack of washout period between treatments for no valid reason, disregard for possible carryover effect, sequence effect, inappropriate statistical analyses, difficulty in interpreting side effect data, etc. Consequently, the Division of Biometrics decided to present this matter to the FDA Biometric and Epidemiological Methodology Advisory Committee (BEMAC) at a meeting on June 23, 1976. This was an open meeting. Statisticians from FDA, the pharmaceutical industry, and academia made presentations at the meeting and a lively discussion ensued. The audience participation, particularly from drug sponsors, was stimulating. Finally, a report on the two-period crossover design and its applicability in trials of clinical effectiveness was issued by the BEMAC. In essence, the BEMAC made the following recommendations.

---

*Presented at the Professional Postgraduate Services Symposium on September 11, 1984. This symposium was held on September 11–12, 1984, at Bethesda Marriott Hotel, Bethesda, MA. The views expressed in this paper are those of the author and not necessarily of the Food and Drug Administration. Also a version of this work appears in Dubey (1986).

B. BEMAC Recommendations

1. General

In general, the two-period crossover design except in some circumstances is not the design of choice in clinical trials when unequivocal evidence of treatment effect is required.

In most cases, the completely randomized (or randomized block) design with baseline measurements will be the design of choice because it furnishes unbiased estimates of treatment effects without appeal to any modeling assumptions save those associated with the randomization procedure itself.

2. Specific

a. Treatment by period interaction. If there is a treatment by period interaction with unequal period effects ($\pi_{AB} \neq \pi_{BA}$) then the estimate of treatment effect is biased. On the other hand, if the period effects are equal ($\pi_{AB} = \pi_{BA}$), then the estimate of treatment effect is unbiased. The assumption of no treatment by period interaction is not justified under any of the following conditions:

- If the drug produces a permanent effect or "cure";
- If the drug is excreted slowly;
- If the drug produces delayed effects beyond the washout period, either beneficial or adverse; or
- If the natural history of the disease being studied undergoes rapid change or evolution.

The BEMAC report further recommends that the agency should encourage experimental designs that yield unbiased estimates of treatment effects that are as model free as possible, and should require persuasive evidence of the validity of any assumptions that are necessary to establish the unbiasedness of the estimates; and in light of the above criterion the crossover experiment should be designed with sufficient sample size to test and detect with high probability an interaction of a specified amount. Such a requirement for power in detecting a departure from the assumption of no interaction would require a large sample size.

The BEMAC report also makes an alternative recommendation concerning the assumption of no interaction. It is: Supply data and arguments, apart from the experiment at hand, that would justify the assumption of no interaction. Given extensive prior experience with the disease, the end points to be used, and the drugs under study, convincing support for the assumption might be marshaled.

b. Baseline, normality, and analysis. The BEMAC report

encourages the use of baseline information in the analysis by employing difference responses of treatment minus baseline changes, use of analysis of covariance procedures if assumptions are met, and use of percentages change from baseline values.

The report recognizes that the assumption of normality may not always be applicable, nor may the variability from treatment to treatment, period to period, or sequence to sequence always be similar. In such instances one may need to resort to less model-dependent approaches, such as randomization tests.

Finally, the report recommends that the crossover experiments should be analyzed as a crossover design. That is, appropriate account should be assigned to period effect, treatment effect, sequence effect, and possible interaction of treatment by period effect. First-period treatment effect should be analyzed separately; a test for interaction should always be performed and a decision should be made to not make a combined estimate of effects over both periods if the data indicate it is not warranted.

C. Impact of the BEMAC Recommendations

1. Post BEMAC Period: Drug Sponsors and FDA Statistical Reviewers

As a result of the BEMAC recommendations a marked drop in the use of crossover designs was experienced. This trend continued for several years. In early 1982, a small survey was conducted among statistical reviewers of the Statistical Evaluation and Research Branch with a view to determining several things. One of the these dealt with the frequency of the use of crossover designs in clinical trials. We obtained a count of 11 crossover designs out of 90 clinical trials in 19 consecutive new drug applications. This gives a figure of 12%. However, recently we have experienced an increasing use of crossover studies in NDA submissions with a number of troublesome problems. Its use ranges between 20% and 50% for some drug classes. Many of these crossover trials have not been designed, analyzed, or interpreted properly, a fact with which other researchers have also been concerned.

2. Post BEMAC Period: Drug Researchers

Possibly because of the BEMAC Report, statistical researchers became active in researching critical research problems in the field of crossover designs. Their research efforts have produced several publications on the topic of crossover designs and analyses in prominent scientific journals.

The main recommendations and results from selected publications are summarized here.

a. Two-by-two crossover Designs. Hills and Armitage (1979) recommended that a crossover trial should always be large enough for it to be analyzed as a parallel group study. The trial should also be large enough for any appreciable interaction to be detected on a between subject basis. Brown (1980a) noted that the crossover experiment can yield great savings in cost if the assumption of no carryover effect is valid. However, the design should not be used if this assumption is in doubt.

Fisher and Wallenstein (1981) indicated that crossover designs can be very valuable to the investigator in those situations where the procedure is valid; that statisticians should be cautioned that the theoretical advantages of crossover designs are frequently not obtained because of nonlinear disease status from one period to another; and that side effects are more informative and easier to interpret in parallel than in crossover studies. Finally, Huitson et al. (1982) observed that:

1. The crossover trial may be designed to detect a possible treatment difference at an early stage of drug evaluation. On the other hand, the parallel-group design may be used to confirm previous indications of efficacy.
2. If it is likely that the treatment will produce an irreversible change in the disease state (e.g., "healing") then the choice of a parallel-group study is mandatory.
3. Patients may be subject to overriding influences, unrelated to treatment, leading even to withdrawal. For example, a major life event (e.g., bereavement) might exert much more effect than the treatment. Under these circumstances, if an appreciable withdrawal occurs, crossover design must not be used.
4. When the estimated interaction effect exceeds the estimated drug effect it will be impossible to deduce which drug is preferable. Consequently crossover design is not helpful in indicating preference for a drug.

b. Research Results on Extended Crossover Designs. Kershner and Federer (1981) considered designs other than the two-by-two. The following definitions are necessary to understand the statements to be made below regarding the research of Kershner and Federer.

A *direct treatment effect* is the effect that a treatment has on the response of an experimental unit during the period of application.

A *residual treatment effect* is an effect of the treatment that lasts beyond the period of application.

There are several types of residual effects.

First-order residual effects are effects that last only one period beyond application. Likewise, second, third, . . . , kth order residual effects last for two, three, . . . , and k periods, respectively, beyond the period of application.

The magnitude of these residual effects is often a function of the length of the treatment period.

The arithmetic sum of the direct treatment effect and the first-, second-, . . . , and kth-order residual effects of the treatment is defined as the *cumulative treatment effect*. The effect so defined requires that there is no interaction between the various treatment effects.

In view of the definitions given above, the following designs

Design number	Design
D 2.3.4	AB
	BA
	BA
D 4.3.1	ABAB
	ABBA
	BABA
D 4.4.1	ABAB
	ABBA
	BABA
	BAAB

provide estimators of contrasts among direct, among residual and among cumulative effects in a variety of settings. In addition, designs D 4.3.1 and D 4.4.1 provide estimators of contrasts among second-order residual effects, among direct by residual interactions, and among direct by period interaction effects under a variety of models. For the two treatment case, the simplest contrast would be difference between two treatment mean effects.

Laska, Meisner, and Kershner (1982) noted that under either the random patient-effect model with sequence effects or the fixed patient-effect model, the usual two-period, two-treatment crossover design, AB, BA, cannot be used to estimate the contrast between direct treatment effects when unequal carryover effects are present. If baseline observations is more efficient. In fact, they show that this design is optimal*

*When there are two treatments, a universally optimal design has the property that the variance of the best linear unbiased estimator (BLUE) of a contrast (difference between two treatment mean effects) is minimum over the class of competing designs.

whether or not baseline observations are available. For experiments with more than two periods, universally optimal designs are found for both models, with and without carryover effects. It is shown that uncertainty about the presence of carryover effects is of little or no consequence, and the addition of baseline observations is of little or no added value for designs with three or more periods; however, if the experiment is limited to only two periods the investigator pays a heavy penalty.

Ebbutt (1984) recommended the following three-period, two-treatment crossover design, which allows carryover effects to be tested against the within-subject variability.

	Sequence 1	Sequence 2	Sequence 3	Sequence 4
Period 1	A	B	A	B
Period 2	B	A	B	A
Period 3	B	A	A	B

It should be noted that (1) if the extra treatment period leads to an excessive number of withdrawals, it will still be possible to analyze the first two periods in the usual way, and (2) extension of the two-period design to three periods would not be practical for all trials because of a variety of reasons (e.g., prolongation of trial may be become unacceptable). Further (3), use of the extended design in a series of trials in a particular therapeutic area might enable a return to the two-period crossover design, with more confidence in its validity.

The last point conveys a scientific hope, designed to provide inspiration to devoted researchers.

D. FDA Clinical Guidelines Relevant to Crossover Designs

The FDA clinical guidelines for the development of drugs for various indications are widely available. They may be used to form the following categories of indications relevant to using crossover designs in clinical trials forming the basis for an NDA for such indications.

Indications for which crossover designs are recommended are analgesics, antianginals, anticonvulsants, antiinflammatories (ankylosing spondylitis), and hypnotics.

Indications for which crossover designs are permitted are antianxiety agents, psychoactive drugs in children, and radiopharmaceuticals.

Indications for which crossover designs are permitted but discouraged are antacids, antiarrhythmics, antidepressants, antidiarrheals, bronchodilators, gastric secretory depressants, g.i. motility modifiers, and laxatives.

Indications for which crossover designs are not recommended are antiinfectives, osteoporosis, dental caries agents, general anesthetics, local anesthetics, and periodontal disease agents.

Overall, the 22 FDA clinical guidelines with respect to the use of crossover designs may be summarized as follows:

Recommendation	Frequency	Percentage
Crossover recommended	5	23%
Permitted	3	13%
Permitted but discouraged	8	36%
Not recommended	6	28%

E. Impact of the FDA Clinical Guidelines

It follows from the above data that a drug sponsor may attempt to use crossover designs in 16 different drug groups out of 22. This comes out to be 73% of cases. Our current experience in the Statistical Evaluation and Research Branch suggests that the crossover designs are being used in the range of 20% to 50% depending on the disease and drug class. Thus one may infer that FDA's BEMAC recommendation regarding the use of crossover designs has some impact on drug sponsors.

F. Recent Experience

Our experience reflects the joint impact of the BEMAC recommendations, the FDA clinical guidelines, and the regular interaction between FDA reviewers and drug sponsors through meetings and review communications. The updating process of the FDA clinical guidelines is a continuing activity at the Center for Drugs and Biologics.

According to the Guidelines for the Clinical Evaluation of Antianxiety Drugs a crossover design may be permitted for antianxiety drugs, but in actuality our statistical reviewers have not seen the use of crossover designs for antianxiety drugs for some time. A crossover design is generally not used for analgesics except in the case of cancer patients where pain is involved. In the case of antiinflammatories, the frequency of use of crossover designs has decreased markedly.

In a motion sickness study a crossover design was used properly and analyzed properly by a drug sponsor. In a chronic skin condition, crossover design has been considered proper and a clinical trial has been conducted. Crossover designs have been used for sleep aid studies and have been found to be inappropriate or incorrectly analyzed. In cancer therapy, several crossover trials were conducted for nausea and vomiting and they were done properly. Also, crossover designs have been used for heartburn studies and they have been found acceptable by our reviewers. Crossover designs have been also used for menopausal flushing and have been handled properly by drug sponsors.

Use of crossover designs in antiarrhythmics has been troublesome from the statistical review standpoint. Patients recruited in antiarrhythmic drug trials are often severely sick. This causes high within-patient variability. Besides, dropout rates are high. Also, the number of patients entered into the trial is not sufficient to verify crucial assumptions of the crossover designs and analyses. FDA's statistical reviewers still find in the NDA submissions data of both periods pooled and a single analysis performed, which is an example of bad statistical practice.

Wrong designs, improper analyses, lack of "washout" between treatments for no valid reason, disregard for possible carryover effect, inadequate number of patients in the trial for detecting true carryover effect, and lack of baseline measurements for each treatment period are some of the common difficulties our statistical reviewers have experienced in reviewing crossover trials.

G. Concluding Comments

Further research has confirmed the soundness of the BEMAC recommendations regarding the use of the two-period crossover designs in clinical trials. Both clinical investigators and clinical statisticians have recognized the virtues of these recommendations. A considerable degree of caution has been exercised by drug researchers in the choice of crossover designs in clinical trials. Nevertheless, critical problems still exist in the use of crossover trials. Some of the problems are:

- Inadequate number of patients to verify crucial assumptions of the crossover designs;
- Lack of baseline measurements for each treatment period;
- Lack of "washout" between treatment periods for no valid reason;
- High dropout of patients;
- Interpretation of side effects data because of possible carryover effect; and
- Inadequate analysis relative to the design.

With more effective and timely communications between FDA reviewers and drug sponsors, I am hopeful that our current problems associated with the crossover trials will be vanishing in a rational way.

I will conclude by making the following constructive suggestions. Crossover designs may be used when:

Objective measurements and interpretable data for both efficacy and safety are obtainable.

Chronic (relatively stable) diseases are under study.

Prophylactic drugs with relatively short half-lives are being investigated.

Relatively short treatment periods are considered.

Baseline and washout periods are feasible.

An adequate number of patients to detect carryover effect with high power, taking into account expected dropouts, is feasible or extra study information is available to rule out carry over effects.

Analyses appropriate to the design are carried out.

Otherwise, parallel designs are preferable.

APPENDIX 1: SURVEY OF USE OF CROSSOVER DESIGNS IN CLINICAL TRIALS DURING LAST *FIVE* YEARS

Name ______________________ (Optional)
Phone ______________________ (Optional)

Design*	Therapeutic indication	Phase of clinical development	Use of washout periods in design? Yes or No	Use of baseline values in analysis? Yes or No	Primary reason for using this design	Year when used	FDA's response, if any	Your suggestions or comments

*Type of crossover designs: (1) 2-treatment, 2-period, (2) 2-treatment, 3-period, (3) 2-treatment, 4-period, (4) 3 × 3 or higher order Latin square. If you used any other design, please specify it in the "design" column.

APPENDIX 2: FDA CLINICAL GUIDELINES

FDA 77-3042 Guidelines for the Clinical Evaluation of Antidepressant Drugs (GPO 017-012-00247-1, $1.00).

FDA 77-3043 Guidelines for the Clinical Evaluation of Antianxiety Drugs (GPO 017-012-00248-0, $1.00).

FDA 77-3044 Guidelines for the Clinical Evaluation of Radiopharmaceutical Drugs (GPO 017-012-00249-8, $1.50).

FDA 77-3046 Guidelines for the Clinical Evaluation of Anti-Infective Drugs (Systemic) (Adults and Children) (GPO 017-012-00250-1, $0.90).

FDA 78-3047 Guidelines for the Clinical Evaluation of Anti-Anginal Drugs (GPO 017-012-00259-5, $0.70).

FDA 78-3048 Guidelines for the Clinical Evaluation of Anti-Arrhythmic Drugs (GPO 017-012-00256-1, $0.80).

FDA 78-3049 Guidelines for the Clinical Evaluation of Antidiarrheal Drugs (GPO 017-012-00257-9, $1.00).

FDA 78-3050 Guidelines for the Clinical Evaluation of Gastric Secretory Depressant (GSD) Drugs (GPO 017-012-00252-8, $0.90).

FDA 78-3051 Guidelines for the Clinical Evaluation of Hypnotic Drugs (GPO 017-012-00253-6, $1.00).

FDA 78-3052 Guidelines for the Clinical Evaluation of General Anesthetics (GPO 017-012-00254-4, $0.90).

FDA 78-3053 Guidelines for the Clinical Evaluation of Local Anesthetics (GPO 017-012-00255-2, $0.80).

FDA 78-3054 Guidelines for the Clinical Evaluation of Anti-Inflammatory Drugs (Adults and Children) (GPO 017-012-00258-7, $1.50).

FDA 78-3065 Guidelines for the Clinical Evaluation of Antacid Drugs (GPO 017-012-00261-7, $0.90).

FDA 78-3066 Guidelines for the Clinical Evaluation of G.I. Motility-Modifying Drugs (GPO 017-012-00262-5, $0.90).

FDA 78-3067 Guidelines for the Clinical Evaluation of Laxative Drugs (GPO 017-012-00263-3, $0.90).

FDA 79-3055 Guidelines for the Clinical Evaluation of Psychoactive Drugs in Infants and Children (GPO 017-012-00281-1, $4.75).

FDA 79-3073 Guidelines for the Clinical Evaluation of Bronchodilator Drugs (GPO 017-012-00271-4, $0.80).

FDA 79-3074 Guidelines for the Clinical Evaluation of Drugs to

	Prevent, Control and/or Treat Periodontal Disease (GPO 017-012-00272-2, $0.80).
FDA 79-3075	Guidelines for the Clinical Evaluation of Drugs to Prevent Dental Caries (GPO 017-012-00273-1, $0.90).
FDA 80-3093	Guidelines for the Clinical Evaluation of Analgesic Drugs (GPO 017-012-00283-8, $1.50).
FDA 80-3094	Guidelines for the Clinical Evaluation of Drugs Used in the Treatment of Osteoporosis (GPO 017-012-00284-6, $1.25).
FDA 81-3110	Guidelines for the Clinical Evaluation of Antiepileptic Drugs (Adults and Children) (GPO 017-012-00292-7, $1.50).

BIBLIOGRAPHY

Albohali, M., and Milliken, G. A. (1984). A practical approach for analyzing repeated measures data with autocorrelated errors. *Am. Stat. Assoc., Proceedings of Biopharmaceutical Section*.

Andersen, A. H., Jensen, E. B., and Geart, S. (1981). Two-way analysis of variance with correlated errors. *International Statistical Review 49:* 153–169.

Anderson, O. D. (1979). The formulae for the expected values of the sample variance and covariances from series generated by general autoregressive integrated moving average processes of order (p, d, q). *Sankhya B, 41:* 177–195.

Armitage, P. and Hills, M. (1982). The two-period crossover trial. *The Statistician, 31:* 119–131.

Azzalini, A. (1984). Estimation and hypothesis testing for collections of autoregressive time series. *Biometrika, 71:* 85–90.

Balaam, L. N. (1965). A two-period designator treatment by period interaction. Paper no. Bu-177-M, Biometrics Unit, Cornell University, Ithaca, NY.

Biometric and Epidemiological Methodology Advisory Committee to the FDA, minutes of the meetings, June 23, December 6, 1976.

Bishop, S. H. and Jones, B. (1984). A review of higher-order crossover designs. *Journal of Applied Statistics, 11:* 29–50.

Boadi-Boateng, F. (1983). A crossover design with "choice." Master's thesis, University of Washington, Seattle.

Bora, A. C. (1985). Changeover design with first-order residual effects and errors following a first-order autoregressive process. *The Statistician, 34:* 161–173.

Box, G. E. P., and Cox, D. R. (1964). An analysis of transformations. *Journal of the Royal Statistical Society, Series B, 26:* 211–252.

Brown, B. W. (1980a). The crossover experiment for clinical trials. *Biometrics, 36:* 69–79.

Brown, B. W. (1980b). Statistical controversies in the design of clinical trials—Some personal views. *Controlled Clinical Trials, 1:* 19–21.

Castellana, J. V. and Patel, H. I. (1985). Analysis of two-period crossover design in a multicenter clinical trial. *Biometrics, 41:* 969–977.

Chassan, J. B. (1970). A note on relative efficiency in clinical trials. *Journal of Clinical Pharmacology*, 359–360.

Ciminera, J. L., Bolognese, J. A. and Gregg, H. H. (1987). The statistical evaluation of a three-period two-treatment crossover pharmacokinetic drug interaction study. *Biometrics, 43:* 713–718.

Cochran, W. G. and Cox, G. M. (1957). *Experimental Designs*, 2nd Ed., New York: John Wiley & Sons.

Cox, D. R. (1958). *Planning of Experiments*. New York: John Wiley & Sons.

Dixon, W. J. (1953). Power functions of the sign test and power efficacy for normal alternatives. *Annals of Mathematical Statistics, 24:* 467–473.

Dubey, J. (1986) Current thoughts on crossover designs. *Clinical Research Practice and Drug Regulation, 4 (no. 2):* 187.

Ebbutt, A. F. (1984). Three-period crossover designs for two-treatments. *Biometrics, 40:* 219–224.

Farewell, V. T. (1985). Some remarks on the analysis of crossover trials with a binary response. *Applied Statistics, 34:* 121–128.

Fava, G. M., and Buhite, S. G. (1981). The analysis of conditional crossover designs. Presented at the *Combined Annual Scientific Sessions of the Society for Clinical Trials and the Eighth Annual Symposium for Coordinating Clinical Trials*, San Francisco.

Fidler, V. (1984). Changeover clinical trial with binary data: Mixed-model-based comparison of tests. *Biometrics, 40:* 1063–1070.

Fisher, A. C., and Wallenstein, S. (1981). Crossover designs in medical research, in *Statistics in the Pharmaceutical Industry* (Buncher and Tsay, eds.). New York: Marcel Dekker, Inc. pp. 139–156.

Fleiss, J. L., Wallenstein, S., and Rosenfeld, R. (1985). Adjusting for baseline measurements in the two-period crossover study: A cautionary note. *Controlled Clinical Trials, 6:* 192–197.

Fleiss, J. L. (1986a). Letter: On multiperiod crossover studies. *Biometrics, 42:* 449–450.

Fleiss, J. L. (1986b). *The Design and Analysis of Clinical Experiments*. New York: John Wiley and Sons.

Fleiss, J. L. (1989). A critique of recent research on the two-treatment crossover design. *Controlled Clinical Trials* (to appear).

Gart, J. J. (1969). An exact test for comparison matched proportions in crossover designs. *Biometrika, 56:* 75–80.

Grieve, A. P. (1985). A Bayesian analysis of the two-period crossover design for clinical trials. *Biometrics, 41:* 979–990.

Grieve, A. P. (1987). A note on the analysis of the two-period crossover design when the period-treatment interaction is significant. *Biometrics Journal, 29:* 771–775.

Grizzle, J. E. (1965). The two-period changeover design and its use in clinical trials. *Biometrics, 21:* 467–480. Corrigenda in *Biometrics, 30:* 727 (1974).

Heydayet, A. and Afsarinejad, K. (1978). Repeat measurements design, II. *Annals of Statistics*, *6:* 619–628.

Hills, M., and Armitage, P. (1979). The two-period crossover clinical trial. *British Journal of Clinical Pharmacology*, *8:* 7–20.

Huitson, A., Polonecki, J., Hews, R., and Barker, N. (1982). A review of crossover trials. *The Statistician*, *31:* 71–80.

Jennrich, R. I., and Schlucter, M. D. (1986). Unbalanced repeated measures models with structured covariance matrices. *Biometrics*, *42:* 805–820.

Johnson, D. E. (1986). Considerations for using extended-period crossover designs. *Proceedings of the 1986 Biopharmaceutical Section of the American Statistical Association*, 183–187.

Jones, B. (1986). Discussion on crossover designs and repeated measures. *Proceedings of the 1986 Biopharmaceutical Section of the American Statistical Association*, 161–162.

Jones, B., and Kenward, M. G. (1987). Modelling binary data from a three-period crossover trial. *Statistics in Medicine*, *6:* 555–564.

Kenward, M. G., and Jones, B. (1987a). A log-linear model for binary crossover data. *Journal of the Royal Statistical Society-C*, *36:* 192–204.

Kenward, M. G., and Jones, B. (1987b). The analysis of data from 2 × 2 crossover trials with baseline measurements. *Statistics in Medicine*, *6:*911–926.

Kershner, R. P. (1986). Optimal three-period two-treatment crossover designs with and without baseline readings. *Proceedings of the 1986 Biopharmaceutical Section of the American Statistical Association*, 152–156.

Kershner, R. P., and Federer, W. T. (1981). Two-treatment crossover designs for estimating a variety of effects. *Journal of the American Statistical Association*, *76:* 612–619.

Klotz, J. H. (1966). The Wilcoxon, ties and the computer. *Journal of the American Statistical Association*, *6:* 772–787.

Koch, G. G. (1972). The use of nonparametric methods in the statistical analysis of the two-period changeover design. *Biometrics*, *28:* 577–584.

Koch, M. (1986). A cost analysis of the two-period crossover with baselines. Presented at the *Meeting of the American Statistical Association*, Chicago.

Kunest, J. (1987). On variance estimation in crossover designs. *Biometrics*, *43:* 833–845.

Lakatos, E. and Raghavarao, D. (1987). Undiminished residual effects designs and their suggested applications. *Communications in Statistics—A*, *16:* 1345–1350.

Laska, E., Meisner, M., and Kushner, H. B. (1981). Designs for carryover and effects. Technical report, Information Sciences Division, Rockland Research Institute, Orangeburg, NY.

Laska, E. M., Meisner, M., and Kushner, H. B. (1983). Optimal crossover designs in the presence of carryover effect. *Biometrics*, *39:* 1087–1091.

Laska, E. M., and Meisner, M. (1985). A variational approach to optimal two-treatment crossover designs: Applications to carryover effect models. *Journal of the American Statistical Association*, *80:* 704–710.

Layard, M. W. J. and Arvesen, J. N. (1978). Analysis of Poisson data in crossover experimental designs. *Biometrics*, *34:* 421–428.

Le, C. T. (1984). Logistic models for crossover designs. *Biometrika*, 216–217.

Lee, C. T. (1984). Prediction and estimation of growth curves with special covariance structures. *Journal of the American Statistical Association*, *83:* 432–440.

Lee, M. L., Kantrowitz, J. L., and Mullis, C. E. (1984). Sample size, crossover trials and the problem of treatment equivalence. *Proceedings of the 1984 Biopharmaceutical Section of the American Statistical Association*, 78–79.

Lehman, E. L. (1975). *Non-Parametrics: Statistical Methods Based on Ranks*. San Francisco: Holden-Day.

Lewis, J. (1983). Clinical trials: Statistical developments of practical benefit to the pharmaceutical industry with discussion and reply. *Journal of the Royal Statistical Society—A*, *146:* 362–393.

Leung, H. M. (1984). Clinical trials in antiarrhythmic drugs: A statistical reviewer's experience. *Proceedings of the 1984 Biopharmaceutical Section of the American Statistical Association*, 87–90.

Louis, T. A., Lavori, Bailar, and Polansky, M. (1981). Crossover and self-controlled designs in clinical research. *New England Journal of Medicine*, 24–31.

Lucas, H. L. (1950). Design and analysis of experiments with milking dairy cattle. Series 18, Institute of Statistics, North Carolina State University, Raleigh, NC.

Lucas, H. L. (1951). Bias in estimation of error in changeover trials with dairy cattle. *Journal of Agricultural Science*, *41:*146–148.

Matthews, J. N. S. (1987). Optimal crossover designs for the comparison of two-treatments in the presence of carryover effects and autocorrelated errors. *Biometrika*, *74:* 311–320.

McHugh, R., and Gomez-Marin, O. (1987). Randomization and additivity in the two-period crossover clinical trial. *Biometrics Journal*, *29:* 961–970.

McNair, D. M. (1971). Antianxiety drugs and human performance. *Archives of General Psychiatry*, *29:*611–617.

McNemar, Q (1947). Note on the sampling error of the difference between correlation proportions of percentages. *Psychometrika*, *12;* 153–157.

Nam, J. (1971). On two tests for comparing matched proportions. *Biometrics*, *27:* 945–59.

O'Neill et al. (1977). FDA Position. BEMAC Report.

O'Neill, R. T. (1978). Subject-own control designs in clinical drug trials: Overview of issues with emphasis on the two treatment problem. Presented at 1978 Annual NCDEU Meeting, Key Biscayne, FL.

Pantula, S. G., and Pollock, K. H. (1985). Nested analysis of variance with autocorrelated errors. *Biometrics*, *41:* 909–920.

Patel, H. I. (1983). The use of baseline measurements in two-period crossover design in clinical trials. *Communications in Statistics—A*, *12:* 2693–2712.

Patel, H. I. (1985). Analysis of incomplete data in a two-period crossover design with reference to clinical trials. *Biometrika*, *72:* 411–418.

Patel, H. I. (1986). Analysis of repeated measures design with changing covariates in clinical trials. *Biometrika*, *73:* 707–715.

Patel, H. I., and Hearne, E. M. (1980). Multivariate analysis for the two-period

repeated measures crossover deign with application to clinical trials. *Communications in Statistics—Theory and Methods*, *18:* 1919–1929.
Patterson, H. P. (1950). The analysis of changeover trials. *Journal of the Royal Statistical Society—B*, *24:* 937–951.
Peace, K. E. (1983). Discussion, Biopharmaceutical Section Proceedings of the American Statistical Association, 27–28.
Petric, A. (1982). The Crossover Design *in The Randomized Clinical Trial and Therapeutic Decisions*. (Tygst, N., Lachin, J. M. and Juhl, E., eds.) New York: Marcel Dekker, Inc.
Pigeon, J. G., and Raghavarao, D. (1987). Crossover designs for comparing treatments with a control. *Biometrika*, *74:* 321–328.
Pocock, S. J. (1983). *Clinical Trials, A Practical Approach*. New York: John Wiley and Sons.
Prescott, R. J. (1981). The comparison of success rates in crossover trials in the presence of an order effect. *Applied Statistics*, *30:* 9–15.
Racine-Poon, A., Grieve, A. P., Fluehler, H., and Smith, A. F. M., (1987). A two-stage procedure for bioequivalence studies. *Biometrics*, *43:* 847–850.
Sato, S. et al. (1982). Valproic acid versus ethosuximide in the treatment of absence seizures. *Neurology*, *32:* 157–163.
Selwyn, M. R., Dempster, A. P., and Hall, N. R. (1981). A Bayesian approach to bioequivalence for the 2×2 changeover design. *Biometrics*, *37:* 11–22.
Shah, B. K. (1980). A note on two period crossover design. Rockland Research Institute, Orangeburg, NY.
Tsai, K. T., and Patel, H. I. (1987). Nonparametric methods for analyzing a two-period crossover design with baseline measurements. *Proceedings of the 1987 Biopharmaceutical Section of the American Statistical Association*, 35–40.
Wallenstein, S. (1979). Abstract: Inclusion of baseline values in the analysis of crossover designs. *Biometrics*, *35:* 894.
Wallenstein, S. (1986). Analysis of crossover design with baseline. *Proceedings of the 1986 Biopharmaceutical Section of the American Statistical Association*, 157–160.
Wallenstein, S., and Fisher, A. C. (1977). The analysis of the two-period repeated measurements crossover design with application to clinical trials. *Biometrics*, *33:* 261–269.
Wallenstein, S., and Fleiss, J. L. (1988). The two-period crossover design with baseline measurements. *Communications in Statistics*, *17:* 3333–3343.
White, B. G. (1979). A class of ethical designs for controlled clinical trials. Doctoral dissertation, Johns Hopkins University, Baltimore, MD.
Willan, A. R., and Pater, J. L. (1986a). Carryover and the two-period crossover clinical trials. *Biometrics*, *42:* 593–599.
Willan, A. R., and Pater, J. L. (1986b). Using baseline measurements in the two-period crossover clinical trial. *Controlled Clinical trials*, *7:* 282–289.
Zimmerman, H. and Rahlfs, V. (1978). Testing hypotheses in the two-period changeover design with binary data. *Biometrical Journal*, *20:* 133–142.
Zimmerman, H. and Rahlfs, V. (1980). Model building and testing for the changeover design. *Biometrical Journal*, *22:* 147–210.

4
Active Control Equivalence Studies

Robert W. Makuch *Yale University, New Haven, Connecticut*

Gordon Pledger *National Institutes of Health, Bethesda, Maryland*

David B. Hall *Centers for Disease Control, Atlanta, Georgia*

Mary F. Johnson *G. H. Besselaar Associates, Princeton, New Jersey*

Jay Herson *Applied Logic Associates, Inc., Houston, Texas*

Jiann-Ping Hsu* *Food and Drug Administration, Rockville, Maryland*

I. INTRODUCTION

Robert W. Makuch

The purpose of this chapter is to discuss a relatively new type of clinical trial that is designed to establish the equivalence between a new and standard treatment. We call this type of study an active control equivalence study (ACES). The reasons for undertaking this type of trial are compelling. In many disease areas, current standard treatments reflect a series of previous successes in the development of new therapies. It is often unethical to design a study where the new treatment of interest is compared to a placebo, or no-treatment, control rather than to a currently effective control. Whereas the discovery that a new treatment is actually superior in efficacy to the active control would be a

**Present affiliation:* Warner-Lambert Company, Ann Arbor, Michigan.

highly desirable result, and one in which standard methodologic principles would apply, achievement of the more modest goal of efficacy "equivalence" while minimizing side effects or reducing the cost of therapy would still render the trial a success.

In Section II, Pledger and Hall emphasize that an ACES yields only *indirect* evidence as to the efficacy of a new treatment because one must depend on data external to the study. This is referred to as the "historical control assumption." They motivate their discussion using some studies submitted to the Food and Drug Administration in support of a labeling revision for cimetidine. In Section III, Makuch and Johnson present their views on a number of topics that are pertinent to the design and interpretation of an ACES. These issues include (1) hypothesis testing versus estimation, (2) sample size for an ACES, (3) "intent-to-treat" versus "efficacy" analysis, and (4) the "historical control assumption." Next, Herson reviews the inferential, operational, and analytic considerations associated with an ACES in Section IV. He also provides some recommendations concerning the appropriate methodology and regulatory practice for these considerations. Finally, Hsu considers the assessment of statistical evidence from ACES in Section V.

II. ACTIVE CONTROL EQUIVALENCE STUDIES: DO THEY ADDRESS THE EFFICACY ISSUE?*

Gordon Pledger and David Hall

The most natural context for an active control clinical trial is one in which the question of interest is whether a test drug is superior in some way to a standard drug. There, the active control study provides direct evidence regarding the question of interest. In this section, we are interested primarily in a situation where positive control studies yield only indirect evidence, that is, the situation in which a new drug is not necessarily expected to represent a therapeutic advancement over existing treatment, but proof of effectiveness is sought. For a variety of reasons, the use of active control studies in this situation, already common, is becoming more frequent. However, the way in which these studies are usually planned, analyzed, and reported indicates that there is a need for a careful consideration of the requirements for demonstrating efficacy by this indirect approach. We attempt to present such a consideration below.

---

*Reprinted from the 1986 Proceedings of the Biopharmaceutical Section of the American Statistical Association.

A. The Problem

There is only one direct test of effectiveness of a new drug therapy. Response of patients treated with the drug are compared to responses of similar (or the same) patients treated with an indistinguishable inactive preparation. However, in many cases, a study design permitting this direct assessment of efficacy may be contraindicated because of considerations involving ethics or feasibility. Generally, examples of the latter involve problems with blinding or with unacceptably high or disparate attrition rates. Another type of example is the situation, as with some dermatological and some aerosol drug products, in which the vehicle has been found to have a deleterious effect on the condition being treated. (In this case, a drug versus vehicle study could still show activity, but this would not necessarily imply effectiveness.)

In order to see exactly what sort of information is lost due to the unavailability, for whatever reason, of a direct test for efficacy in a study, it is useful to begin by considering what information is gained with an "ideal" study design. Therefore, consider a design allowing comparisons among three treatments: a test drug (A), an active control (B), and placebo (P). This design not only permits a direct test for efficacy of A but also places the hypothesis test in context by allowing an internal check on the detectability of activity of the positive control drug B. The possible outcomes of the study can be listed by means of a shorthand notation in which left-to-right order indicates decreasing sample means (assume bigger is better) and > indicates a "statistically significant" paired difference. Thus, AB > P means that the observed mean for treatment B was less than that for A and more than that for P, with the A versus P and the B versus P comparisons being statistically significant. Using this convention, the possible outcomes and likely explanations are given in Table 4.1.

We are interested primarily in the situation where the goal is to show that the experimental drug A and the tested dose of B are "equally effective." Thus, Table 4.1 assumes that an attempt was made to adjust the dose of B to a level that would produce a response similar to the expected response to A.

The case in which A is expected to be effective but less so than B is similar but less common, while the case in which the goal is to show A superior to B is essentially different and is analytically similar to a placebo control study. In this context, the only successful outcomes of the study are AB > P and BA > P, that is, only these two outcomes are truly consistent with pretrial expectations. Any other outcome is, to some extent, a study failure and should provide information useful in modifying the design for future studies.

TABLE 4.1 Possible outcomes of A versus B versus P study[a]

Outcome	Explanation/Comment
AB > P	Expected result
BA > P	Expected result
ABP, A > P	Expected result or insensitivity
BAP, B > P	Insensitivity or dose of B too high
A > BP	Insensitivity or dose of B too low
B > AP	Failure of test drug
A > B > P	Dose of B too low
B > A > P	Dose of B too high
APB, A > B	Insensitivity or dose of B too low
BPA, B > A	Insensitivity or failure of test drug
AP > B	Inconsistent B vs. P result
BP > A	Insensitivity and failure of test drug
A > PB	Insensitivity or dose of B too low
B > PA	Failure of test drug
A > P > B	Inconsistent B vs. P result
B > P > A	Failure of test drug
PAB, P > B	Inconsistent B vs. P result
PBA, P > A	Insensitivity and failure of test drug
PA > B	Inconsistent B vs. P result
PB > A	Insensitivity and failure of test drug
P > AB	Inconsistent B vs. P result
P > BA	Inconsistent B vs. P result
P > A > B	Inconsistent B vs. P result
P > B > A	Inconsistent B vs. P result and failure of test drug
PAB	Insensitivity
PBA	Insensitivity
ABP	Insensitivity
APB	Insensitivity
BAP	Insensitivity
BPA	Insensitivity

[a] A = test drug, B = active control, P = placebo. Left to right order indicates decreasing improvement; > denotes a statistically significant difference.

Now consider this study without the placebo control. Table 4.2 shows the observable outcomes of this restricted study together with the corresponding, now unobservable, outcomes from Table 4.1. It is clear from Table 4.2 that a finding of no significant difference, that is, AB or BA, does not justify an inference that A is effective. (This seems a very elementary point, but exactly that inference is made in study after study

TABLE 4.2 Possible outcomes of A versus B study without placebo versus with placebo[a]

Outcome of A vs. B study	Corresponding outcomes of A vs. B vs. P study
AB	AB > P; ABP, A > P; PAB, P > B; P > BA; APB; ABP; PAB
BA	BA > P; BAP, B > P; PBA, P > A; P > BA; BPA; BAP; PBA
A > B	A > BP; A > B > P; A > PB; ABP, A > B; AP > B; A > P > B; PA > B; P > A > B
B > A	B > AP; B > A > P; B > PA; BPA, B > A; BP > A; B > P > A; PB > A; P > B > A

[a] A = test drug; B = active control; P = placebo. Left to right order indicates decreasing improvement; > denotes a statistically significant difference.

submitted to the Food and Drug Administration and in published studies.) The logical case for efficacy of A requires supplementary extra-study information that would allow one to eliminate those corresponding (unobservable) outcomes that do not support efficacy. Thus, there is a

TABLE 4.3 Results of six trials comparing an experimental antidepressant (NEW), imipramine (IMI), and placebo with placebo data concealed; Hamilton depression scale (HDS) mean scores[a] at last visit[b]

	Common baseline	Drug	Sample size	HDS	*p* Value
Study 1	23.9	NEW	33	13.4	0.78
		IMI	33	12.8	
Study 2	26.0	NEW	39	13.0	.86
		IMI	30	13.4	
Study 3	28.1	NEW	11	19.4	.81
		IMI	11	20.3	
Study 4	29.6	NEW	7	7.3	0.63
		IMI	8	9.5	
Study 5	37.6	NEW	7	21.9	1.00
		IMI	8	21.9	
Study 6	26.1	NEW	37	11.2	0.85
		IMI	32	10.8	

[a] Scores adjusted by analysis of covariance.
[b] Score at 4 weeks or, if none available, last score available prior to 4 weeks.

need for a basis on which to eliminate the possibility that neither A nor B was effective in the study as well as the possibility that the study was not sensitive enough to detect important differences between A and B.

Leber (1983) has presented a specific example illustrating the point made abstractly in Tables 4.1 and 4.2. He discussed six trials, each of which compare a new (potential) antidepressant drug to both a positive control (imipramine) and placebo.

Patients in these trials were classified as moderately-to-severely depressed by standard criteria, including a Hamilton Depression Scale score of at least 18 at baseline. The study results presented by Leber are restricted to (adjusted) Hamilton Depression Scale mean scores, and he indicates that these results are quite representative of results using other

TABLE 4.4 Results of six trials comparing an experimental antidepressant (NEW), imipramine (IMI), and placebo: Hamilton Depression scale (HDS) mean scores[a] at last visit[b]

	Common baseline	Drug	Sample size	HDS
Study 1	23.9	NEW	33	13.4
		IMI	33	12.8
		PBO	36	14.8
Study 2	26.0	NEW	39	13.0
		IMI	30	13.4
		PBO	36	13.9
Study 3	28.1	NEW	11	19.4
		IMI	11	20.3
		PBO	13	18.9
Study 4	29.6	NEW	7	7.3
		IMI	8	9.5
		PBO	7	23.5[c]
Study 5	37.6	NEW	7	21.9
		IMI	8	21.9
		PBO	8	22.0
Study 6	26.1	NEW	37	11.2
		IMI	32	10.8
		PBO	36	10.5

[a]Scores adjusted by analysis of covariance.

[b]Score at 4 weeks or, if none available, last score available prior to 4 weeks.

[c]NEW, IMI better than PBO, $p < 0.001$.

summary measures, such as global physician improvement scores and severity ratings.

Table 4.3 represents only the scores of patients treated with imipramine (IMI), the standard antidepressant, or the experimental drug (NEW). In all six trials mean scores decreased (i.e., improved) over the course of 4 weeks and results for the two drugs were almost identical. Moreover, it appears that both the new drug and the positive control had a sizable effect; Leber states that the patients in studies 1, 2, 4, and 6 "would be considered either recovered or very substantially improved."

The results from the placebo-treated group, included in Table 4.4, change the overall interpretation drastically. Only in study 4, the smallest of the six, was the active control drug distinguished from placebo. The other five trials did not indicate even a favorable trend for imprimine, even though, as Leber points out, "Imipramine is an established standard drug, considered by many expect clinicians to be the drug of choice for the treatment of depressions of this type, and there is no doubt of its effectiveness."

B. Current Approaches

Inattention to details of study design and implementation, while not necessarily a fatal flaw in direct comparison situations, takes on added importance in positive control studies. Methodologic deficiencies that simply diminish the value of a placebo control study can render a positive control study useless. The positive control clinical trial presents a complicated research problem of indirect inference. Current approaches to this difficulty can be characterized as statistical salvage procedures, because rather than rethink the whole experimental inference framework, researchers have concentrated on statistical calculations aimed at assuring "power" with adequate sample sizes and new statistical methods.

If there is any discussion at all of inferential problems in connection with positive control trials it is generally a somewhat superficial consideration of the ability of the study to distinguish between A and B. Usually this discussion involves the statistical power (with either the planned or the actual sample size) to detect some subjectively chosen difference, say D, considered "clinically significant." Sufficient statistical power is taken as grounds for concluding that a nonsignificant difference between A and B implies efficacy of A. This power approach is inadequate for several reasons:

1. It encourages limiting study size, using insensitive measures of response, and allowing study characteristics that needlessly increase variation or obscure A versus B differences. The underly-

ing statistical methodology, hypothesis testing, is asymmetric. It treats a Type I error, incorrectly rejecting the null hypothesis of equivalence of study treatments, as being much more serious than a Type II error, incorrectly failing to reject the null hypothesis. This statistical framework results in an incentive to study adequate numbers of subjects, use precise methods, etc. when the goal of the trial is the rejection of the null hypothesis, as in a placebo control study. However, these incentives are reversed when failure to reject the null hypothesis is taken as evidence of effectiveness.

Temple (1982) points out that an idea of what one should expect when hypothesis testing is misused in this way can be gained from past experience with chronic animal testing and the experience in this area is not reassuring. "In such animal studies, lack of difference from placebo is the 'favorable' outcome, just as it is in the positive control clinical trial. It is clear that in the past, even major pharmaceutical houses tolerated very poor studies, sometimes in their own laboratories and more often in the laboratories of their contractors." Generally, this might have been unintentional, simply a consequence of the absence of the strong push toward excellence which is required to produce a good study.

2. The power approach makes little use of the observed results of the study. As practiced, the observed difference is not considered except as part of a test statistic and the actual observed response rates are given little or no consideration. Neither the observed difference nor the observed variance is scrutinized, compared to historical or theoretical standards, or examined for heterogeneity and other deviations from assumptions.
3. The power approach depends on a quantity D that cannot be empirically validated. The selection of D is usually based on some subjective impression of what would be a meaningful difference in a clinical practice setting. This difference may be quite lacking in relevance to the clinical trial setting in which treatment effects are assessed under rigidly controlled and highly artificial conditions. Generally, there is no basis for relating to clinical practice the magnitude of drug effects seen in a especially chosen group of patients treated under double-blind conditions with a variety of other unusual restrictions on dosage, concomitant medication, scheduled examinations, etc. The choice of an important difference in a clinical trial should be based not on what would be considered important in clinical

practice but on what has been observed previously in similar controlled studies.

There has been some recent work [see Blackwelder and Chang (1982) and references therein] apparently motivated by a recognition of problems (1) and (2) but ignoring (3). The basis of these methods is that a clinically meaningful difference D can be specified and then a null hypothesis constructed, in terms of D, having the form "A and B differ by a clinically significant amount." Then an indication of the effectiveness of A is taken to correspond to rejection of the null hypothesis. This approach, while representing a step in the right direction, still does not go far enough. It is content to answer the question, "Are A and B equivalent?" without addressing the possibility that neither A nor B would have beaten placebo had a placebo group been included in the trial.

C. Alternative Approach

As we have tried to demonstrate, the isolated positive control clinical trial is not an effective research tool. While emphasis should be on better design and implementation, it is also useful to consider statistical approaches that are more properly focused on the relevant questions.

One such approach can be exemplified using some studies submitted to the Food and Drug Administration in support of a labeling revision for cimetidine. The material presented here is from the December 16, 1983 statistical review of the studies written by David Zucker. Cimetidine is approved and widely used in the United States for the treatment of active duodenal ulcer. At the time of these studies, the insert for cimetidine stated that the recommended adult oral dosage of cimetidine for active duodenal ulcer was 300 mg four times a day. The 300 mg q.i.d. regimen was the regimen used in the U.S. clinical trials included in the original New Drug Application submission, although the standard regimen overseas was 200 mg t.i.d. plus 400 mg h.s. There was interest in adding to the package insert a statement that a regimen of 400 mg b.i.d. is also effective and that similar rates of effectiveness have been observed with the 400 mg b.i.d. regimen as with the 300 mg q.i.d. regimen.

The situation here is complicated beyond even the usual positive control situation, because the proposed b.i.d. regimen is compared to the approved U.S. regimen not directly but through a "middleman," the standard European (SE) regimen. Therefore, for purposes of this illustration we will consider only the question of whether there is any statistical evidence that the b.i.d. dosage regimen is effective, in any population. The primary statistical basis for addressing the efficacy question consists of confidence intervals for differences in 4-week healing rates, shown in Table 4.5.

These confidence intervals are based on randomized, endoscopically monitored studies. In each case, concomitant antacids were allowed. The data show reasonable consistency, for example, the SE versus placebo PBO intervals for the two populations are similar, and each of the studies going into computing these intervals numerically favored the SE cimetidine regimen over the placebo with many of the comparisons being statistically significant.

It does not seem reasonable to conclude from the last two intervals that the proposed b.i.d. dosage is equivalent to the SE dosage. In one case, the interval is very wide and in the European studies the results tilt strongly in favor of the active control treatment.

On the other hand, the results of all of these studies taken in combination may provide some statistical evidence that the b.i.d. regimen is superior to placebo with respect to 4-week healing. For example, in the European population, the probability of healing by 4 weeks with the b.i.d. regimen may be reasonably regarded as at worst 0.12 lower than the corresponding probability with the SE regimen, which in turn may be reasonably regarded as at worst 0.29 higher than the corresponding probability with placebo. Consequently, the probability of healing by 4 weeks with the b.i.d. regimen might reasonably be regarded as at worst 0.17 higher than the corresponding probability with placebo. Similarly, in Latin American patients, the probability of healing by 4 weeks with the b.i.d. regimen might reasonably be regarded as at worst 0.14 higher than the corresponding probability with placebo.

However, the evidence has to be viewed with some caution. Although the SE versus PBO difference with respect to probability of healing in 4 weeks appears from the previous studies to be approximately at least 0.28, there is no guarantee that the SE versus PBO difference

TABLE 4.5 Confidence intervals for differences in 4-week ulcer healing rates from controlled cimetidine trials[a]

Comparison	Setting	95% CI
SE minus PBO	Europe, antacids allowed	(0.29, 0.40)
SE minus PBO	Latin America, antacids allowed	(0.28, 0.52)
SE minus BID	Europe, antacids allowed	(0.00, 0.12)
SE minus BID	Latin America, antacids allowed	(−0.13, 0.14)

[a]SE = 200 mg t.i.d. plus 400 mg h.s., BID = 400 mg b.i.d., PBO = placebo.

under the circumstances of the b.i.d. versus SE studies would not be less. In addition, the b.i.d. versus SE studies may have been affected by "positive-control study upward bias." That is, because both patients and physicians knew that every patient was receiving an active drug, patients may have been more likely to feel better or at least claim to feel better, and physicians may have been more likely to find that a patient is healed, than in a double-blind placebo-control study.

The preceding example demonstrates reasoning focused on the efficacy question, and it recognizes that the clinical trial context is different from the clinical practice context. This example also makes clear the "historical control" nature of positive control trials. The presence of the positive control group enabled us to use historical information on the difference between the positive control and placebo response rates, rather than on the placebo rate alone. Hopefully, the difference in response rates will be more stable across trials. In this connection, a useful area for statistical research would be the identification of measures of relative efficacy that combine cross-trial stability and low vulnerability to "positive control bias."

D. Discussion

We wish to avoid overemphasis on methodologic aspects of interpreting data from positive control trials. There is no specific method of analysis that provides "the solution" to the problems presented by these indirect comparisons. The best-intentioned statistical analyses can be invalidated by various characteristics of the design and implementation of the trial.

The comparative clinical trial can provide an internal comparison between treatments, but even when all goes well and the available direct comparisons are what is desired, the results must be interpreted carefully. They mean little or nothing unless there is a frame of reference, a wider context within which the trial and its results can be fit. At a macro level medical research is extraordinarily thorough in establishing a frame of reference. Medical researchers work long hours keeping up with the latest developments in their field of expertise. Unfortunately, seldom is anyone on the research team paying the same attention to establishing a frame of reference at the micro level. To interpret the results of any clinical trial one must have a frame of reference concerning the investigator, the treatment and the measuring instrument. Clearly, the state of the art for positive control clinical trials does not represent good research practice. Measuring instruments are not calibrated and investigators are not trained in their use. Normal course of the disease with all of the treatment regimen except the drug is not documented. The action of the active control is not adequately documented. The research history of the investigator is not documented. Each of these shortcomings is more important than the difficulties in statistical analysis that are usually the subject of discussion of positive control studies.

In an active control study, the comparison is between two therapeutic regimens, and the contributions of various components in the regimens cannot be evaluated. When patients with the same disease are all treated similarly in terms of concomitant therapy, medical attention, and instructions for study compliance, the additional effect of medication may be overwhelmed. Equivalence of the two therapeutic regimens under examination may be due to the therapeutic equivalence of the components that are different or due to the action of the components which are common to both regimens.

An example was a recent trial that compared a new nonsteriodal antiinflammatory drug with indomethicin, when each was added to aspirin in patients with rheumatoid arthritis. During the study there was little change in the test drug or Indocin-treated patients, and, in fact, during a 2-week placebo period at the end of the study there was again little change. Nonetheless, the sponsor concluded from the study that his test drug was effective because it was as effective as Indocin. In fact, such a study could probably not prove anything even if both drugs had been associated with improvement, because it would inevitably be difficult to separate time, placebo, and drug effects and because the effectiveness of Indocin under those circumstances has never been established.

With respect to statistical analysis, the widely held philosophy of conservativeness, fairly straightforward in its application to analysis of placebo control studies, requires rethinking in the case of active control trials. For instance, an approach frequently used for placebo control survival studies is sometimes referred to as an "intent-to-treat analysis" and simply compares survival patterns, from entry to end of study, for all patients randomized to the treated group versus those for placebo patients, regardless of protocol compliance. This approach guards against inflating the Type I error probability, but at the expense of a loss in sensitivity. As discussed previously, there is motivation to minimize this loss of sensitivity and, thus, to adhere to the protocol as closely as possible. Use of this approach in analysis of active control trials measuring survival time would exacerbate the power shortage present in most such studies. Moreover, it would not be conservative in the sense of affording protection at a specified level against concluding that the test drugs are equivalent when, in fact, they are not.

We are not suggesting that the philosophy of "analyze what you randomize" is not applicable to positive control studies. Virtually every clinical trial has deviations from the protocol, for example, patients who miss visits or miss doses of study medication, patients who drop out or are withdrawn for various, possibly treatment-related reasons. There is no clearly proper way to include such patients in the analysis; rather, one should be looking for consistency of results among the different ways which suggest themselves in a given case. For a further discussion of this topic (as well as difficulties in the interpretation of a particular active control trial), see Pledger and Hall (1982).

Similarly, the conservative approach to subgroup analyses is turned about to be anticonservative in active control trials. Limiting the number of subgroup analyses and making corrections for multiplicity will reduce power and help insure the desired "nonsignificant result."

E. Conclusions

Whatever the motivation for choosing an active control design, the issues involved in inferring efficacy from such studies must be dealt with. In particular, we would stress the following points:

1. The positive control trial offers no direct evidence of effectiveness of the test drug and, therefore, requires supplementary information.
2. Generally, the appropriate source for this supplementary information is previous studies conducted under a design similar in all important aspects, for example, patient population, dosage requirements, response assessment methods, control of concomitant therapy. This is because comparisons between a test and a control therapy are made within the context of study. The subjective concept of what would be a "clinically significant difference" in medical practice may have little relevance to the research situation.
3. The degree to which the results of an active control trial support the test drug's efficacy depends on the level of confidence that the observed response is beyond what could be attributed to a placebo. This usually involves comparison of the observed response, both absolute and relative, to the analogous quantities in previous studies.

The criteria we have described for concluding that an active control study indicates efficacy of the test drug seem, and are, rigorous. This merely reflects the fact that it is much harder in most cases to show effectiveness this way than with a placebo control study that addresses the question directly. Moreover, it is important that the difficulties discussed above be addressed explicitly and with care in each case where an active control design is used. Otherwise, there will be a general degradation in the quality of evidence over time, because after all, today's new drugs are tomorrow's positive controls.

In light of the inferential problems involved it would seem prudent, before embarking on a positive control study, to consider other alternatives to the standard placebo control design. For instance, options such as a dose-response design or an early-escape placebo control design may be preferable, in many circumstances, to an active control design.

III. ACTIVE CONTROL EQUIVALENCE STUDIES: PLANNING AND INTERPRETATION

Robert W. Makuch and Mary Johnson

A. Introduction

One of the most critical stages in the evaluation of new therapies involves the planning of comparative clinical trials. Careful attention to study design helps to ensure that reliable, unbiased information required to determine the efficacy of a new treatment is captured. Also, a good study design can ultimately simplify data analysis and strengthen interpretation of results. By so doing, results are obtained that are statistically valid and convincing to others. Numerous statistical designs are available for the vast majority of traditional clinical trials whose purpose is the demonstration of superiority of a new treatment relative to a standard therapy (Byar et al., 1976; Gehan and Freirich, 1974; Zelen, 1979, 1982; Peto, 1978; Schoenfeld and Gelber, 1979; Makuch and Simon, 1978b).

For a variety of reasons, including the fact that current standard treatments reflect a series of previous successes in the development of new therapies, a relatively new type of clinical trial design has grown popular. Rather than being oriented toward detecting a significant difference between two treatments, these new trials are directed toward showing that an experimental treatment is "equivalent" in efficacy to a standard therapy. The latter is referred to as an active or positive control therapy.

The reasons for undertaking this type of trial are compelling. In many disease areas, current standard treatments reflect a series of previous successes in the development of new therapies. It is often unethical to design a study where the new treatment of interest is compared to a placebo, or no-treatment, control rather than to a currently effective control therapy. Whereas the discovery that a new treatment is actually superior in efficacy to the active control would be a highly desirable result, and one in which standard methodologic principles would apply, achievement of the more modest goal of efficacy "equivalence" while minimizing side effects or reducing the cost of therapy would still render the trial a success. Examples of these types of trials, referred to hereafter as active control equivalence studies (ACES), include (1) radiation therapy plus lumpectomy versus radical mastectomy for early-stage breast cancer, (2) extracorporeal shock wave lithotripsy versus percutaneous lithotripsy for the elimination of kidney stones, and (3) low-dose versus standard-dose azidovudine (AZT) therapy for patients with acquired immunodeficiency syndrome (AIDS) and advanced AIDS-related complex.

Active control equivalence studies often present difficulties in their design and interpretation that are not fully recognized or appreciated. A recent example of claimed equivalence involved a published report by Wharton and his colleagues (Wharton et al., 1986), who concluded that trimethoprim-sulfamethoxazole and pentamidine isethionate were equally effective for the treatment of *Pneumocystis carinii* pneumonia in patients with AIDS. Objections to this conclusion were raised by several individuals (Bégin and Hanley, 1987; Polis and Blackwelder, 1987; Erban, 1987), who indicated that the data did not support efficacy equivalence because the sample size was inadequate to estimate the difference in response rates with an acceptable degree of precision.

Inadequately small sample sizes are not the only difficulty seen in ACES. Perhaps because of its resemblance to traditional clinical trials designed to demonstrate the superiority of a new treatment, many statistical aspects of ACES have received relatively little scrutiny. In these studies an experimental treatment is compared to a standard treatment that has been established as being effective in other clinical settings. Thus there is no placebo group for internal study validation. This implies that an extra step is required beyond the primary experimental–control group study comparison. One must have a reliable external estimate of the efficacy of the active control to ensure that it is more effective than placebo within the current study. This initial validation process may focus attention on inadequacies of the current study that could affect the interpretation of the primary study comparison. The purpose of this section is to discuss this and other issues that are pertinent to the design and interpretation of ACES.

B. Some Issues in ACES

1. Hypothesis Testing versus Estimation

An objective of ACES is the selection of the new treatment when it is not worse than the active control by more than some difference judged to be acceptable by the clinical investigator. A successful demonstration of equivalence for any specified end point of interest will usually demand that the observed difference between treatments be relatively small and that this difference be estimated with adequate precision (Makuch and Johnson, 1986). A simple significance test may fail to reject the standard null hypothesis H_0 of equality in treatment efficacy between two treatments although the true difference may be considerable. Reasons include (1) limited sample size, (2) use of insensitive measures of response to therapy, (3) selection of a suboptimal drug dose or treatment delivery scheme for the active control group, and (4) introduction of extraneous variability or "noise" into the trial due to the inclusion of inevaluable patients, poor patient compliance, or excessively broad eligibility criteria.

Because the Type II (false negative) error is not explicitly reflected in the reporting or performance of a significance test, this approach to analysis invites false confidence in the null result (Makuch et al., 1978a). An example of this phenomenon is seen in Table 4.6 below. Because nonsignificant p values only imply that the data remain consistent with the null hypothesis of treatment equality and not that equivalence has been demonstrated, confidence intervals are preferred since they indicate how large a true treatment difference may exist with reasonable likelihood.

The use of confidence intervals as opposed to hypothesis testing also is becoming increasingly popular in traditional trials to show treatment superiority (e.g., Bulpitt, 1987; Gardner and Altman, 1986; Simon, 1986). Cox states that "It is necessary to calculate so-called confidence limits for the magnitude of effect and not just values of p. This is of crucial importance. It is very bad practice to summarize an important investigation solely by a value of p" (Cox, 1984). This issue also has received considerable attention in bioequivalence studies. There, it is widely accepted that establishment of a confidence interval rather than standard hypothesis testing of no treatment difference is appropriate to their analysis (Mandallaz and Mau, 1981; Shirley, 1976; Westlake, 1972, 1976, 1979).

To illustrate the distinction between estimation and hypothesis testing for accepting a claim of treatment equivalence, assume an investigator requires that the response rate to the active control therapy (C) not exceed by more than 10% the response rate to the experimental

TABLE 4.6 Comparison of confidence intervals and hypothesis testing for accepting a claim of treatment equivalence

Results of experiment	95% Confidence limits (lower, upper)	Confidence limit acceptance criterion	Decision based on hypothesis test
Observed difference (C − E) in response Rates between control (C) and experimental (E) groups		Upper limit must be 0.10 or less	$\alpha = 0.05$
0.00	(−0.10, 0.10)	Acceptable	Acceptable
0.00	(−0.20, 0.20)	Unacceptable	Acceptable
0.08	(0.06, 0.10)	Acceptable	Unacceptable
0.08	(0.02, 0.14)	Unacceptable	Unacceptable

therapy (E) in order to declare that two treatments are similar in efficacy. Table 4.6 shows that conclusions regarding drug equivalence from the traditional hypothesis-testing and confidence-interval viewpoint do not always coincide. Let the observed difference in response rates between C and E be zero. With a broad confidence interval of (−0.20, 0.20), the investigator would not claim equivalence of C and E using the 10% criterion. However, a simple test of significance would give a large, nonsignificant p value, and one might falsely claim equivalence when the true treatment difference is considerable. In summary, while confidence interval estimation is no more a special requirement in equivalence studies than it is in conventional studies designed to show the superiority of a new treatment compared to a standard, we believe its use in ACES is especially appropriate because it should reduce the likelihood of misinterpreting a "nonsignificant" difference between two treatments as an indication of their "equivalence."

2. Sample Size for ACES

Blackwelder and Chang (1982), Makuch and Simon (1978a), and Spiegelhalter and Freedman (1986), among others, have reckoned with the special problems posed by ACES as they relate to the estimation of anticipates will occur. A value (d) is selected such that if the two Makuch and Simon (1978a), primarily because it was the first to provide sample size estimates for the design of ACES using a normal theory confidence interval approach. Use of this method therefore ensures consistency between the initial design and final analysis based on confidence intervals for estimation.

Their method assumes a binary outcome (e.g., responder versus nonresponder, alive versus dead at 1 year). The method also requires careful judgment about P, the overall proportion of successes that one anticipates will occur. A value (d) is selected such that if the two treatments are equally effective, an upper $100 \times (1-\alpha)\%$ confidence limit for the difference in the proportion of successes on the two treatments will exceed d with probability $(1-\beta)$, where α is the probability of committing a Type I error (false positive) and β is the probability of committing a Type II error (false negative). Once the anticipated overall proportion of successes is specified, along with the values of d, α, and β, the required number of patients (N) per treatment group is given by $2P(1-P)(z_\alpha + z_\beta)^2/d^2$, where z_α is the upper α tail point of the standard normal distribution (e.g., $z_{0.05} = 1.645$).

To illustrate the calculations, assume $P = 0.80$ and we wish the sample to be large enough so that with a high degree of confidence $(1-\beta = 0.80)$ one can conclude the two treatments differ at 2 years by no more than $d = 0.05$. For $\alpha = 0.05$, one would need 791 patients per group. Using the same values for α, β, and d, the number of patients required per group is 235, 445, 630, 927, and 1038 for $P = 0.95$, 0.90, 0.85, 0.75, and 0.70, respectively. Sample sizes for lower values of P are not included because medical attention would be more likely to focus on the identification of more efficacious treatments instead. These sample sizes show that large numbers of patients often are needed in well-designed ACES to avoid the risk of reaching a false-negative result. Pocock (1983), who also recommended the Makuch–Simon sample size approach for equivalence studies, emphasized this point as well.

3. "Intent-to-Treat" and "Efficacy" Analysis

Schwartz and Lellouch (1967) described the "intent-to-treat," or pragmatic, approach as one that allows the comparison of "two treatments under the conditions in which they would be applied in practice. It is characteristic of the pragmatic approach that the treatments are flexibly defined and absorb into themselves the contexts in which they are administered" (Schwarz and Lellouch, 1967). Using this approach, the analysis includes efficacy assessments obtained from patients initially randomized into the trial, regardless of protocol deviations such as noncompliance, use of disallowed concomitant medications, or early withdrawal. Biases introduced through exclusion of patient data for reasons that may directly or indirectly be related to treatment response also are prevented.

Thus the trialist is motivated during the conduct of the study to eliminate any practices that would increase the variability of response measurements and ultimately contribute to a failed trial outcome (nonrejection of the traditional null hypothesis). Because one hopes to show a treatment difference, there are obvious incentives to minimize the effects of interfering concomitant treatments, and to have an adequate number of subjects, so that differences are not obscured. In general, the "intent-to-treat" approach represents a conservative approach to the interpretation of traditional trials by making it more difficult to reject H_0 and to accept the hoped-for alternative hypothesis H_A that the new treatment is superior. This emphasis on guarding against false positive conclusions also is reflected in the asymmetric error rates associated with tests of H_0. The maximum allowable probability of a Type I error is usually selected to be smaller than that of a Type II error, typically 5% versus 20%.

In ACES, however, the new treatment is often accepted as efficacious (and the trial considered a success) if the classic null hypothesis of treatment equivalence is *not* rejected. This mistaken objective runs counter to the error specifications for classic study design in terms of H_0 and H_A. In ACES, the equivalence hypothesis is the alternative hypothesis that requires demonstration, and not the standard null hypothesis. Use of the standard hypothesis-testing framework in ACES reverses the usual incentives for meticulous trial conduct and monitoring. Researchers are not penalized for the use of inadequately small sample sizes, insensitive measures of response to therapy, or other influences that will tend to obscure treatment differences. Thus, the standard intent-to-treat approach is anticonservative for ACES in the sense that trial "noise" inflates the p value, leading to nonrejection of H_0 and acceptance of the new treatment. Finally, the asymmetric error rate structure makes it more difficult to reject the traditional null hypothesis of therapeutic equivalence. The reversal of the standard hypothesis-testing framework has been recognized by a few authors in the design and analysis of equivalence studies (Blackwelder et al., 1982; Dunnett et al., 1977). Hauck and Anderson (1983, 1984) recognized this problem in the context of testing for equivalence in comparative bioavailability trials.

An alternative strategy to the widely used intent-to-treat approach is the "efficacy" or "explanatory" approach (Schwartz and Lellouch, 1967). One might prefer an efficacy analysis is establishing treatment equivalence on the grounds that "noise" is considerably reduced. Another reason is that the explanatory approach provides information on the effects of key components of the treatment and that valuable information is thereby gained at the biological level. However, because some advocates of this approach claim it is reasonable to exclude certain patients and events from the primary analysis of efficacy, one may be faced with the problematic issue of bias in the treatment comparison unless certain precautions are taken (Schwartz and Lellouch, 1967).

Sackett and Gent (1979) proposed an attractive middle ground between these two approaches that depends on specific elements of the individual trial, including the nature of the questions posed, the perspective from which the hypotheses were developed, and the avoidance of specific bias. The rules and criteria for excluding certain patients and events should be clinically sensible, established during the protocol's development, operationally feasible, and applied in a demonstrably unbiased way. There must also be full disclosure on all patients and events in the final report. Because many clinical trials are complex experiments that contain both explanatory and pragmatic elements, such reasoned compromise seems warranted and, indeed, necessary.

4. The Historical Control Assumption

A special feature of ACES, and one that is commonly overlooked or unrecognized in their planning and analysis, is reliance on an implicit "historical control assumption." One cannot automaticallly assume that the active control drug, by virtue of the fact that it was previously proven to be efficacious for a given indication, will be effective under a new set of trial conditions. This is particularly true when the disease is highly variable or ambiguously defined, or when the efficacy of the active control is not firmly established (Leber, 1983; Temple, 1982). If this assumption is not satisfied, ACES can become a source of misinformation about the efficacy of an experimental treatment, even if in the primary analysis clinically important differences between the experimental and active control groups can be ruled out with a high degree of confidence. Thus, demonstration of the superiority of the active control relative to placebo represents an additional step in the analysis of ACES that often is made implicitly or goes totally unrecognized.

To examine the effect in ACES of excluding a placebo or no-treatment control against which superiority of C and E is hypothesized, we examine what possible study outcomes could occur if a concurrent placebo group were in fact included. Assume upon study completion that E and C are very similar to one another. This finding would be consistent with any one of the following outcome types: (1) both E and C are superior to placebo (the hoped-for result), (2) neither E nor C is superior to placebo (an insensitive study), or (3) both E and C are inferior to placebo (an unexpected outcome based on prior knowledge). Likewise,

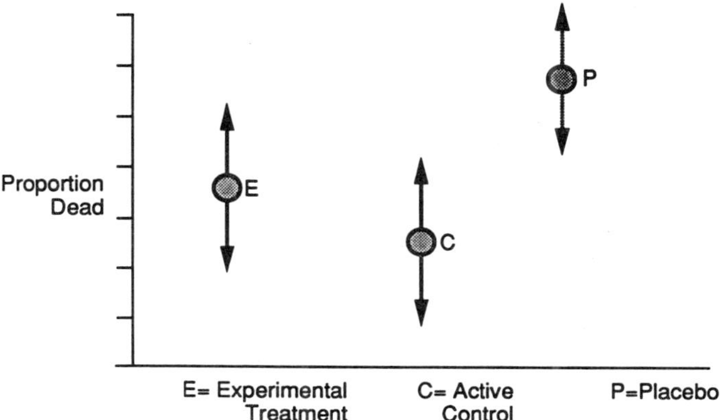

FIGURE 4.1

because the observed similarity between E and C does not necessarily imply that they are truly equivalent to one another, it would also be possible that (4) E is superior to the placebo, but C is not, or (5) C is superior to the placebo, but E is not. Figure 4.1 illustrates the dilemma. In a hypothetical ACES comparing death rates in patients receiving E or C, the 95% confidence limits around the estimated death rate on E could include the observed death rate on C and yet still overlap with confidence bounds for the placebo estimate, had a placebo been included in the study. Thus, there are many categories of study outcome consistent with an observed similarity between E and C that, if a placebo group had been included, would not support the efficacy of E relative to placebo.

If one bypasses a placebo as an internal study reference point on ethical or other grounds, one must be prepared to make crucial assumptions concerning its unobserved effect based on data external to the study. Steps to verify this assumption should be taken prior to initiation of ACES because their goal (to prove that E and C are equivalent) is only meaningful if the observed effect of C is beyond that expected of a placebo. If this fundamental "historical control assumption" of the active control study cannot be made, the design must be considered suspect.

C. Discussion

Active control equivalence trials obviously should be designed to reduce excess "noise," and so yield precise estimates of relative drug effects. For the primary study outcome, confidence intervals can be used to evaluate differences between the experimental and active control groups. But a second step that is made implicitly or goes totally unrecognized is also required to firmly establish the activity of the experimental therapy. Supplementary information must be enlisted from previous studies of similar design in order to estimate the placebo effect relative to the active control drug. To properly interpret an active control trial, one must have some assurance that the active control treatment is as efficacious under the new experimental conditions as it was in previous placebo-controlled trials. A technique called meta-analysis (Glass, 1977; Sacks et al., 1987) should be useful in this regard, since it provides a well-defined structure for combining results across studies and avoids the systematic bias that can arise when just a few trials (especially the positive ones) become the most well known. The degree to which the results of ACES support the efficacy of the new treatment will depend on the level of confidence that the observed response is beyond what could be attributed to a placebo.

The search for historical estimates of the placebo effect in relation to that of the active control has some merit both in the planning and in the interpretation of an active control trial. Nevertheless, the limitations of basing efficacy conclusions on indirect arguments and interstudy comparisons must be recognized (Farewell and D'Angio, 1981; Pocock, 1977). Only if the effects of the active control are demonstrably superior to placebo will such historical estimates offer a rationale, albeit an indirect one, for inferring the efficacy of a new drug from the completed study.

If one proposes to establish the effectiveness of a new drug by demonstrating its equivalence to a known effective agent, one must assume the burden of verifying this fundamental historical control assumptions of ACES. Steps to be taken might include the following. First, one undertakes a systematic, unbiased review of previous placebo-controlled studies of the active control drug to show that the drug can be shown superior to a placebo. Second, close attention should be given to the design and conduct of the completed studies in which the proposed active control was shown to be effective. Study planners can then incorporate similar design features in the new study (such as eligibility criteria, dosage, schedule, and response measurements) that facilitate comparisons with previous work and improve the chances that the active control drug will be effective.

ACKNOWLEDGMENT

This work was supported by grants CA-08341 and CA-16359 from the National Cancer Institute.

IV. CONSIDERATIONS IN THE INTERPRETATION OF ACTIVE CONTROL EQUIVALENCE STUDIES

Jay Herson

A. Introduction

Active Control Equivalence Studies (ACES) are defined as those clinical trials where investigators wish to demonstrate that a new experimental treatment (E) is equivalent to a marketed standard treatment (S). The purpose of this section is to present recommendations for the conduct and interpretation of such studies that are consistent with the highest scientific and regulatory standards.

B. Problems in Conducting Active Equivalence Studies

Table 4.7 summarizes objections to ACES that have been made by FDA reviewers as well as academic and industry clinical trials professionals. The table considers four areas—inference, design, conduct of the trial, and analysis.

In spite of the problems cited above, it is important in some cases that ACES be undertaken.

1. There is considerable demand for less expensive, less toxic, and more humanizing treatments for certain diseases, even though these treatments are equivalent in efficacy to marketed treatments.
2. Pharmacologic development often requires that analogs of existing marketed drugs be tested. The positive control trial appears appropriate in this case.
3. It is considered unethical to perform placebo-controlled trials of beta blockers, treatments for moderate to severe hypertension, and certain malignancies.

C. Recommended Methodology

1. Creating an Incentive to Conduct a First-Rate Trial

One of the major problems in ACES is that a hastily and poorly conducted trial is likely to result in E and S appearing equivalent even when, in fact, they are not equivalent. To have credibility, positive control trials must be conducted under the highest scientific standards. In addition, if positive control trials are not required to be of high quality and expensive to conduct, sponsors will not bear the considerable cost to bring new treatments to market through placebo-controlled trials when

TABLE 4.7 Problems in conducting active control equivalence studies[a]

I. Inference
   A. Inherent inference problem in "proving" equivalence
   B. Specification of alternative hypothesis
   C. Difficulty in deciding how effects compare to placebo effect—historical control problem
II. Design
   A. No incentive for conducting a high-quality trial because a sloppily conducted trial is more likely to result in E and S looking equivalent
   B. Imprecision of measurement
   C. Inappropriate patient population—treatment-resistant, low level of disease at baseline
   D. Inappropriate diagnostic procedures
   E. Subpotent dose
   F. Problem of designing appearance of E and S so that they look alike (capsule vs. tablet, laser vs. drug, contact lenses, surgery or radiotherapy in conjunction with drugs, differential number of visits, differential side effects)
III. Conduct of the trial
   A. S might not be effective in this trial
   B. Spontaneous improvement in study population
   C. Delay in effects (antidepressants)
   D. Side effects cause interruption in treatment
   E. Interfering concomitant treatments
   F. Noncompliance
IV. Analysis
   A. Overstratification
   B. Conservative statistical methods are used that make it less likely to find statistical significance
      1. Small significance levels are used to adjust for multiple comparisons
      2. Intent to treat
   C. Multivariate methods (e.g., Hotelling's t^2) are used to test significance for multiple end points, rather than univariate methods
   D. Subgroup analysis

[a]E = Experimental treatment, S = standard treatment.

another sponsor can then come along and do an inexpensive sloppy trial and get to market on the basis of equivalence.

There are various ways to motivate a high-quality trial:

a. Require sponsor of E to contract with sponsor of S to conduct a trial to show that S is superior to E. If the trial fails to show superiority the conclusion of equivalence is likely to have more credibility than if the sponsor of E reached this conclusion on the basis of a sloppily conducted trial. This option is, in most cases, grossly impractical but it leads us to the following two approaches.

b. Sponsor of E contracts trial operations to a third party such as a contract research firm or university. The third party is instructed to conduct the trial to show that S is superior to E.
c. Sponsor of E conducts the trials but under the auspices of a blue-ribbon panel of academic researchers who oversee trial operations. This panel will report progress to the FDA periodically.

The contract research organization or blue-ribbon panel would also be charged with making sure that the protocol for the trial is appropriate for the treatments and indications under considerations. They would also certify the appropriateness of the statistical methods to be utilized in analysis.

2. Is S Effective in This Trial?

The major question to be answered in an active control equivalence study is whether S is displaying a level of efficacy above the placebo level. Although S has shown efficacy in past clinical trials there is no guarantee that it will show efficacy in this trial. Historical control considerations and varying eligibility requirements make use of previous data on efficacy of S difficult to justify.

ACES should only be performed where medical practice has found standard treatments whose efficacy is generally accepted. To perform such a trial with S treatments whose efficacy is not generally accepted or where substantial placebo effects are possible is not only bad science, it is bad business.

Investigators may wish to conduct a one-arm open-label trial of treatment S prior to conducting the randomized trial. The purpose of this preliminary trial is to gather evidence on response to treatment S in the proposed protocol.

In the randomized trial, early termination rules that stop the trial when early evidence shows S to be ineffective would be appropriate. When a trial terminates with lack of evidence that S is effective, the trial should be repeated.

For certain diseases an open-label "run-in" period can precede randomization. Here all patients must respond to S in order to enter the randomized phase of the trial. This approach could be used with relatively few diseases (e.g., chronic skin rash, dysmenorrhea, chronic pulmonary obstruction, etc.) and suffers from the weakness of the "run-in" phase being uncontrolled.

3. Analysis: Confidence Intervals versus Support Intervals

At the conclusion of ACES, investigators must evaluate the relative effects of E and S.

Let θ_E be the response proportion on treatment E and θ_S be the response proportion on treatment S. Makuch and Simon (1978) have indicated that a confidence interval for $\Delta = \theta_E - \theta_S$ is the appropriate tool for treatment evaluation. The range of plausible values for Δ afforded by a 95% confidence interval is vital to the best case–worst case type analysis dictated by regulatory considerations.

Confidence intervals, however, have a repeated-sampling interpretation. While repeated-sampling concepts are vital in pretrial planning, likelihood concepts are our chief basis of inference in posttrial evaluation. The likelihood function conditions on the sample actually observed and specifies the relative likelihood for any value of parameters being estimated. Edwards (1972) has introduced the notion of k-unit support intervals based on log likelihoods. The 2-unit support intervals for the unknown parameter often approximate 95% confidence intervals. An inversion rule has been developed to produce an appropriate support interval for $\Delta = \theta_E - \theta_S$. This interval is approximate because the inversion rule ignores a nuisance parameter.

D. Regulatory Practice

1. Therapeutic Index

An important question regulators must ask relative to the decision they must make in ACES is what is to be lost from:

a. Concluding that E is equivalent to S when it is actually inferior.
b. Concluding that E is inferior to S when it is actually equivalent.

The answer to this question should be based on the therapeutic index of S. Figure 4.2 displays a graphical definition of the therapeutic index for a curative cancer treatment. A separate definition exists for palliative treatments.

Assume that E actually reduces risk but efficacy data are equivocal. If S has a low TI then there may be little to be lost if error a. is committed and is uncovered by postmarketing experience.

If S has a moderate TI there is more to be lost in error a than if S has a low TI, even though postmarketing experience will eventually uncover the error.

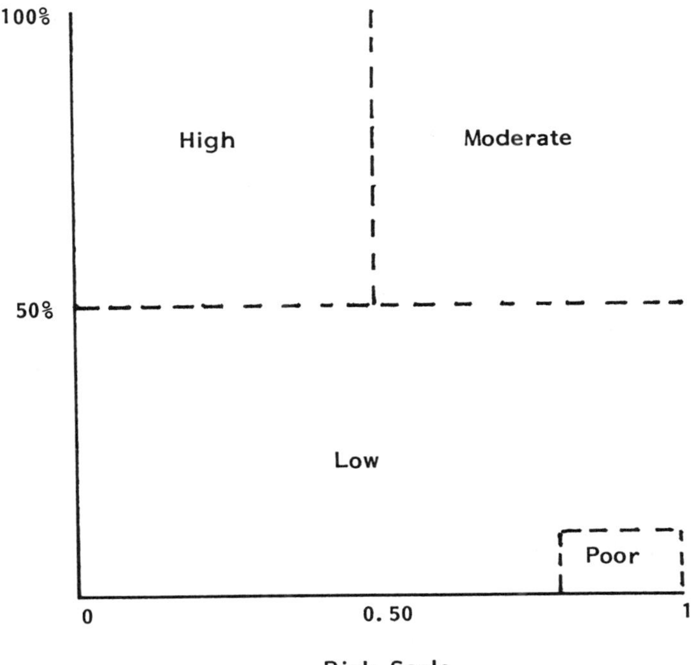

FIGURE 4.2 Therapeutic Index for curative cancer therapy.

When error b. is committed no postmarketing arena will be opened for further evaluation but the degree of seriousness in the error depends on the degree of risk reduction afforded by E.

In general in the face of equivocal efficacy data, the lower the TI the more attractive is a conclusion of equivalence. For higher TIs an equivalence conclusion becomes attractive only in the case of substantial risk reduction.

2. Type of Evidence Required

The clinical trial–FDA review process is far from perfect in the case of placebo-controlled trials. If it were, the question of "Is S effective in this trial?" would be irrelevant because S was presumably licensed though placebo-controlled trials. However, the placebo-controlled trial yields information that lends itself more to regulatory decision making than positive controlled trials. Perhaps it is reasonable for us to require placebo-controlled trials to show efficacy "beyond shadow of a doubt" but for ACES to show equivalence only through a "preponderance of evidence", that is, a series of well-conducted studies most of which yield evidence of equivalence.

E. Conclusions

ACES are not examples of faultless scientific practice but a necessary consequence of the real-world medical regulatory decisions that must be made.

ACES should be conducted:

1. When the S treatment is a generally recognized treatment of choice for the disease under investigation.
2. Under the auspices of a third party or blue-ribbon panel.
3. Using confidence intervals or likelihood methods for inference.
4. With the therapeutic index of E and S in mind and an appropriate role for post marketing experiences. In the face of equivocal results, a tendency to lean toward equivalence is recommended when the TI is low and/or when a large reduction in risk is afforded.
5. Under the realization that regulators are seeking a preponderance of evidence of efficacy rather than a "beyond shadow of a doubt" level of evidence. This will usually imply more investigator sites with larger numbers of patients than are generally used in placebo-controlled trials.

Adherence to these principles will not result in a "proof" of equivalence, but to deny the implications of trials conducted and regulatory decisions made under these principles is to deny our ability to reason from experience. Clinical trials are merely a formalization of the empirical nature of medicine. ACES are needed. The challenge before us is to select the appropriate empirical arena for their conduct.

V. THE ASSESSMENT OF STATISTICAL EVIDENCE FROM ACTIVE CONTROL CLINICAL TRIALS*

Jiann-Ping Hsu

A. Introduction

New single-ingredient drugs usually have to be tested in controlled clinical trials to demonstrate their therapeutic effects. A basic design for

*A version of this paper was presented at the ASA Annual Joint Meeting, August 1983, Toronto, Canada. At that time the author was a member of the Biometrics Division of the FDA. The views expressed herein are those of the author and not necessarily those of the Food and Drug Administration.

this purpose is a randomized double-blind trial comparing the test drug to the placebo in parallel groups of patients. If the patients respond more favorably to the test drug and the study is unbiased, then the observed difference in response would be attributed to the effect of the test drug. In new drug applications submitted to FDA, it is also common to find clinical trials conducted with an active control drug instead of a placebo.

The active control seems to have become increasingly popular. Its foremost appeal over the placebo control is mainly based on ethical considerations. The option of receiving a drug approved for its safety and efficacy or a new drug with the potential for approval will ease the difficulty in recruiting clinicians and patients to participate in the study. Blinding may be maintained more effectively, and probably fewer patients will withdraw due to lack of efficacy.

Drugs indicated for diseases such as terminal cancers and severe infections usually can not be tested against a placebo for ethical reasons. Active controls are thus an alternative to historical control or no control at all. Active controls are also widely used in clinical evaluation of certain drugs for chronic diseases when the duration of the trial is too long to make the placebo control plausible.

As more drugs are being approved for marketing, possibly more and more drugs will be tested against a greater variety of control agents. Yet, can active control trials serve the purpose for demonstrating the therapeutic effect of the new drug? The merits of the active control trials are readily recognized. However, the limitations have not been given due consideration. Temple, Pledger, and Hall (1983) have pointed out many problems in active control trials intended to establish efficacy of new drugs.

This section discusses some of the difficulties encountered in reviewing and evaluating statistical evidence from the active control equivalence studies in new drug applications. Most of the controlled drug trials evaluate both the beneficial effects and the undesirable effects of the test drug. Evaluation of the beneficial effects of the drug always has a specific goal, namely, to prove that the test drug is effective, while the evaluation of adverse drug effects usually involves exploratory and descriptive analysis. This section focusses on the evaluation of the therapeutic effects of the test drug.

B. Approach of Analysis

In an ordinary active control trial the response to the test drug is compared to the response to the control drug. Without loss of generality, let us assume that the larger the value of the response variable, the more desirable the therapeutic effect of the drug.

Suppose that R_t and R_c are the random variables denoting the responses to the test drug and the control drug and they follow the distributions F_t and F_c, respectively. The patients' responses in each group are assumed to be independent and identically distributed observations when the patient population is homogeneous with respect to factors relevant to the response.

For purpose of discussion, we need to introduce a fictitious concurrent placebo control in the trial. Denote the response to the placebo by R with distribution function F.

The goal of the study is to demonstrate the therapeutic effect of the test drug, namely, to infer

$$R_t > R \tag{4.1}$$

based on the result of

$$R_t > R_c$$

on R_t and R_c being statistically and clinically "equivalent."

Incidentally, the procedure is stated in terms of stochastic ordering for generality and completeness. Random variable A is stochastically greater than random variable B if the distribution function of A is less than the distribution of B at every sample point. In practice, relation of stochastic ordering is simplified to expressions involving only parameters such as means or medians, by imposing assumptions on the distribution functions.

The analytic approach contains three components:

1. To show that

   $$R_t > R_c$$

   or, that R_t and R_c are "equivalent."
2. To assume

   $$R_c > R \tag{4.2}$$

3. To imply equation (4.1), given 1 and 2.

If the test drug is expected to outperform the control drug, then the null hypothesis

$$F_t \geq F_c$$

will be tested against the alternative

$$F_t < F_c$$

The circumstances are almost the same as those involved in testing against a placebo control except that an adequate dose level of the control drug is crucial to the study outcome. Components 2 and 3 become less critical.

More frequently the beneficial effect of the drug is anticipated to be at most as good as, but not better than, that of the control drug. The conventional method to establish that R_t and R_c are "equivalent" is to test the null hypothesis of $F_T = F_c$ in anticipation of finding an insignificant p value. This scheme is inappropriate and unfruitful because the null hypothesis can be disproved but not proved. Failure to reject the null hypothesis does not prove that the null hypothesis is correct, but calls for examination of the type II error.

Some clinicians and statisticians also view the hypothesis $F_t = F_c$ as unrealistic. They would consider F_t and F_c "equivalent" if they did not differ "too much."

The idea of "equivalence" is similar to that in bioequivalence studies where a test drug is judged to be bioequivalent to the reference drug if the difference or the ratio of the mean bioavailability of the two drugs in population fall within a prespecified range. For reference, see Westlake (1976) and Schuirmann (1982).

To revise the conventional method, Dunnett and Gent (1977), Patel and Gupta (1981), and Blackwelder and Chang (1982) propose to define equivalence between two treatments by a constant Δ. Assume that F_t and F_c belong to the same family of distributions and the difference between the effects of the two drugs is measured by the difference between the two population means θ_t and θ_c. Then the statistical hypotheses are stated as

$$H\colon \theta_c - \theta_t \geq \Delta$$

versus

$$K\colon \theta_c - \theta_t < \Delta$$

or in two-sided form,

$$H\colon |\theta_c - \theta_t| = \Delta$$

versus

$$K: |\theta_c - \theta_t| < \Delta$$

The advantage of their approach is that it controls the error of claiming equivalence when in fact the effects are not equivalent. Nevertheless, the advantage is offset by the difficulty in determining the value of Δ.

Furthermore, all these various versions of hypothesis testing focus only on demonstrating "equivalence," but equivalence does not necessarily imply "equally effective." To show that the test drug is "as effective as" the control drug, it is necessary to look into 2 and 3.

Although the active control drug is indicated for its therapeutic effect, there is no assurance that the significant result is replicable in every clinical testing against the placebo. The test may fail due to chance. More importantly, biases in design, execution, and analysis can deprive it of strength in demonstrating the drug effect. Therefore it is necessary to verify the assumption of equation (4.2),

$$R_c > R$$

Since R is a fictitious variable, validity of (4.2) can not be confirmed within the trial. It seems that the only recourse is to enlist information from historical studies involving the control drug and the placebo. In doing so, any further result will inevitably be subject to the same concerns inherent in the use of historical controls.

One may question the need to examine the magnitude of the effect of an active control while the magnitude of the placebo effect has not been a big issue. Indeed, for some extensively researched diseases the level of the placebo effect is predictable and unusual results can be spotted easily. Yet, there are other reasons for the lax attitude toward the placebo effect.

Consider a randomised, double-blind, placebo-controlled trial. To ensure that the placebo effect will be accurately represented, the study must have at least:

a. Adequate sample size
b. Appropriate enrollment criteria and patient selection procedure
c. Low dropout rate
d. Limited and controlled use of concomitant medication
e. Precise measurement of the response variables.

These items constitute part of the requirement for an adequate, controlled clinical trial. Absence of any one of them will reduce the study's ability to achieve its goal. Severe deficiencies may result in study failure. Thus the conductor of the trial is motivated to safeguard against these potential pitfalls by enrolling a sufficient number of patients, minimizing withdrawals, etc. Subsequently biases are likely to be reduced or minimized in the observed data.

The situation is the opposite for active control trials. Deficiencies with respect to a–e tend to obscure the difference between F_t and F_c and make it easier to demonstrate the closeness of F_t and F_c. Therefore when the responses in the two groups are shown to be equivalent, it is important to examine various sources of biases that would operate in favor of the result. It is desirable, but usually difficult to estimate the magnitude of biases. Nevertheless, if the biases were large enough to invalidate the assumption (4.2), the result of equivalence would be of no value. Validity of condition (4.2) should thus be confirmed before proceeding to the third component of the analysis.

Now suppose that the comparison of F_t to F_c produces an estimate for the difference between F_t and F_c, in addition to the claim of F_t and

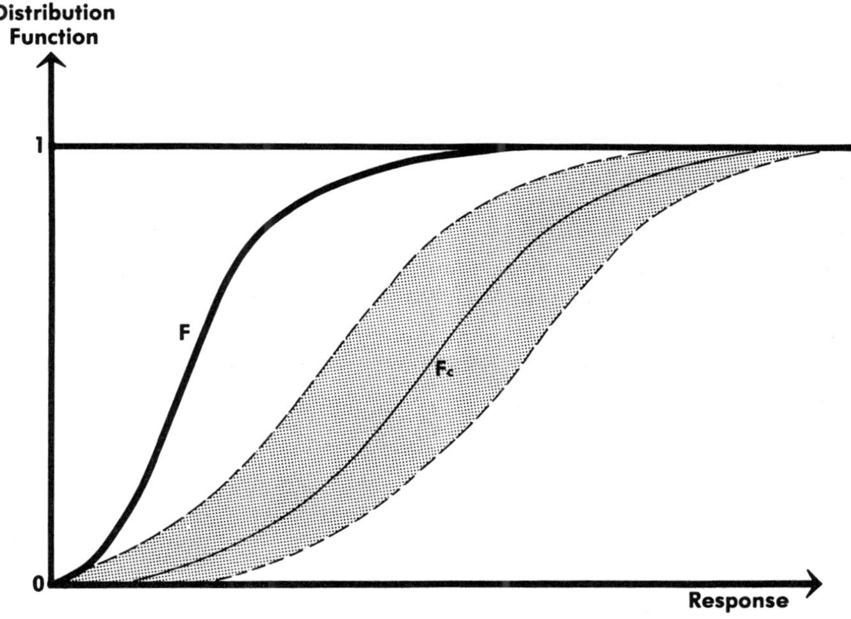

FIGURE 4.3

F_c being equivalent, and there is sufficient evidence for

$$F_c < F$$

We want to know whether

$$F_t < F \tag{4.3}$$

can be accepted at a given level of significance. Let us describe the analytic problem in Fig. 4.3 where F_t (not shown) lies in the shaded region around F_c and F_c is a distance away from F. With the shaded area being narrow and F_c being farther away from F, this picture would be convincing that the data could support the conclusion (4.3).

However, if the difference between F_t and F_c is large or the estimation for the difference is imprecise, that is, the shaded region is large, or, if the distance between F_c and F is small, then it will be difficult to verify the validity of (4.3). These situations arise frequently in the active control equivalence studies. An example is given next.

C. Example

The data in this example are taken from two clinical trials in a new drug application for a nonsteroidal antiinflammatory drug. The response variable examined is reduction of the number of swollen joints after 4 weeks of experiment.

Both trials are randomized and double-blind. In order to obtain homogeneous patient groups, only patients with 30 or more swollen joints at the baseline are included in the evaluation for this example. In one trial, 82 patients who received the test drug will be compared to the 86 patients who received an active control drug. Fifteen placebo controls from another trial are selected. No more than three patients have dropped out in each of the three groups.

Figure 4.4 shows that the empirical distribution for the active control almost always lies below that for the test drug. Undoubtedly the two curves can be shown to be "equivalent" with a proper definition of equivalence.

Another trial is introduced to provide a comparison to the active control trial data. At lower response level, say 0–15, the empirical distribution for the placebo well supercedes the distributions for the active control drug and the test drug. At response level 15 or greater, the empirical distribution for the test drug becomes much closer to the placebo distribution than does the active control distribution and crosses

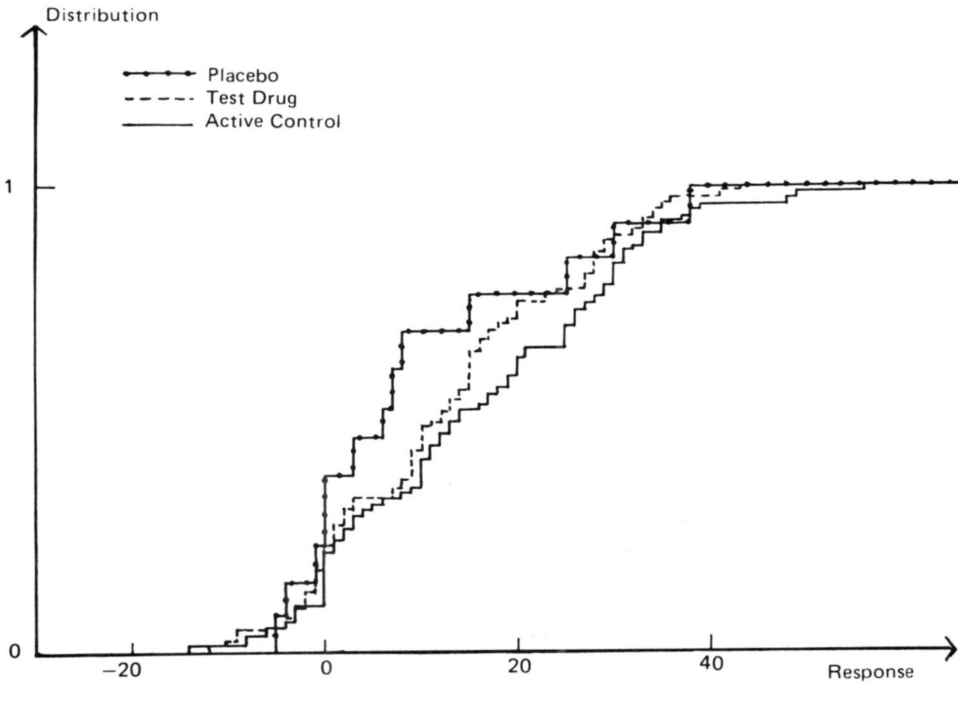

FIGURE 4.4

the placebo curve many times as they approach unity. The placebo data, in spite of the fact that the number of patients is relatively small, has given us insight on the therapeutic effect of the test drug that is not obtainable by the conventional analysis of drug "equivalence."

D. Summary and Prospect

Active control equivalence studies have an undeniable position in clinical research and the demand is growing stronger. However, they have not always produced clear results for evaluation of new drug efficacy.

The mechanism of demonstrating drug efficacy through active control trials differs entirely from that through placebo control trials. The determination of drug efficacy from comparative study of the test drug and the control drug is not straightforward. The design, analysis, and assessment of the trial demand great effort to assure adequacy of study results.

Some points need to be considered in planning active control equivalence studies:

1. Selection of the control drug—Only drugs with a predictable, consistent, and easily detectable therapeutic effect are desirable choices for the control.
2. Dosage—The potential for underdosing the controls should be prevented. Whether the drugs will be administered at fixed dosage or at each individual's optimal dose level and how the dose regimen will affect interpretation of study results should be considered.
3. Supplementary data on the control drug—The trial will require supplementary data or knowledge on the control drug. This may become a criterion for selecting the control drug.
4. Sample size—The active control trials usually require a large number of patients to achieve adequate statistical accuracy and precision. Consequently the cost will increase.
5. Study biases—Proper precautions must be taken to minimize biases that work in favor of the test drug or against distinguishing the two drugs. The effects of these biases on the results of study need to be examined.
6. "Equivalent" versus "equally effective"—"Equivalence" of the drug responses does not imply that the drugs are "equally effective." Further analysis is needed to establish the efficacy of the test drug even if the "equivalence" has been shown.

REFERENCES

Bégin, P., and Hanley, J. Letter to the Editor. *Ann. Intern. Med.*, *106:* 474–475, 1987.

Blackwelder, W. C., and Chang, M. A. "Proving the null hypothesis" in clinical trials. *Controlled Clinical Trials*, *3:* 345–353, 1982.

Bulpitt, C. J. Confidence intervals. *Lancet*, *1:* 494–497, 1987.

Byar, D. P., Simon, R. M., Friedewald, W. T., Schlesselman, J. J., DeMets, D. L., Ellenberg, J. H., Gail, M. H., and Ware, J. H. Randomized clinical trials. *N. Engl. J. Med.*, *295:* 74–80, 1976.

Cox, D. R. Statistical significance tests, in *Current Problems in Clinical Trials* (D. M. Chaput de Saintong and D. W. Vere, eds.). Boston, Blackwell, 1984, pp. 41–47.

Dunnett, C. W., and Gent, M. Significance testing to establish equivalence between treatments, with special reference to data in the form of 2 × 2 tables. *Biometrics*, *33:* 593–602, 1977.

Edwards, A. W. F. *Likelihood*. Cambridge, Cambridge University Press, 1972.

Erban, J. K. Letter to the Editor. *Ann. Intern. Med.*, *106:* 475, 1987.

Farewell, V. T., and D'Angio, G. J. A simulated study of historical controls using real data. *Biometrics*, *37:* 169–176, 1981.

Gardner, M. J., and Altman, D. G. Confidence intervals rather than *P* values: Estimation rather than hypothesis testing. *Br. Med. J.*, *292:* 746–750, 1986.

Glass, G. Integrating findings: The meta-analysis of research. In *Review of Research in Education* (L. Schulman, ed.). Itasca, IL, Peacock, 1977.

Hauck, W. W., and Anderson, S. A new procedure for testing equivalence in comparative bioavailability and other clinical trials. *Commun. Stat. A.*, *12:* 2663–2692, 1983.

Hauck, W. W., and Anderson, S. A new statistical procedure for testing equivalence in two-group comparative bioavailability trials. *J. Pharm. Pharmacol.*, *12* 83–91, 1984.

Leber, P. The implicit assumptions of active control trials. Invited FDA Case Study, Annual Meeting of the Society for Clinical Trials, San Diego, 1983.

Makuch, R. W., and Johnson, M. F. Some issues in the design and interpretation of 'negative' clinical trials. *Arch. Intern. Med.*, *146:* 986–989, 1986.

Makuch, R., and Simon, R. Sample size requirements for evaluating a conservative therapy. *Cancer Treat. Rep.*, *62:* 1037–1040, 1978a.

Makuch, R. W., and Simon, R. M. A note on the design of multiinstitution three-treatment studies. *Cancer Clin. Trials*, *1:* 301–303, 1978b.

Mandallaz, D., and Mau, J. Comparison of different methods for decision making in bioequivalence assessment. *Biometrics*, *37:* 213–222, 1981.

McNeer, J. F., Wagner, G. S., Ginsburg, P. B., et al. Hospital discharge one week after acute myocardial infarction. *N. Engl. J. Med.*, *298:* 229–232, 1978.

Patel, H. I., and Gupta, G. D. (1981). A problem of equivalence in clinical trials. Presentation at the Spring ENAR Meeting, Lexington.

Peto, R. Clinical trial methodology. *Biomedicine*, *28:* 24–36, 1978.

Pledger, G., and Hall, D. Withdrawals from drug trials. *Biometrics*, *38:* 276–77, 1982.

Pocock, S. J. Randomized clinical trials (letter). *Br. Med. J.*, *1(6077):* 1661, 1977.

Pocock, S. J. *Clinical Trials: A Practical Approach*. New York, John Wiley, 1983, pp. 129–130.

Polis, M. A. and Blackwelder, W. C. Letter to the Editor. *Ann. Intern. Med.*, *106:* 475, 1987.

Sackett, D. L., and Gent, M. Controversy in counting and attributing events in clinical trials. *N. Engl. J. Med.*, *301:* 1410–1412, 1979.

Sacks, H. W., Berrier, J., Reitman, D., et al. Meta-analysis of randomized clinical trials. *N. Engl. J. Med.*, *316:* 450–455, 1987.

Schoenfeld, D., and Gelber, R. Designing and analyzing clinical trials which allow institution to randomize patients to a subset of the treatments under study. *Biometrics*, *35:* 825–829, 1979.

Schuirmann, D. J. (1987). Fixed sample tests for internal hypothesis associated with bioequivalence trials. Presentation at the Annual American Statistical Association Meeting, San Francisco.

Schwartz, D., and Lellouch, J. Explanatory and pragmatic attitudes in therapeutic trials. *J. Chron. Dis., 20:* 637–648, 1967.

Shirley, E. The use of confidence intervals in biopharmaceutics. *J. Pharm. Pharmacol., 28:* 312–313, 1976.

Simon, R. Confidence intervals for reporting results of clinical trials. *Ann. Intern. Med., 105:* 429–435, 1986.

Spiegelhalter, D. J., and Freedman, L. S. A predictive approach to selecting the size of a clinical trial, based on subjective clinical opinion. *Stat. Med., 5:* 1–14, 1986.

Temple, R. Government viewpoint of clinical trials. *Drug Inform. J., 1:* 10–17, 1982.

Temple, R. J., Pledger, G., and Hall, D. (1983). On positive control clinical drug trials intended to establish efficacy. Unpublished manuscript.

Westlake, W. J. Use of confidence intervals in analysis of comparative bioavailability trials. *J. Pharm. Sci., 61:* 1340–1341, 1972.

Westlake, W. J. Symmetric confidence intervals for bioequivalence trials. *Biometrics, 32:* 741–744, 1976.

Westlake, W. J. Design and statististical evaluation of bioequivalence studies in man, in *Principles and Perspectives in Drug Bioavailability*. Basel, Karger, 1979, pp. 192–210.

Wharton, J. M., Coleman, D. L., Wofsky, C. B., et al. Trimethoprim-sulfamethorazole or pentamidine for *Pneumocystis carinii* pneumonia in the acquired immunodeficiency syndrome: A prospective randomized trial. *Ann. Intern. Med., 105:* 37–44, 1986.

Zelen, M. A new design for randomized clinical trials. *N. Engl. J. Med., 300:* 1273–1275, 1979.

Zelen, M. Strategy and alternate randomized designs in cancer clinical trials. *Cancer Treat. Rep., 66:* 1095–1100, 1982.

5
Optimization in Clinical Trials and Combination Drug Development

Donald M. Stablein and Joel W. Novak *The EMMES Corporation, Potomac, Maryland*

Karl E. Peace* *Biopharmaceutical Research Consultants, Inc., Ann Arbor, Michigan*

Eugene M. Laska and Morris J. Meisner *Nathan S. Kline Institute for Psychiatric Research, Orangeburg, New York and New York University Medical Center, New York, New York*

I. OPTIMIZATION IN CLINICAL TRIALS

Donald M. Stablein and Joel W. Novak

A. The Drug Testing Framework

Therapeutic clinical research takes on many varied forms specific to the disease entities and treatment regimens being assessed. A common pattern to much of these efforts can be elicited, a strategy that is marked by Phase I, Phase II, and Phase III trials (Burdette and Gehan, 1970). The goal of the first stage or Phase I trials is the ascertainment, with but a few patients, of the maximum tolerable dose. Although regimen activity is examined, the purpose of Phase I trials is more one of

**Previous affiliation:* Warner-Lambert Company, Ann Arbor, Michigan.

determination of safety rather than testing for efficacy. The level of activity is examined specifically in the Phase II trial. From the results of the Phase I trial a dose and treatment schedule is selected and, in the Phase I setting, tested to determine whether it is likely that a certain level of activity or response rate exists. If sufficient activity is evident, then one pursues further study in the form of a Phase III trial. This trial is a study intended to provide information regarding the comparative effectiveness of the test item with reference to standard treatment given for a specific disease.

In some sense the Phase I, II, III framework of testing has been institutionalized. Regulations developed by the Food and Drug Administration that set forth minimum standards for those engaged in drug development and evaluation incorporate this strategy. Thus, the methodology permeates clinical research efforts and drug development programs.

Statisticians have made minimal contributions to the design of Phase I trials, where clinical considerations dominate the procedures employed. We have developed a methodology, such as it is, to support Phase II trials. While it may be impossible to find a statistician who is content with available Phase II methodology, we sort of "play along" with clinical colleagues on the grounds that this is only a screen and that a truly rigorous evaluation of the test item is just around the corner. Clearly, it is in Phase III comparative trials that important statistical contributions to the methodology of modern clinical research have been made.

It is beyond the scope of this paper to discuss the decades of statistical developments related to the study of Phase III clinical trials methodology. Suffice it to say that by using a combination of techniques for evaluating different dependent variables—hypothesis testing, specification of Type I and Type II errors, and the like—statisticians give confidence and even authority to study results in which treatment A is compared to treatment B. That the statistician does not have an abiding interest in the treatments being evaluated has served to underscore the integrity of the analysis and enhance the degree of confidence that the clinician places in the statistical findings. Further, these developments can be described as being more closely associated with hypothesis testing than with estimation.

B. The Problem of Dose

Unfortunately, there is a flaw in this framework that has to do with the manner in which test items are selected for trial. As suggested, the test items that are subjected to the rigorous evaluation of a Phase III clinical trial are generally administered in doses that were selected in Phase I trials, often because they were maximally tolerable and not because they were maximally effective. In fact, when standard treatment is no therapy (or a dose of zero) of the new treatment, then a paradox exists. For if the maximally effective dosage were known, it is unlikely that a comparative study with a no-treatment control arm (or a zero dose level) would be necessary. This is because it is hard to imagine knowing the location of the optimal treatment if it is not known whether such a location exists. This is of particular concern when combinations of cytotoxic agents are under study. For example, Hollander and Harlan (1973) reported that significant therapeutic benefit could not be ascribed to antacid therapy in the treatment of duodenal ulcers. Later, Peterson et al. (1977) showed just the opposite. As Peterson pointed out in his discussion of the later trial, several factors may explain the inconsistent results of these two studies, including the fact that he used an effective dose that was nearly eight times that used in the Hollander study. Peterson, of course, was persistent in his feeling that antacid therapy has more than a palliative benefit to patients with duodenal ulcers. Many, if not most, investigators would have dropped any such interest on reading the first report, thereby forfeiting their opportunity to discover what could have been a useful therapy.

Certainly the question can be raised regarding the frequency with which most effective treatment has been discarded because the dose levels chosen for evaluation in the clinical trial were not maximally effective. An answer to such a question is certainly not available, although it may not be a particular problem where single agents are concerned. Clinicians are well-trained observers, and a clinically important difference between a recommended dose and an effective dose may sooner or later become apparent to someone like Peterson, at least for single-agent therapies.

The matter of ascertaining whether suboptimal doses or schedules have been employed when multiple agents or multimodality therapies are used clearly presents a different problem. In the first place, most individual clinicians do not have experience with a sufficient number of dose or schedule combinations to ascertain their relationship to outcome. Second, even if the clinician does have a large enough pool of information available, the ability to observe such relationships in the three, four, or five dimensions required is not what it is for single-agent therapy. Notwithstanding this limitation, we do see reports in the clinical literature that posit dose/response relationships in multiple agent therapy. Such reports should raise questions about what is the optimal treatment for a given disease. Moreover, they raise questions about the adequacy of the research methods used to select dose assignments in multiagent trials.

Two examples of recent reports that raise questions about the dose levels selected and used in multiagent cancer clinical trials can be cited. Bonadonna et al. (1981), in a breast cancer trial, noted that patients who received high doses of drug fared better than those whose treatment was scaled downward or terminated early. While his results are subject to misinterpretation because of the confounding of certain variables, we must acknowledge that he has raised an important question. Perhaps more important, Frei and Cannellos (1980) report dose/response relationships across a number of protocol studies that included a number of different drug combinations used to treat a number of different tumors. In one of the intriguing conclusions that emerge from this study, Frei and Cannellos raise questions on what is the optimal dose of 5-FU, a chemotherapeutic agent that has been in widespread use for over 20 years. With hundreds of thousands of patients that have been treated with 5-FU, and with the tens of thousands of patients that have been entered into clinical trials utilizing 5-FU therapy, it is incredible that its optimal dosage level is still unknown.

C. The Development of Dose Optimization Methods

Statisticians have, of course, been interested in problems associated with optimization for some time. Optimum-seeking experimental designs likewise are not new, although their application in the field of biomedicine has been slow.

Mantel (1958) and NCI biologist Abe Goldin et al. (1957) were among the first to see the need to consider optimum-seeking designs. Goldin had demonstrated what is now pretty much taken for granted with cytotoxic therapies: that in animal experiments there is an optimal dose of a single drug with respect to survival. The logic behind Goldin's observation is simple and compelling. If the dose of an active chemotherapeutic agent is too small, its use is ineffective and the animal dies of disease. On the other hand, if the dose is too high, the therapy is likely to cause treatment-related death. Theoretically, for each substance there is an optimal dose that maximizes cures. Clearly, the search for that optimal dose is the suitable objective of experimentation.

Mantel, along with Goldin, Vendetti, and others (1957), undertook a series of experiments beginning in the mid-1950s to find optimum doses in two-drug combination therapies where survival was the endpoint of interest. In one such experiment, 33 groups of subjects were allocated to both single and combination treatments that involved five different ratios of dose level, for two different drugs. The analytical procedure employed, which was based on visual inspection, was concerned with identifying that combination that was maximally effective. That combination, defined in terms of dose levels for the two agents, was considered to be the optimum treatment. This research led to assessments of the concept of therapeutic synergy—that is, combination treatment gives results superior to that of component drugs.

Recognizing that there are levels of sublethal toxicity that are of significance, Mantel anticipated that study designs would be required that provide for the determination of optimum treatments that include consideration of important constraints such as tolerable toxicity. In a review of the Mantel paper, Box (1958) agreed with him, pointing out that response-surface methodology, which was designed for problems seen in the chemical industry, lends itself to the evaluation of combination therapies—that is, optimum-seeking experimental designs might be utilized where the test points are defined by various doses of the drugs included in the combination treatment. In his discussion, Box reminds us that the real objective of the combination therapy experiment is to find that dose of each agent that leads to maximally effective therapy.

From a methodological point of view, optimum-seeking experiments in biomedicine did not see another advance until Addelman et al. (1966) proposed a scheme for determining optimal combinations of two drugs for treating mice with experimental leukemias. The schema that they suggested included a sequence of up to three experiments. In each experiment, the optimal combination is approached via a least-squares polynomial analysis of resulting survival times, with information from earlier experiments incorporated into later analyses. Addelman, for the first time, offered a truly rigorous methodology for analyzing experiments designed to find optimum drug combinations.

At about the same time, Goldin, Vendetti, Mantel et al. (1968) began their work on the substantially more complicated three-drug combination problem. These experiments were based on a equilateral triangle in which the vertices represented single drugs, points on the side of the triangles represented two-drug combinations, and points in the interior of the triangle represented dose levels of three drugs in the combination. Using five mice for each of 148 experimental combinations, the study required in excess of 700 subjects. Since the analysis was limited to visual inspection of the resulting median survival times, a large experiment was required in order to ensure that the treatment space had been adequately explored. This effectively prevented experiments with more drugs in the combination.

The next advances incorporated improved analytic methods through explicit modeling of the dose response surface. Carter et al. (1977) used the logistic function to model the relationship between the probability of a favorable outcome and the levels of treatment in a two-drug combination. The model was a complete quadratic in the drug dosages to account for toxicity and drug interactions. After establishing the adequacy of the model, response-surface methods were used to estimate the dosage levels of the drugs in combination associated with maximum probability of a favorable outcome. Since the optimal treatment estimate could vary with the definition of favorable outcome, Carter, Stablein, and Wampler (1979) successfully used Cox's proportional hazard model quadratic in the dosage levels to relate dosage levels to the survival distributions of treated animals. After determining that there was no significant lack of fit, response-surface techniques were used to explore the fitted surface and the treatment combination with minimum estimated hazard was determined. If the assumption of proportionality is valid, the optimum obtained in this manner is independent of time. However, Stablein, Carter, and Wampler (1980) have shown that this may not always be the case by considering treatment by time interactions in a study of two drugs and showing that they do exist. In such cases the optimum combination is time dependent.

The approach taken by these authors is easily extended to combinations of three or more drugs. An important advantage associated with the use of such models is realized in the design of experiments to yield the information required to estimate the model parameters. As a result of the predictive ability of the model, fewer treatment combinations can be considered than in the case of an analysis dependent on a visual inspection of the data. However, in animal experiments it is important to make the treatment region large enough to contain toxic combinations so that the estimated optimum combination can be found in its interior.

D. Ethical Concerns

As may be expected, all of the examples of optimum-seeking studies that have been described were animal experiments. Such studies use relatively homogeneous subjects that have had relatively homogeneous experimental tumor systems carefully grafted into them. Certainly, experiments of this type present simpler design and analysis problems than are likely to be met in clinical trials, where patients and tumors alike are more variable and where the period of follow-up time required by the study is considerably lengthened.

Notwithstanding these and other arguments, optimal-seeking clinical trials can be designed that meet technical as well as ethical standards. One example of the diversity of the acceptable dose range can be seen in the design of new single-agent treatment studies for relatively rare disease. As no single investigator has a sufficient patient pool, some type of multiinstitutional cooperative study is required. Attendance at the protocol design sessions almost invariably shows that the dose selected is a result of clinical compromises. Dose selection is arbitrary in a statistical sense, and if one considers that doses larger than that ultimately selected and no dose of the drug are both contemplated, it appears that the ethical dose range is substantially wider than that tested.

The ethical requirement may be to design the clinical experiment so that the true optimum is near the edge of design regions. This avoids causing overt therapy-induced toxicities, which may be ethically unacceptable. It will also reduce the ability to estimate curvature and thus locate the optimum of the surface. Constrained optimization methods and confidence bounds for constrained optima provide effective tools that would find real application in clinical studies (Wampler et al., 1978 and Stablein et al., 1983).

E. Conclusion

It is important that our understanding of how to design and analyze such clinical studies be expanded. We can no longer afford to use and study a drug as intensively as 5-FU has been for 20 years and still have little knowledge about its optimal use. The increasing costs and competition for clinical research funding will not permit us the luxury of comparing all possible dose levels of drug A with all possible dose levels of drug B in the context of present-day Phase III clinical trials methodology. And, given the trend to combination and multimodality therapies, we cannot rely any longer on the casual observation and intuitive analysis of the astute clinician to identify optimum doses and/or schedules for complex treatment programs.

The time has come to deliberately seek out ways of adapting and extending available statistical methodology to these problems in clinical research. This will require developments in two related areas. First, we must rethink the framework within which we conduct clinical trials research. While the Phase I, II, and III framework as currently defined may (or may not) serve the needs of the FDA, it clearly is limited as a methodological framework for the broader needs of clinical research. Specifically, we need to make provisions within the framework for rationally selecting optimum dose levels and schedules, particularly for multiagent therapies.

It has been remarked that while there may be a place for optimum-seeking strategy in clinical research, it certainly was not in Phase III trials. This is certainly the case. Phase III clinical trials as presently conceived provided clear and unambiguous information about the effectiveness of treatment A relative to treatment B and should not be changed. However, it is clear that classical Phase III trials are also limited insofar as the questions they can answer. Hence, we would propose that the use of such trials be limited, and further, that together with our clinician colleagues we seek to define a more meaningful framework for evaluating new clinical therapies.

Modification of the FDA framework for evaluating new therapies will require new and innovative experimental designs and analyses, particularly if we are to meaningfully attack the problem of identifying optimal combinations of the complex regimens being considered in biomedicine today. Both sets of these requirements present the statistician with unusual opportunities to contribute to a useful redirection of modern clinical research.

II. CONSIDERATIONS IN COMBINATION DRUG DEVELOPMENT

Karl E. Peace

A. Introduction

The definition of a combination drug is, "Two or more drugs, each in a fixed amount, which are formulated as one dosage form and administered together." The combination drug policy, as stated in the *Federal Register* (300.5021 CFR), is, "Two or more drugs may be combined in a single dose form when each component makes a *contribution* to the *claimed effects* and the dosage of each component is such that the combination is safe and effective for a significant patient population requiring such concurrent therapy. . . ." This policy, as stated, applies to the development of combination drugs for human consumption. The policy statement for the development of drugs for animal consumption is similar. It is fair to say that these policy statements form the basis for regulatory approval of combination drugs to be marketed in the United States.

There are many issues and questions inherent in the development of combination drugs. Some are discussed in this section.

B. Issues or Questions

Some of the issues or questions appear explicitly in the Statement of Policy. For example, (1) what is meant by the term "contribution"? Other questions are: (2) Should combination drug trials be placebo-controlled? (3) What are the hypotheses to be tested? (4) What is the most efficient or appropriate experimental design to address the hypotheses? (5) What are the most appropriate analyses of data collected from the experiment? (6) To what extent are answers to the previous five questions influenced by the phrase "claimed effects"—which appears in the policy statement? (7) To what extent does the clinical development approach depend on the number of components in the combination? Appropriate consideration of these questions poses a final one: (8) Should policy requirements be modified?

C. Discussion

To shed some light on the first question, "What is meant by the term 'contribution'?" one interpretation for a two component combination (AB) is that it must be superior to component A and also superior to component B. But what do we mean by "superior"? Does this mean statistical significance at the 0.05 level? Or statistical significance at some other less stringent level? Or perhaps statistical significance at a more stringent Type I error level? The combination AB compared to A and AB compared to B being the *only* requirements says that there is no interest in the effectiveness of A or B alone.

In addition, the *combination may be effective* yet not statistically significantly better than either component alone. Further, neither component may be significantly better than placebo. In this case, it would appear from the policy statement that the combination (AB) could not be marketed—even though it was effective! Ultimately, effectiveness of the combination should be the main concern.

On the question "Should combination drug trials be placebo-controlled?" they should, providing ethical considerations are not prohibitive. Because with an appropriate design, the effectiveness of each component alone may be assessed—which from a scientific perspective would have to be of interest. More importantly, however, the crucial question of effectiveness of the combination may be addressed. The contrast for the effectiveness of the combination is the estimate of the effect of AB minus the estimate of the effect of placebo: $\widehat{AB} - \hat{P}$. One may algebraically express the contrast as:

$$\tfrac{1}{2}[(\widehat{AB} - \hat{B}) + (\hat{A} - \hat{P})] + \tfrac{1}{2}[(\widehat{AB} - \hat{A}) + (\hat{B} - \hat{P})]$$

That is, the contrast for the effectiveness of the combination is the sum of the estimate of the net effect of A and the estimate of the net effect of B—without consideration of interaction between A and B.

Viewing the effectiveness of the combination in this manner reflects the need to include a placebo group in the clinical trial and that the associated experimental design should be a 2×2 factorial. Two other points are germane. The first is that addressing the effectiveness question and expressing it as contributions from the individual components projects the most proper interpretation of the term "contribution" as used in the policy statement. The single components of the combination should be viewed as making contributions to the effectiveness of the combination in an estimation sense. If the estimate of the effect of either component is zero, then the other component would essentially drive the effectiveness of the combination—if, in fact, the combination were effective. The second point is that it is possible for the sum of the effect of A and the effect of B to be effective when neither component individually is effective.

Now one may also write the effectiveness contrast as:

$$(\hat{A}-\hat{P})+(\hat{B}-\hat{P})+\hat{I}, \quad \text{where } \hat{I}=[(\widehat{AB}-\hat{B})-(\hat{A}-\hat{P})]$$

That is, the effectiveness of the combination contrast is also the sum of the estimates of the effects of A and B when compared to placebo plus the estimate of the magnitude of the interaction between A and B.

Viewing the effectiveness contrast of the combination in this manner again reflects proper interpretation of the term "contribution" in the policy statement. For it is possible for the individual components when compared to placebo to not be effective or to be marginally effective yet synergistic and still guarantee the effectiveness of the combination. In such settings, it should be important to assess the degree to which the individual components contribute jointly—in terms of synergistic effects.

Turning to the question of what are the hypotheses to be tested, one could interpret testing the individual null hypotheses H_{01}: $\mu AB = \mu A$ and H_{02}: $\mu AB = \mu B$ versus the respective individual alternative hypotheses H_{a1}: $\mu AB > \mu A$ and H_{a2}: $\mu AB > \mu B$ as being consistent with the policy statement—that is, require AB to be better than A at the Type I error level α and AB to be better than B also at level α in order for regulatory approval to market the combination to be given.

The policy statement may also be interpreted as testing the null hypothesis H_{03}: $H_{01} \cup H_{02}$ versus the joint alternative hypothesis H_{a3}: $H_{01} \cap H_{02}$ at the Type I error level α^* ($=0.05$, say). That is, the null hypothesis is that AB is no different from A *or* AB is no different from B, and the alternative hypothesis is that AB is better than A *and* AB is better than B at the α^* level. As Laska and Meisner point out in Section III, if one adopts the point of view that this hypothesis framework is appropriate, then the sample size per group would be on the order of 20% greater than the sample size per group for the individual hypotheses

(H_{01}, H_{02}). The 20% greater increase in sample size assumes 5% error levels of both types. The interpretation most often given to the policy statement as to what hypotheses to be tested is the individual hypotheses (H_{01}, H_{02}) setting or the joint hypotheses (H_{03}) setting. Again, the crucial question really should be the effectiveness of the combination as compared to placebo; although this is not to gainsay interest is assessing the degree to which each component alone is superior to placebo, the extent to which the effect of A (in combination with B) is significant and the extent to which B (in combination with A) is significant and the extent to which the interaction between A and B is significant. Therefore, other hypotheses of possible interest are:

$$H_{04}\colon \mu AB = \mu P \quad \text{versus} \quad H_{a4}\colon \mu AB > \mu P$$

$$H_{05}\colon \mu A = \mu P \quad \text{versus} \quad H_{a5}\colon \mu A > \mu P$$

$$H_{06}\colon \mu B = \mu P \quad \text{versus} \quad H_{a6}\colon \mu B > \mu P$$

$$H_{07}\colon \tfrac{1}{2}\{(\mu AB - \mu A) + (\mu B - \mu P)\} = 0 \quad \text{versus} \quad H_{a7}\colon \tfrac{1}{2}\{(\mu AB - \mu A) + (\mu B - \mu P)\} > 0$$

$$H_{08}\colon \tfrac{1}{2}\{(\mu AB - \mu B) + (\mu A - \mu P)\} = 0 \quad \text{versus} \quad H_{a8}\colon \tfrac{1}{2}\{(\mu AB - \mu B) + (\mu A - \mu P)\} > 0$$

$$H_{09}\colon I = 0 \quad \text{versus} \quad H_{a9}\colon I > 0$$

Whether exploration of any of these hypotheses should exact a penalty on the overall type I error is debatable.

Considering the question of what is the most efficient design, the design of choice should be the full 2×2 factorial. This is clearly the case in the absence of trying to define the levels of A and B that should be used in the combination through response-surface methodology (cRSM) (Myers, 1971) techniques. Other possible designs would be less than the full 2×2 factorial. For example, excluding placebo would be consistent with the policy statement. Including placebo and excluding A and B would permit assessment of the effectiveness of the combination alone, but would not allow exploration of how A and B contribute to the effectiveness.

In the development of new combination drugs, particularly in Phase II trials, we should have larger factorial experiments or other appropriate response-surface methodology (RSM) designs with several levels of components A and B. This would enable drug developers to define the optimal levels of the two factors that should be combined in a single formulation. Examples of this position and associated methods are addressed in Section IV. Such a Phase II program could then be followed by a definitively designed, confirmatory Phase III trial. The Phase III trial would employ a completely randomized design of only the combination at the optimal levels of the components and placebo.

Now, concerning the question of what the most appropriate analyses are, the design chosen, the hypothesis framework, the effectiveness measures, and their behavior will dictate appropriate statistical methodological analyses. The completely randomized design with AB, A, B, and P permits one to exploit the factorial nature of the experiment and to address the effectiveness questions. In addition, comparison among any of the four treatment groups could be made. Laska and Meisner present in Section III most powerful tests for the hypothesis framework H_{03} versus H_{a3}. The role of estimation should also be explored. It is of interest to know, regardless of the underlying experimental design, what the estimate of the effectiveness of the components alone is and, in addition to just those point estimates, what corresponding interval estimates are. In my view, if the design is the full 2×2 factorial, then the only hypothesis that should be tested is the combination versus placebo. It should command the full experimentwise Type I error. All other contrasts should be estimated without any penalty on the Type I error for the combination compared to placebo.

In addition, there are situations where one would want to test hypotheses regarding the effectiveness of the combination as compared to placebo and the superiority of the combination as compared to one component but also provide an interval estimate on the combination versus the other component as well. An example would be in the development of combinations for use in treating a condition where one component would be expected to ameliorate one symptom and the other component would be expected to ameliorate another symptom.

Now addressing the question of to what extent answers to the previous five questions are influenced by the claimed effects, the interpretation of the policy statement in Section III reflects the situation where there is one primary response measure that both components enhance. However, what are the appropriate hypotheses, what are the appropriate analyses, and what are the appropriate comparisons in a situation where there is only one primary response measure and one component enhances but the other does not? An example would be where an inactive compound is added to an active compound to reduce the toxicity caused by the active compound. There is also the situation alluded to in the previous paragraph where there are two primary response measures (Y_1, Y_2) that you hope the combination will ameliorate but you know that one component (A) enhances one response measure (Y_1) and not the other and vice versa. Parenthetically, this situation is fairly common in proving efficacy of drugs which were on the market prior to the Kefauver–Harris Amendment of 1962 and the Drug Efficacy and Safety Implementation (DESI) Review that followed that amendment. In this particular setting, what are the appropriate hypotheses? There are two individual alternative hypotheses that are appropriate: $H_{AY1}: \mu AB > \mu P$ and $\mu AB > \mu B$ and $H_{AY2}: \mu AB > \mu P$ and $\mu AB > \mu A$. One would furnish individual confidence intervals comparing AB to A in terms of the response measure Y_1 and comparing AB to B in terms of the response measure Y_2. However, these intervals should not exact a penalty on the Type I decision risk regarding approval of effectivenessness of the combination.

Now focusing on the penultimate question of to what extent the development approach is dependent on the number of components, one can easily envision situations where more than two drugs at individual dosages are desired. Antineoplastic drugs are a prime example. What would be the interpretation of the combination drug policy in these situations? If the combination contained three components (A, B, or C), would the sponsor have to demonstrate that ABC is better ($>$) than A, that $ABC > B$, that $ABC > C$, that $ABC > AB$, that $ABC > AC$, and that $ABC > BC$? And would the appropriate hypotheses be the implied six individual hypotheses or just one joint hypothesis? In either case, what would be the appropriate experimentwise Type I error rate?

Finally, and meriting much attention, is the choice of the levels of the drugs that go into the eventual combination. As alluded to before, drug developers should conduct RSM experiments that would enable one to choose a combination that contains levels of the factors which are optimal at some clinical definition of optimality. The methodology of Carter et al. (1977, 1979, 1983), Stablein et al. (1980, 1983), and Wampler et al. (1978) is useful in this regard. However, the methodology, based on the state of the art of experimentation, may be more readily applied to the development of animal drugs than to the development of drugs for human consumption. This is in part due to size and logistical difficulties in conducting clinical trials. However, there are many indications for human consumption where response surface methodology could be used to identify the optimum levels of the drugs to be placed in combination. Having performed those trials, which would likely be viewed as exploratory but which should provide adequate evidence as to the choice of the particular components and their levels, then follow-up, confirmatory, Phase III efficacy trials should only be required to confirm the effectiveness of the combination at those levels. This could be done with a single placebo-controlled trial against the combination at the optimum levels.

III. HYPOTHESIS TESTING FOR COMBINATION TREATMENTS

Eugene M. Laska and Morris J. Meisner

The FDA's regulations for combination treatments require that "each component makes a contribution to the claimed effects." In the case of a univariate response measure this leads to the statistical problem of testing whether a combination treatment is *better* than each of its component treatments. Suppose there are univariate tests S_i that contrast the combination treatment with component treatment i. The min test is defined to be the procedure that rejects the null hypothesis that the combination treatment is not better than each component if each S_i rejects the hypothesis that the combination treatment is not better than the ith component. Restricting attention to test statistics that are monotone nondecreasing functions of S_i, the min test is an optimal α-level test. For normal random variables the min test is also the likelihood ratio test. For combination drugs treating more than one symptom, one of several possible translations of the FDA regulation is given. By analogy to the definition of admissibility, we say that each component contributes if none of the components is at least as good as the combination for every symptom. A test procedure is suggested for this multivariate formulation.

A. Introduction

Combination therapies are in wide use and are appropriate in many circumstances. This approach to treatment is not limited to combinations of pharmacological agents. For example, psychiatrists have been interested in the question of the relative merits of the combination of psychotherapy and medication therapy compared to its components alone. To fix ideas in the sequel, however, we shall refer to the treatments as drugs. We assume that there are two component drugs, B and C, and a combination of the two that will be labeled A. Before a drug consisting of several component drugs can be approved the U.S. Food and Drug Administration regulations require that "each component makes a contribution to the claimed effects . . ." (21CFR, 300.50). This requirement is appropriate for nonpharmacological components as well. There are two distinct frameworks in which the problem of translation of this sentence into a statistical hypothesis can be considered. The first relates to combination drugs that affect a single target symptom, that is, a drug in which the outcome measure is a univariate random variable. The second relates to a combination drug in which the drugs treat more than one target symptom, that is, the outcome measure has several components and so the response variable is multivariate. Clearly, the Food and Drug Administration regulations imply that the drug should not be prescribed if one of the constituents is at least as effective as the combination because there may be increased cost as well as risk of adverse effect from the combination yet no additional benefit from exposure to the second constituent. In the univariate case, this requirement is translated into the need to demonstrate that the combination is more effective than each of its constituents. In the multivariate case, the FDA regulation may be interpreted in several different ways, which correspond to different hypothesis tests.

B. Optimal Tests for the General Univariate Case

Let X_0, X_1, and X_2 be three random variables that respectively characterize the effects of treatments A, B, and C. The distribution of X_i has parameter μ_i, $i=1, 2$, or 3, which generally is a location parameter, and we assume that larger values of the parameters indicate greater efficacy and are more desirable. Letting $\gamma=\mu_0-\mu_1$ and $\theta=\mu_0-\mu_2$, the null hypothesis corresponding to 21CFR, 300.50 may be described as

$$H_0\colon \mu_0 \le \mu_1 \quad \text{or} \quad \mu_0 \le \mu_2$$

which is equivalent to $\gamma \le 0$ or $\theta \le 0$, and the alternative hypothesis that the combination treatment is best is

$$H_1\colon \mu_0 > \mu_1 \quad \text{and} \quad \mu_0 > \mu_2$$

which is equivalent to $\min(\gamma, \theta) > 0$.

The problem of testing whether the combination is best is thus framed in terms of testing whether the parameters (γ, θ) lie in a particular region in the two dimensional parameter plane. The points in the interior of the first quadrant excluding the positive axes comprise the alternative hypothesis H_1. All of the points in quadrants two, three, and four, as well as those on the axes of quadrant one, comprise the null hypothesis H_0. In some applications (such as cases in which the outcome is binomial) the parameters (e.g., the probability of response) may be constrained to lie in a bounded subset.

We begin by supposing that there are two univariate test statistics, S for testing $H_{0B}\colon \gamma \le 0$ versus $H_{1B}\colon \gamma > 0$ and T for testing $H_{0C}\colon \theta \le 0$ versus $H_{1C}\colon \theta > 0$ that possess some desirable properties. For example, S and T may be uniformly most powerful (UMP) or likelihood ratio tests. We assume further that the univariate distribution of S, say, $F_1(s; \gamma)$ does not depend on the parameter θ, and similarly, the univariate distribution of T, $F_2(t;\theta)$, does not depend on γ. The distribution of the underlying random variables X_0, X_1, and X_2 will in general determine the joint distribution $F(s, t; \gamma, \theta)$ of the random variables S and T. We shall assume that larger values of S and T provide more evidence in favor of H_{1B} and H_{1C}, respectively. To test H_{0B} univariately the rejection region is of the form $S > k_1$. Similarly, for H_{0C} the rejection region is $T > k_2$ where k_1 and k_2 are the smallest scalar values that yield α-level tests. Thus

$$\alpha = \sup_{\gamma \le 0} \int_{k_1}^{\infty} dF_1(s;\gamma) = \sup_{\theta \le 0} \int_{k_2}^{\infty} dF_2(t;\theta)$$

We shall restrict attention to the family of monotone test statistics, that is, statistics that are generated by functions $g(s, t)$ that are monotone nondecreasing in s and t in both arguments. We shall discuss the justification for this restriction below. A test that is monotone has the property that if a given value of the test statistic rejects the null hypothesis, so do all values that are larger.

We have previously shown (Laska and Meisner, 1989) that the test that rejects H_0 when both S and T reject their respective null hypothesis H_{0B} and H_{0C} is the uniformly most powerful α-level test of H_0 versus H_1 among the family of monotone tests.

Theorem 1: Let G be the family of all monotone nondecreasing functions of two variables. Let us test statistics S and T for H_{0B} and H_{0C}, respectively, be specified. For each $g \in G$ let k, depending on g, be chosen such that

$$\sup_{H_0} P_{\gamma,\theta}(g > k) \le \alpha$$

If for all $g \in G$,

(A) F has the property that $P_{\gamma,\theta}(g > k)$ is a monotone nondecreasing function of γ for each fixed θ and of θ for each fixed γ,

(B1) $$\lim_{\theta \to \infty} P_{0,\theta}\{g > k\} = \int_{g(s,\infty) > k} dF_1(s;0)$$

and

(B2) $$\lim_{\gamma \to \infty} P_{\gamma,0}\{g > k\} = \int_{g(\infty,t) > k} dF_2(t;0)$$

then the rejection region of the uniformly most powerful α-level test of H_0 versus H_1 within the family G is given by $M = \min(S - k_1, T - k_2) > 0$.

We shall call this test the min test.

The conditions (A), (B1), and (B2) on Theorem 1 concern the behavior of the joint distribution F of the test statistics S and T. It is easy to verify the truth of condition (A) simply by checking if $P_{\gamma,\theta}(S > s, T > t)$ is monotone nondecreasing in γ and θ. In the special case when the joint distribution is a translation parameter family, that is, $F(s, t; \gamma, \theta)$ is of the form $F(s - \gamma, t - \theta)$, the conditions follow immediately. The conditions of Theorem 1 also hold for the case when S and T each follow the t distribution.

Condition (A) of the theorem, which requires that the probability measures of the set $g > k$ are increasing in γ and θ, implies that the size of the test α, defined as the supremum over H_0 of the probability of rejection, occurs at either the parameter point $(0, \infty)$ or $(\infty, 0)$. Since P is increasing, $P_{0,0}$ is usually well below α, and therefore the min test is biased. Lehmann (1952) proved that nonrandomized unbiased monotone tests of the hypothesis H_0 do not exist.

If S and T are independent and each gives rise to an α-level test, then for points close to the origin in H_1 the power of the min test is approximately α^2. Mathematically, the difficulty of bias may be remedied to some extent by utilizing tests that are not necessarily monotone. For the translation parameter case, with S and T independent, Guttman (1987) has explicitly constructed a test that is more powerful than the min test. Although Guttman's procedure is an α-level test, at each point (γ, θ) in H_0 the probability of a Type I error exceeds that of the min test. More generally, Cohen, Gatsonis, and Marden (1983) proved that the min test in the translation parameter case is admissible. Berger (1989) also developed a nonmonotone test in the normal case with known covariance matrix, whose power exceeds that of the min test. In fact, Berger's test is more powerful than Guttman's (1987) test.

However, in the application under consideration, the use of nonmonotone tests can lead to seriously unacceptable consequences. The most compelling argument for restricting attention to monotone tests relates to the fact that larger values of either or both of the test statistics, S and T, lend more credence to the alternative hypothesis, H_1. If the monotonicity condition is eliminated it is possible to be in a situation that is difficult or impossible to defend. For example, suppose two drug companies wish to market the same combination drug, and they each provide evidence to the FDA in support of their new drug application. If use of the nonmonotone test were permitted it could happen that the company with the less persuasive evidence has their application approved while the application of the company with the more persuasive evidence is denied. A judicial review of such an FDA decision could only conclude that the regulatory agencies' approach (that is, statistical procedure) is unfair and perhaps irrational. For such reasons the restriction to monotone tests can be considered a rather natural requirement. (However, nonmonotone tests are mathematically interesting. They are theoretically important and there may be applications in which their use makes sense.)

C. The Normal Case

For the normal case the natural candidates for S and T are the sample means in the case of known variance and t statistics in the case of unknown variance. The conditions of Theorem 1 hold so that the min test is the UMP among all monotone nondecreasing functions of the sample means and the t statistics.

It has been shown that the likelihood ratio of H_0 for a multivariate normal distribution with known Σ is identical to the min test (Inada, 1978; Sasabuchi, 1981).

Theorem 2: Let $(Y_1, Y_2)'$ be normally distributed with mean $(\theta, \gamma)'$. If the covariance matrix Σ is known, then the likelihood ratio Λ of H_0 is given by the expression

$$\log \Lambda = \begin{cases} 0 & \overline{Y_1} \leq 0 \quad \text{or} \quad \overline{Y_2} \leq 0 \\ -\min(Y_2^2/\sigma_{11}, Y_2^2/\sigma_{22}) & \overline{Y_1} > 0 \quad \text{and} \quad \overline{Y_2} > 0 \end{cases}$$

In the special case where $\Sigma = \sigma^2 I$ and σ^2 is unknown, the results of Theorem 2 also holds with the pooled estimate of variance replacing σ^2. Sasabuchi (1988) has recently found that if Σ is unknown, the likelihood ratio is the min of two t statistics.

As an application to the combination problem, consider a one-way layout design with three groups, each receiving one of the treatments A, B, or C. If there are n subjects per group, the test statistics

$$S = \sqrt{n/2}(\overline{X_0} - \overline{X_1}) \qquad T = \sqrt{n/2}(\overline{X_0} - \overline{X_2})$$

are bivariate normal with mean $\sqrt{n/2}(\gamma, \theta)$ and covariance matrix

$$\sigma^2 \begin{pmatrix} 1 & 1/2 \\ 1/2 & 1 \end{pmatrix}$$

Applying the theorem above for σ^2 known, it follows that the min test is the likelihood ratio test. If σ^2 is unknown the likelihood ratio test is the min test formed by taking $S' = S/\hat{\sigma}$ and $T' = T/\hat{\sigma}$ where S and T are given above the $\hat{\sigma}^2$ is the pooled mean-squared error term from a one-way ANOVA.

D. Other Cases

Although Theorem 1 is formulated in the continuous case, the conclusion may also be applied in the discrete case. Here, of course, not all significance levels are attainable. We consider two special cases, the Wilcoxon and binomial.

1. Wilcoxon Rank Test

Let X_0, X_1, and X_2, the response to treatments A, B, and C, be respectively distributed as $F(x)$, $F(x-\gamma)$, $F(x-\theta)$. For a three-group one-way layout with n subjects per group, let U_{X_0,X_1} and U_{X_0,X_2} be Mann–Whitney U statistics. Thus, $U_{X,Y}$ is the number of i, j such that $X_i < Y_j$. The discrete analog of the outcome space represented by the plane in Theorem 1 is now the integer lattice points $0 \le i \le n^2$, $0 \le j \le n^2$. The conditions of Theorem 1 may be shown to hold when the variables S and T are U statistics. For condition A, the crux of the proof, omitted here, follows the lines of Lehmann's (1975) proof of the monotonicity of the power functions of the U statistic. The proof rests upon the fact that $F(\cdot)$ has a translation parameter form. We introduce $V = X_1 + \gamma_1 - \gamma$ where $\gamma_1 > \gamma$. Then V has distribution $F(x-\gamma_1)$, and $X_1 \le V$ implying $U_{X_0,X_1} \le U_{X_0V}$. Therefore nondecreasing g, $g(U_{X_0,X_1}, U_{X_0,X_2})$ is less than or equal to $g(U_{X_0,V}, U_{X_0,X_2})$. Thus, $P_{\gamma,\theta}(g > k) \le P_{\gamma_1,\theta}(g > k)$, $\gamma_1 \ge \gamma$, establishing condition (A) of Theorem 1. Conditions (B1) and (B2) follow since $U_{X_0X_1}$ converges almost surely to n^2 as γ goes to infinity. Thus, the min test is UMP among all nondecreasing functions of U_{X_0,X_1} and U_{X_0,X_2}.

2. Binomial Model

Suppose one group of n subjects is given both A and B, and let γ denote the chance that A is preferred to B. Suppose that another n subjects are given both A and C, with θ denoting the probability that A is preferred. Here S denotes the number of successes (A preferred) in the first group and T the number of successes (B preferred) in the second. Under this design S and T are independent. The parameter space is the unit square $0 \le \gamma \le 1$, $0 \le \theta \le 1$. The alternative hypothesis is the square with vertices (1/2, 1/2), (1, 1/2), (1/2, 1), and (1, 1). The point (1/2, 1/2) corresponds to the origin of the parameter space in Theorem 1. The conditions of Theorem 1 apply. To show that condition (A) holds, it must be shown that $P_{\gamma,\theta}(g(S, T) > k)$ is increasing in γ and θ. However for each fixed s, $P_{\gamma,\theta}(g(s, T) > k)$ is equivalent to $P_\theta(T > k_1)$ with $k_1 = k_1(s)$ chosen appropriately. The expression $P_\theta(T > k_1)$ is increasing in θ since the binomial distribution has a monotone likelihood ratio (Lehmann, 1959). Thus, $P_{\gamma,\theta}(g(S, T) > k)$ is a weighted sum with weights $(P_\gamma(S = s))$ of increasing functions of θ, establishing condition (A) for θ. Similarly, $P_\gamma(S > k_1)$ is increasing in γ, establishing condition (A) for γ. Formally taking the limit as θ goes to the boundary in H_1 yields

$$\lim_{\theta \to 1} P_{1/2,\theta}(g(S, T) > k) = P_{1/2}(g(S, n) > k)$$

establishing the condition (B1); (B2) is established similarly.

E. Power and Sample Size in the Univariate Case

For the min test whose components are Student's t or Wilcoxon, for a 5% level test, a table of sample sizes per group necessary to achieve 50%, 80%, 90%, and 95% power is given in Laska and Meisner (1989). For example, 27 subjects per group are required to achieve 80% power with $\alpha = 0.05$ power when $\gamma/\theta = 0.07$ and $\theta/\sigma = 0.10$. There is, however, a simple rule of thumb whose derivation is given in Laska and Meisner (1986) that enables a choice of sample size for the normal and Wilcoxon to be made on the basis of widely available power tables. To guarantee at least 80% power at a point $(\gamma/\sigma, \theta/\sigma)$ in the alternative space H_1, first set $\delta = \min(\gamma/\sigma, \theta/\sigma)$ and, using usual univariate normal tables find the sample size, say m, needed to achieve power 0.80 or better at δ in a test of differences between two treatments. The rule indicates that the sample size n for the combination problem is approximately $1.25m$. Thus, from a power perspective, 25% more subjects per treatment group are required to test the combination hypothesis than are required for the usual comparison of two treatments.

F. Multivariate Case

We now consider the situation in which the combination treatment affects, say, two different symptoms. The response measures are therefore bivariate observations. Components one and two of the random variable respectively correspond to the responses with respect to symptoms one and two. The question of how to translate the phrase "each component makes a contribution to the claimed effect" into a statistical hypothesis is no longer obvious. We give only one of several possible interpretations.

Let (X_0, Y_0), (X_1, Y_1), (X_2, Y_2) be the three bivariate random variables that respectively characterize the response to treatments A, B, and C of the two symptoms. Let (X_i, Y_i) have parameters (μ_i, λ_i), $i=0, 1,$ and 2, with larger values of the parameter corresponding to the more desirable effects. Set

$$\gamma_1(\mathrm{B}) = \mu_0 - \mu_1 \qquad \gamma_2(\mathrm{B}) = \lambda_0 - \lambda_1$$

$$\gamma_1(\mathrm{C}) = \mu_0 - \mu_2 \qquad \gamma_2(\mathrm{C}) = \lambda_0 - \lambda_2$$

Thus, for example, $\gamma(\mathrm{B}) = (\gamma_1(\mathrm{B}), \gamma_2(\mathrm{B}))'$ denotes the increment in effect of the combination treatment A over treatment B, with the effect on symptom i being denoted by the component $\gamma_i(\mathrm{B})$.

The classical statistical definition of admissibility suggests an interpretation of "each component makes a contribution." We shall say that the combination treatment A is admissible if A is superior to each component treatment for at least one symptom. That is, neither B alone nor C alone is at least as good as A for each symptom. If A is superior to B for at least one symptom, then $\max(\gamma_1(\mathrm{B}), \gamma_2(\mathrm{B})) > 0$; if A is superior to C for at least one symptom, then $\max(\gamma_1(\mathrm{C}), \gamma_2(\mathrm{C})) > 0$. To show that each component treatment contributes it is necessary to show that both conditions hold. Thus, the alternative hypothesis to admissibility, which we denote by (a), is

$$H_1(\mathrm{a})\colon \max(\gamma_1(\mathrm{B}), \gamma_2(\mathrm{B})) > 0 \quad \text{and} \quad \max(\gamma_1(\mathrm{C}), \gamma_2(\mathrm{C})) > 0$$

and the null hypothesis is

$$H_0(\mathrm{a})\colon \max(\gamma_1(\mathrm{B}), \gamma_2(\mathrm{B})) \le 0 \quad \text{or} \quad \max(\gamma_1(\mathrm{C}), \gamma_2(\mathrm{C})) \le 0$$

We note that the forms of these hypotheses are similar to the form of univariate H_0 considered above. $H_1(\mathrm{a})$ is the intersection of the two hypotheses $\max(\gamma_1(\mathrm{B}), \gamma_2(\mathrm{B})) \le 0$ and $\max(\gamma_1(\mathrm{C}), \gamma_2(\mathrm{C})) \le 0$. Thus, if there were statistics, say, S to test $\gamma(\mathrm{B})$ and T to test $\gamma(\mathrm{C})$, then according to a minor variant of Theorem 1, the test statistic, $\min(S, T)$ is UMP among all monotone nondecreasing functions of S and T. A modification of Theorem 1 is necessary as four parameters are involved, with S depending on $\gamma_1(\mathrm{B})$ and $\gamma_2(\mathrm{B})$ and T depending on $\gamma_1(\mathrm{C})$ and $\gamma_2(\mathrm{C})$.

The problem of finding statistics to test $\max(\gamma_1(B), \gamma_2(B)) > 0$ has been discussed by Miller (1981), who calls it the "many one" testing problem. Typically, it arises from a comparison of many treatments with a single control to determine if any are better than the control. In a certain sense the problem is dual to the combination drug problem. For the many one problem with parameters, say, β_1 and β_2, H_0 is the third quadrant and $H_1 = \max(\beta_1, \beta_2) > 0$ is quadrants one, two, and four. If U_1 is a test of $\beta_1 > 0$ and U_2 is a test of $\beta_2 > 0$, a reasonable test statistic for the many one problem is $\max(U_1, U_2)$. Returning to the combination problem, suppose S_1 tests $\gamma_1(B) > 0$, S_2 tests $\gamma_2(B) > 0$, T_1 tests $\gamma_1(C) > 0$, and T_2 tests $\gamma_2(C) > 0$. Let $S = \max(S_1, S_2)$ and $T = \max(T_1, T_2)$. In order to apply Theorem 1 and construct a min test, we require an α-level test based on S and an α-level test based on T. Although in many applications the distribution of S_1 and S_2 may be known, generally the distribution of $S = \max(S_1, S_2)$ is unknown or more precisely depends on nuisance parameters. Therefore, an α-level test may be difficult to determine. Several suggestions appear in the literature to circumvent such problems, of which we mention just two.

In the first, a simple expedient to choosing a cut point k is to use Bonferroni's inequality. Let $S = \max(S_1 - k_1, S_2 - k_2)$ and $T = \max(T_1 - k_3, T_2 - k_4)$ where k_1, k_2, k_3 and k_4 are respectively chosen to make each univariate rejection region $S_1 > k_1$, $S_2 > k_2$, $T_1 > k_3$, and $T_2 > k_4$, in $(\alpha/2)$-level test. Then, by the Bonferroni inequality, S and T are each at most α-level tests and therefore the test $\min\{\max(S_1 - k_1, S_2 - k_2), \max(T_1 - k_3, T_2 - k_4)\} > 0$ is at most an α-level test of $H_0(a)$. This test is likely to be reasonably efficient, but it must be recognized that because of the use of the Bonferroni inequality, Theorem 1 cannot be invoked to declare the test to be optimal.

The second approach is asymptotic and assumes that the joint distribution of S_1 and S_2 is known up to a nuisance parameter. The data are used to obtain a consistent estimator of the nuisance parameter, and hence an estimate of the distribution of $S = \max(S_1, S_2)$ is obtained. The latter is used to obtain the α-level test based on S. As with the Bonferroni procedure, this method also cannot be said to yield an optimal test.

Acknowledgement

This work was supported in part by National Institutes of Mental Health grant no. MH42959.

IV. RESPONSE SURFACE METHODOLOGY IN THE DEVELOPMENT OF ANTIANGINAL DRUGS

Karl E. Peace

A. Introduction

Stablein makes the point in Section I that little use of response surface methodology (RSM) and optimization techniques has been made in the clinical development of drugs for human consumption. This is indeed true, even though the relative merits of applying the methods and techniques in the clinical trial setting have been recognized for 30 years. A recent survey I made of the pharmaceutical industry, in preparation for chairing an invited paper session on the topic at the 1986 Midwest Biopharmaceutical Workshop (Muncie Conference), revealed only two companies where the approach had been tried. One application was in the anticancer drug development area. The other was in the antianginal drug development area.

The main focus of this section is the use of RSM techniques in Phase II antianginal trials. Such techniques may be used in this area as well as in Phase II programs of drugs for a variety of indications to more objectively guide the selection of dose and frequency of dosing to be used in confirmatory Phase III programs.

B. RSM Review

In applying RSM techniques, one is interested in studying the influence of certain factors $x_1, x_2, \ldots, x_r$, say, on a measurable response Y, where most often the functional form of Y on the x_i, $i = 1, 2, \ldots, r$, is unknown. So an experiment is conducted over some region of the factor space with Y being measured at points (levels of the factors) in the space.

Once the experiment is conducted and the data gathered, a response surface f is fitted to the data. That is, a model of the form

$$Y = f(x_1, x_2, \ldots, x_r) + e$$

is fitted by least-squares techniques. After acceptance of reasonable fit within the region of interest, the fitted surface,

$$\hat{y} = \hat{f}(x_1, x_2, \ldots, x_r)$$

may be explored as a function of the factors, using search methods or classical optimization techniques.

The functional form chosen for f may be dependent on prior knowledge of the expected relationship between Y and the x_i; however, usually low-order polynomials are adequate to describe the relationship in the region of interest. For example, a second-order polynomial response surface is given by

$$f(x_1, x_2) = \beta_0 + \beta_1 x_1 + \beta_2 x_2 + \beta_{12} x_1 x_2 + \beta_{11} x_1^2 + \beta_{22} x_2^2$$

In vector/matrix notation, the response surface may be written as

$$f(x_1, x_2) = \beta_0 + \mathbf{Xb} + \mathbf{X}B\mathbf{X}'$$

where

$$\mathbf{X} = (x_1, x_2)$$

$$\mathbf{b}' = (\beta_1, \beta_2)$$

$$B = \begin{bmatrix} \beta_{11} & \beta_{12}/2 \\ \beta_{12}/2 & \beta_{22} \end{bmatrix}$$

and where the prime denotes vector transposition. Written in this form, the stationary point or point at which relative minima or maxima may occur is given by

$$\mathbf{X}_0 = -B^{-1}\mathbf{b}'/2$$

where the -1 superscript denotes the inverse matrix. Substituting $\mathbf{X}_0$ into the equation for f yields the candidate for the relative optimum:

$$f(\mathbf{X}_0) = \beta_0 + \mathbf{X}_0\mathbf{b}'/2$$

There are many experimental designs that may be used that permit RSM techniques to be used. To some extent the form of the response surface f is constrained by the experimental design and vice versa. Some designs are factorial in nature—for example, two-factor or three-factor designs, each at k levels, 2^k or 3^k, respectively. There are also composite designs, particularly central composite ones (a 2^k augmented by $2K+1$ center points) as well as equiradial or uniform precision designs. Myers (1971) has a good discussion of the relative merits and properties of such designs.

In the antianginal drug development example that follows, an equiradial hexagonal design is used.

C. Phase II Antianginal Trials

1. Background and Objective

Response surface methodology was incorporated into Phase II clinical trials that sought to estimate dose and frequency of dosing of a new development compound thought to have antianginal efficacy prior to embarking on Phase III antianginal trials. The primary efficacy measure considered for this purpose was time to exercise induced anginal onset. An equiradial hexagonal design—two equilateral triangles with a common center point—and a second-order response model were used. Design and analysis aspects of these trials are reviewed.

The original objective of the Phase II program was to obtain dose-comparison information on measures reflecting possible antianginal efficacy when given b.i.d. and to compare the top b.i.d. regimen with a t.i.d. regimen with the same total daily dose. At the time of bebinning consultation, two draft protocols existed. Aspects of these follow.

2. Protocols

Protocol 1:

- Regimens
    - 0 mg b.i.d.
    - 4 mg b.i.d.
    - 6 mg b.i.d.
    - 4 mg t.i.d.
- The first three regimens furnish dose response or dose comparison information for b.i.d. administration.
- The last two regimens address the question, "Is it better to administer 12 mg per day as 6 mg b.i.d. or as 4 mg t.i.d.?"

Protocol 2:

- Regimens
    - 2 mg b.i.d.
    - 8 mg b.i.d.
    - 6 mg t.i.d.
- The 2 mg b.i.d. regimen was felt to be a "no effect" dose.
- The last two regimens address the question "Is it better to give 16 mg per day as 8 mg b.i.d. or according to the t.i.d. regimen 4 mg, 6 mg, and 6 mg?"

For each protocol, the measures of efficacy were:

- Time to anginal onset (primary)
- Total exercise time

- Double product (heart rate × systolic pressure) at the onset of angina and at the end of the exercise time
- Maximal *St* depression
- Time to maximal *St* depression
- Weekly anginal frequency
- Nitroglycerin use

Dosing and stress test considerations in the protocol were:

- Dosing
  - b.i.d. or t.i.d. for 16 days
  - plus 0 or 1 tablet on the 17th day dependent on dose groups and timing of stress test on day 17
- Stress test
  - first, training/familiarity
  - second, baseline on day 0
  - third, 2 h after last dose on day 17
  - fourth, 7 h after last dose on day 17
  - fifth, 12 h after last dose on day 17

3. Design and Model

At the initial consultation, it was observed that if protocol 2 also included a 4 mg b.i.d. regimen, then the two protocols could be amalgamated under a single equiradial–hexagonal design. This design is essentially two equilateral triangles with a common center point (Table 5.1, Figure 5.1). It is one of the class of uniform precision designs and is also rotatable and orthogonal. It permits exploration of response (endpoints) via second-order RSM techniques as a function of total daily dose (0–16 mg) and time of stress test after dosing. The design may be augmented to assess block (or investigator) differences.

The response surface model is given by

$$\text{Response} = \beta_0 + \beta_1 x_1 + \beta_2 x_2 + B + \beta_{12} x_1 x_2 + \beta_{11} x_1^2 + \beta_{22} x_2^2 + \text{error}$$

where B denotes (center or investigator) block effect and error represents the random error component in measuring response. The errors are assumed to be independent and identically normally distributed random variables with mean 0 and unknown but common variance.

TABLE 5.1 Basic design an equiradial, hexagonal design with center point in two equilateral triangular blocks (centers or investigators)[a]

Center I		Center II	
Coded vertices	Uncoded vertices	Coded vertices	Uncoded vertices
$(1/2, -\sqrt{3}/2)$	(12 mg, 2 h)	$(-1/2, \sqrt{3}/2)$	(4 mg, 2 h)
$(1/2, +\sqrt{3}/2)$	(12 mg, 12 h)	$(-1/2, +\sqrt{3}/2)$	(4 mg, 12 h)
(0, 0)	(8 mg, 7 h)	(0,0)	(8 mg, 7 h)
(−1, 0)	(0 mg, 7 h)	(1, 0)	(16 mg, 7 h)

[a] Dose is now reflected as total daily dose.

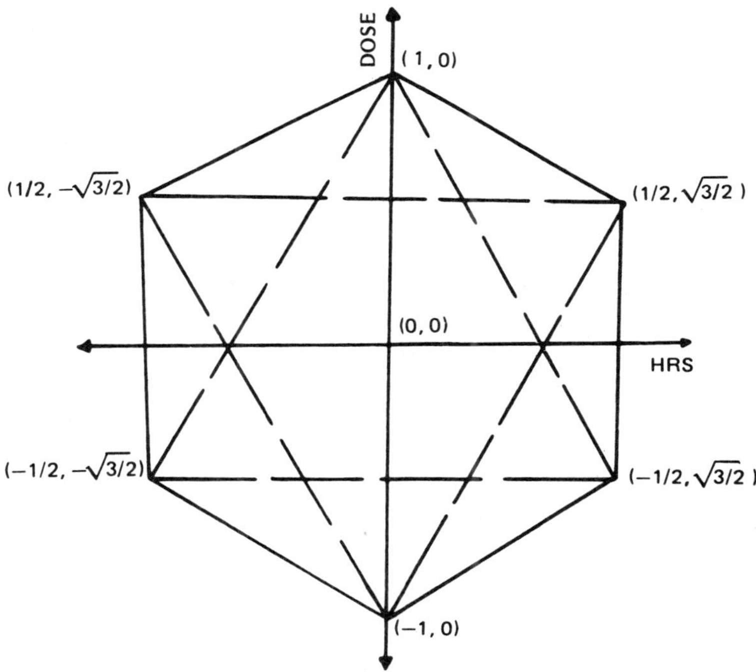

FIGURE 5.1 Equiradial hexagonal design or two equilateral triangles with a common center point.

The design matrix X is

$$X = \begin{bmatrix} x_0 & x_1(\text{dose}) & x_2(\text{time}) & \text{Blocks} & x_1x_2 & x_1^2 & x_2^2 \\ 1 & +1/2 & +\sqrt{3}/2 & +1 & +0.433012 & 1/4 & 3/4 \\ 1 & -1/2 & +\sqrt{3}/2 & -1 & -0.433012 & 1/4 & 3/4 \\ 1 & -1/2 & -\sqrt{3}/2 & -1 & +0.433012 & 1/4 & 3/4 \\ 1 & +1/2 & -\sqrt{3}/2 & +1 & -0.433012 & 1/4 & 3/4 \\ 1 & +1 & 0 & -1 & 0 & 1 & 0 \\ 1 & -1 & 0 & +1 & 0 & 1 & 0 \\ 1 & 0 & 0 & -1 & 0 & 0 & 0 \\ 1 & 0 & 0 & +1 & 0 & 0 & 0 \end{bmatrix}$$

The inverse of $X'X$ is

$$(X'X)^{-1} = \begin{bmatrix} \beta_0 & \beta_1 & \beta_2 & B & \beta_{12} & \beta_{11} & \beta_{22} \\ 0.5 & 0 & 0 & 0 & 0 & -0.5 & -0.5 \\ 0 & 0.33 & 0 & 0 & 0 & 0 & 0 \\ 0 & 0 & 0.33 & 0 & 0 & 0 & 0 \\ 0 & 0 & 0 & 0.125 & 0 & 0 & 0 \\ 0 & 0 & 0 & 0 & 1.33 & 0 & 0 \\ -0.5 & 0 & 0 & 0 & 0 & 1 & 0.33 \\ -0.5 & 0 & 0 & 0 & 0 & 0.33 & 1 \end{bmatrix}$$

Estimates of the parameters are given by

$$\hat{\boldsymbol{\beta}}' = (X'X)^{-1}(X'Y)/N$$

where $\hat{\boldsymbol{\beta}}' = (\hat{\beta}_0, \hat{\beta}_1, \hat{\beta}_2, \hat{B}, \hat{\beta}_{12}, \hat{\beta}_{11}, \hat{\beta}_{22})$, Y is the vector of responses, and N is the number of observations per design point = 6(2 investigators per center by 3 evaluatable patients per dose group).

The variance/covariance matrix of the estimates is given by

$$\text{Var}(\hat{\boldsymbol{\beta}}) = (X'X)^{-1}\, V(\text{error})$$

where V(error) is the estimate of the error variance, which is determined from the mean-square error from an analysis of variance reflecting the model. The variance/covariance matrix of the estimates may be used to construct 95% confidence intervals on the parameters.

4. Analysis Strategy

The data are summarized descriptively. Tables 5.2 and 5.3 reflect summarization of end points from Protocol 1.

Tables 5.4 and 5.5 reflect summarization of end points from Protocol 2. Further, data from the cells of Table 5.5 are used with data from the cells of Table 5.3 of Protocol 1 in second-order response-surface analyses aimed at finding dose and time after dose for which there exists acceptable efficacy for a chronic dosing regimen with total daily doses of 0, 4, 8, 12, and 16 mg. There are three response-surface (RSM) analyses. These are:

	Protocol 1	Protocol 2
Analysis 1:	Cells 12, 22, 31, 33	Cells 11, 13, 22, 32
Analysis 2:	Cells 11, 12, 41, 43	Cells 11, 13, 22, 32
Analysis 3:	Cells 12, 22, 31, 33	Cells 11, 13, 22, 42

Analysis 1 reflects dose and hour search over 0–16 mg total daily dose given b.i.d. chronic dosing. Analysis 2 reflects dose and hour search over 0–16 mg total daily dose given the 12-mg total daily dose was 4 mg t.i.d. instead of 6 mg b.i.d. The difference between the results in these two analyses will reflect differences between 6 mg b.i.d. and 4 mg t.i.d. or differences among subjects between the 6 mg b.i.d. group and the 4 mg t.i.d. group. Analysis 3 reflects dose and hour search over 0–16 mg total daily dose given the 16 mg total daily dose is given as 4 mg, 6 mg, 6 mg. The difference between the results in Analysis 1 and Analysis 3 will

TABLE 5.2 Numbers reference cells of the table

	Test 2 (baseline)	Test 3	Test 4	Test 5
0 mg b.i.d.	11	12	13	14
4 mg b.i.d.	21	22	23	24
6 mg b.i.d.	31	32	33	34
4 mg t.i.d.	41	42	43	44

TABLE 5.3 Numbers reference cells of the table

	Test 3 − Test 2 (2 h post dose)	Test 4 − Test 2 (7 h post dose)	Test 5 − Test 2 (12 h post dose)
0 mg b.i.d.	11	12	13
4 mg b.i.d.	21	22	23
6 mg b.i.d.	31	32	33
4 mg t.i.d.	41	42	43

TABLE 5.4 Numbers reference cells of the table

	Test 2 (baseline)	Test 3	Test 4	Test 5
2 mg b.i.d.	11	12	13	14
4 mg b.i.d.	21	22	23	24
8 mg b.i.d.	31	32	33	34
6 mg t.i.d.[a]	41	42	43	44

[a]4 mg, 6 mg, and 6 mg.

TABLE 5.5 Numbers reference cells of the table

	Test 3 − Test 2 (2 h post dose)	Test 4 − Test 2 (7 h post dose)	Test 5 − Test 2 (12 h post dose)
2 mg b.i.d.	11	12	13
4 mg b.i.d.	21	22	23
8 mg b.i.d.	31	32	33
6 mg t.i.d.[a]	41	42	43

[a]4 mg, 6 mg, and 6 mg.

reflect differences between 8 mg b.i.d. and 4 mg, 6 mg, 6 mg, or differences among subjects between the 8 mg b.i.d. group and the 4 mg, 6 mg, 6 mg group. Subject differences may be assessed using baseline measurements.

5. Results

The raw data reflecting time to exercise induced anginal onset appear in Tables 5.6 and 5.7 for Protocols 1 and 2, respectively. A descriptive analysis of these data appears in Table 5.8. A descriptive analysis of the change from baseline of the data in Tables 5.6 and 5.7 appears in Table 5.9. Plots of these changes appear in Fig. 5.2. Table 5.10 and Fig. 5.3, Table 5.11 and Fig. 5.4, and Table 5.12 and Fig. 5.4 reflect the three RSM analyses. Each table of the three pairs represents the standard analysis of variance (ANOVA) of the quadratic model. Each table is standard default output from the SAS PROC RSREG. Each figure of each pair represents a contour plot of the fitted quadratic model. These plots are also standard output from the RSREG PROC. Tables 5.13 and 5.14 present descriptive analyses of time to anginal onset at baseline of

TABLE 5.6 Raw data: Protocol 1, endpoint is time (min) to anginal onset

Group	PAT	INV	(BTIMEAO)	(TIMEAO2)	(TIMEAO7)	(TIMEAO12)
0 mg b.i.d.	1101	1	5.1	5.3	5.8	6.1
	1102		6.1	5.4	6.5	7.1
	1103		5.8	6.2	7.0	6.5
4 mg b.i.d.	1104		6.2	8.5	8.1	7.1
	1105		5.4	8.4	7.7	6.1
	1106		6.2	6.8	6.9	5.9
6 mg b.i.d.	1107		4.8	8.1	7.6	5.2
	1108		5.1	7.6	7.1	6.1
	1109		5.9	8.5	7.2	6.8
4 mg t.i.d.	1110		6.0	6.5	6.1	5.6
	1111		5.2	8.2	7.6	6.3
	1112		6.2	7.6	7.8	6.9
0 mg b.i.d.	1201	2	5.1	6.5	6.2	6.4
	1202		6.1	5.8	6.1	6.9
	1203		4.8	5.6	5.2	6.2
4 mg b.i.d.	1204		5.0	7.6	7.1	6.1
	1205		4.4	8.2	7.6	6.4
	1206		5.4	6.1	5.6	5.7
6 mg b.i.d.	1207		5.6	8.2	7.8	7.1
	1208		4.8	7.8	6.2	5.1
	1209		6.0	7.0	7.1	6.4
4 mg t.i.d.	1210		5.4	6.0	6.2	5.8
	1211		5.1	7.2	6.3	5.8
	1212		5.7	5.6	4.9	5.6

TABLE 5.7 Raw data: protocol 2, endpoint is time to anginal onset

Group	PAT	INV	(BTIMEAO)	(TIMEAO2)	(TIMEAO7)	(TIMEAO12)
2 mg b.i.d.	2101	1	5.1	6.1	4.8	6.2
	2102		4.8	6.0	5.3	4.7
	2103		5.1	4.8	6.1	5.2
4 mg b.i.d.	2104		4.8	6.1	6.3	5.4
	2105		5.2	7.2	6.9	5.9
	2106		5.4	5.6	5.9	5.0
8 mg b.i.d.	2107		5.2	6.4	7.8	7.1
	2108		6.1	8.2	8.5	7.4
	2109		5.8	7.5	7.4	6.9
6 mg t.i.d.	2110		5.2	7.4	7.1	5.8
	2111		5.3	7.8	8.0	6.1
	2112		5.4	6.5	6.2	5.0
2 mg b.i.d.	2201	2	5.4	6.2	6.4	5.1
	2202		5.1	5.4	4.4	5.8
	2203		6.1	7.4	7.6	6.4
4 mg b.i.d.	2204		4.7	5.1	5.1	5.9
	2205		4.8	6.1	6.4	5.4
	2206		6.2	7.0	7.5	6.1
8 mg b.i.d.	2207		4.1	7.0	8.5	6.1
	2208		5.5	7.2	7.9	6.0
	2209		5.3	6.0	6.1	6.7
6 mg t.i.d.	2210		5.1	6.2	6.1	5.4
	2211		5.4	7.2	7.1	6.1
	2212		5.2	6.4	6.7	6.1

TABLE 5.8 Descriptive summary: mean ± SD, time to anginal onset

Group	BTIMEAO	TIMEAO2	TIMEA07	TIMEAO12
0 mg b.i.d. $n = 6$	5.50 ± 0.57	5.80 ± 0.47	6.13 ± 0.61	6.53 ± 0.39
2 mg b.i.d. $n = 6$	5.77 ± 0.45	5.98 ± 0.87	5.77 ± 1.17	5.57 ± 0.67
4 mg b.i.d. $n = 12$	5.31 ± 0.62	6.89 ± 1.33	6.76 ± 0.92	5.92 ± 0.54
6 mg b.i.d. $n = 6$	5.37 ± 0.54	7.78 ± 0.53	7.17 ± 0.55	6.12 ± 0.82
8 mg b.i.d. $n = 6$	5.33 ± 0.69	7.05 ± 0.78	7.53 ± 1.27	6.70 ± 0.55
4 mg t.i.d. $n = 6$	5.68 ± 0.44	6.85 ± 0.99	6.57 ± 1.07	6.80 ± 0.51
6 mg t.i.d. $n = 6$	5.27 ± 0.12	6.92 ± 0.64	6.87 ± 0.70	5.75 ± 0.46

[a]4 mg, 6 mg, and 6 mg.

TABLE 5.9 Descriptive summary: mean ± SD, time to anginal onset/change from baseline

Group	TAO2HR	TAO7HR	TAO12HR	Overall average
0 mg b.i.d. $n = 6$	0.30 ± 0.75	0.63 ± 0.46	1.03 ± 0.27	0.65 ± 0.53
2 mg b.i.d. $n = 6$	0.63 ± 0.81	0.40 ± 0.66	0.37 ± 0.64	0.47 ± 0.71
4 mg b.i.d. $n = 12$	1.58 ± 1.15	1.45 ± 0.89	0.61 ± 0.68	1.21 ± 0.93
6 mg b.i.d. $n = 6$	2.50 ± 0.79	1.80 ± 0.65	0.75 ± 0.47	1.68 ± 0.65
8 mg b.i.d. $n = 6$	1.77 ± 0.75	2.70 ± 1.50	1.37 ± 0.55	1.95 ± 1.02
4 mg t.i.d. $n = 6$	1.25 ± 1.15	0.97 ± 1.17	0.40 ± 0.56	0.87 ± 0.75
6 mg t.i.d.[a] $n = 6$	1.65 ± 0.61	1.60 ± 0.68	0.48 ± 0.48	1.24 ± 0.60

[a]4 mg, 6 mg, and 6 mg.

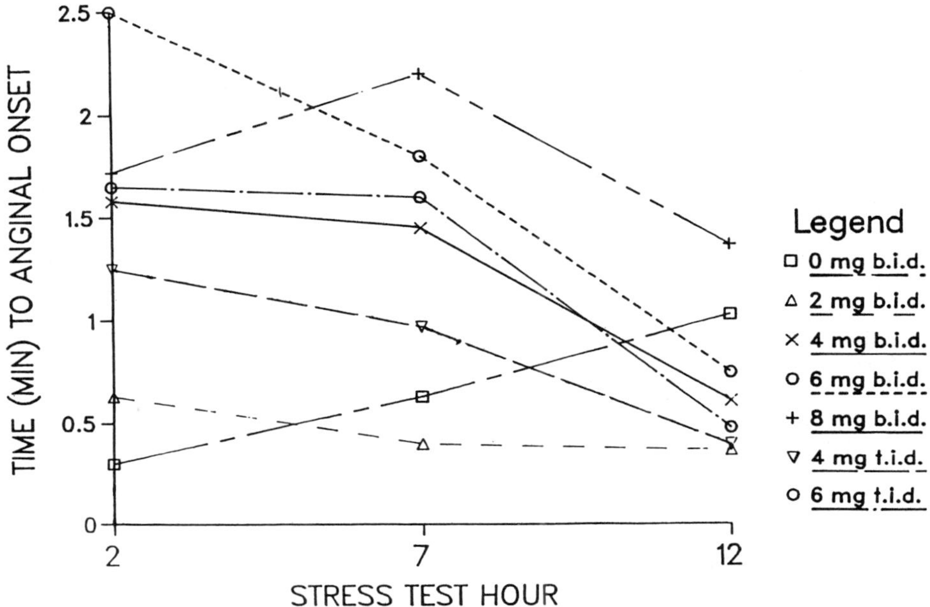

FIGURE 5.2 Time to anginal onset and change from baseline.

TABLE 5.10 Anova summary for RSM analysis 1: 0, 2, 4, 6, and 8 mg b.i.d.

Response mean	1.2458				
Root MSE	0.83334971				
R-square	0.46792738				
Coef. of variation	0.66890906				
Regression	DF	Type I SS	R-square	F-ratio	Prob.
Linear	2	21.4422	0.3911	15.44	0.0001
Quadratic	2	1.5425	0.0281	1.11	0.3389
Crossproduct	1	2.6667	0.0486	3.84	0.0567
Total regress	5	25.6514	0.4679	7.39	0.0001
Residual	DF	SS	Mean square	F-ratio	Prob.
Lack of fit	1	0.44444444	0.44444444	0.634	0.4303
Pure error	41	28.7233	0.70056911		
Total error	42	29.1678	0.69447090		
Parameter	DF	Estimate	SD	T-ratio	Prob.
Intercept	1	1.4333	0.24056719	5.96	0.0001
χ_1	1	0.89444444	0.19642229	4.55	0.0001
χ_2	1	−0.62546279	0.19642224	−3.18	0.0027
$\chi_1 * \chi_1$	1	−0.01666667	0.34021339	−0.05	0.9612
$\chi_1 * \chi_2$	1	−0.76980036	0.39284458	−1.96	0.0567
$\chi_2 * \chi_2$	1	−0.48333333	0.34021339	−1.42	0.1628
Factor	DF	SS	Mean square	F-ratio	Prob.
χ_1	3	17.0689	5.6896	8.19	0.0002
χ_2	3	11.1100	3.7033	5.33	0.0033

TABLE 5.11 ANOVA summary for RSM analysis 2: 0, 2, 4, 8 mg b.i.d., 4 mg t.i.d.

Response mean	1.0458				
Root MSE	0.89328773				
R-square	0.33237050				
Coef. of variation	0.45413966				
Regression	DF	Type I SS	R-square	F-ratio	Prob.
Linear	2	9.5006	0.1893	5.95	0.0053
Quadratic	2	6.9025	0.1375	4.33	0.0196
Crossproduct	1	0.28166667	0.0056	0.35	0.5556
Total regress	5	16.6847	0.3324	4.18	0.0036
Residual	DF	SS	Mean square	F-ratio	Prob.
Lack of fit	1	0.87111111	0.87111111	1.094	0.3017
Pure error	41	32.6433	0.79617886		
Total error	42	33.5144	0.79796296		
Parameter	DF	Estimate	SD	T-ratio	Prob.
Intercept	1	1.4333	0.25786995	5.56	0.0001
χ_1	1	0.62777778	0.21054994	2.98	0.0048
χ_2	1	−0.36565517	0.21054994	−1.74	0.0898
$\chi_1 * \chi_1$	1	−0.01666667	0.36468319	−0.05	0.9638
$\chi_1 * \chi_2$	1	−0.25018512	0.42109987	−0.59	0.5556
Factor	DF	SS	Mean square	F-ratio	Prob.
χ_1	3	7.3772	2.4591	3.08	0.0375
χ_2	3	8.8900	2.9633	3.71	0.0186

subjects not common to all three RSM analyses. These tables suggest that any differences between the three RSM analyses are not likely to be due to subject differences.

6. Summary and Recommendation

In the ANOVA summarized in Tables 5.10–5.12, χ_1 denotes total daily dose and χ_2 denotes time of stress test (STESTHR) following the last dose administered. Generally, all RSM analyses reflect that both factors are significant, that the significance is due primarily to the linear components of the model, and that there is significant interaction between the factors. Specific results from each RSM analysis appear below and in Table 5.15.

a. RSM Analysis 1. Estimated delay of anginal onset increases as total daily dose increases and time of postbaseline stress test decreases. A maximal delay of 2.98–3.16 min (55–59% above baseline) at 16 mg and

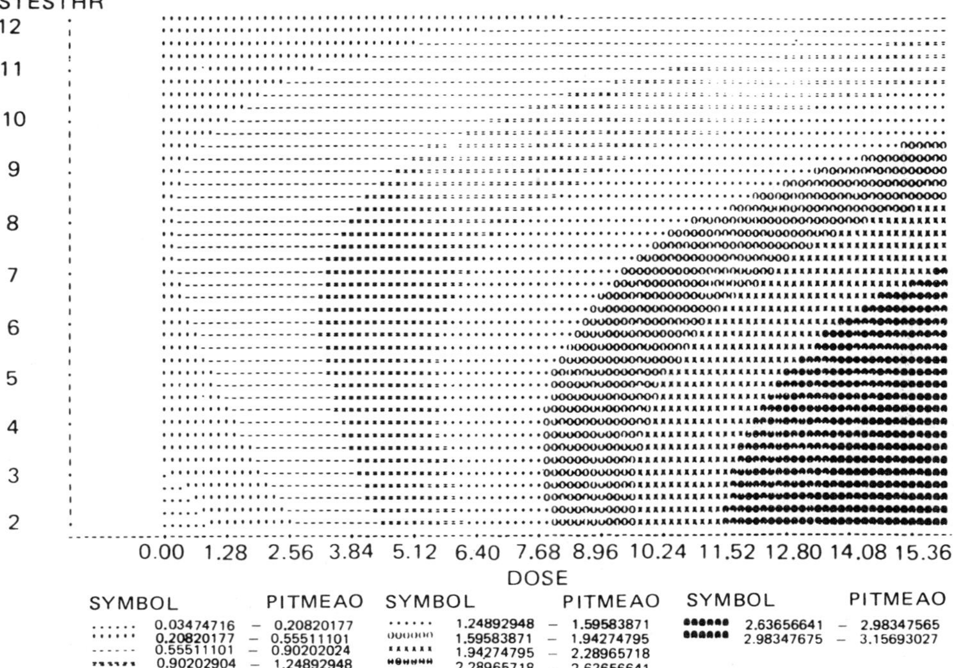

FIGURE 5.3

stress test at 2 h is predicted. To achieve a clinically significant predicted delay of at least 1.60 min (30% above baseline), a total daily dose of at least 8 mg must be given. However, this effect at a total daily dose of 8 mg would be predicted to be maintained only for 2–5 h. To maintain this predicted effect out to 8.5–9.5 h maximally requires 16 mg.

b. RSM Analysis 2. Estimated delay of anginal onset increases as total daily dose increases and time of postbaseline stress test decreases. A maximal delay of 2.02–2.14 min (38–40% above baseline) at 16 mg and stress test at 3-7 h is predicted. To achieve a clinically significant predicted delay of at least 1.60 min (30% above baseline), a total daily dose of at least 14 mg is required.

c. RSM Analysis 3. Estimated delay of anginal onset increases as total daily dose increases and time of postbaseline stress test decreases. A maximal delay of 2.58–2.73 (48–51% above baseline) at 16 mg and stress

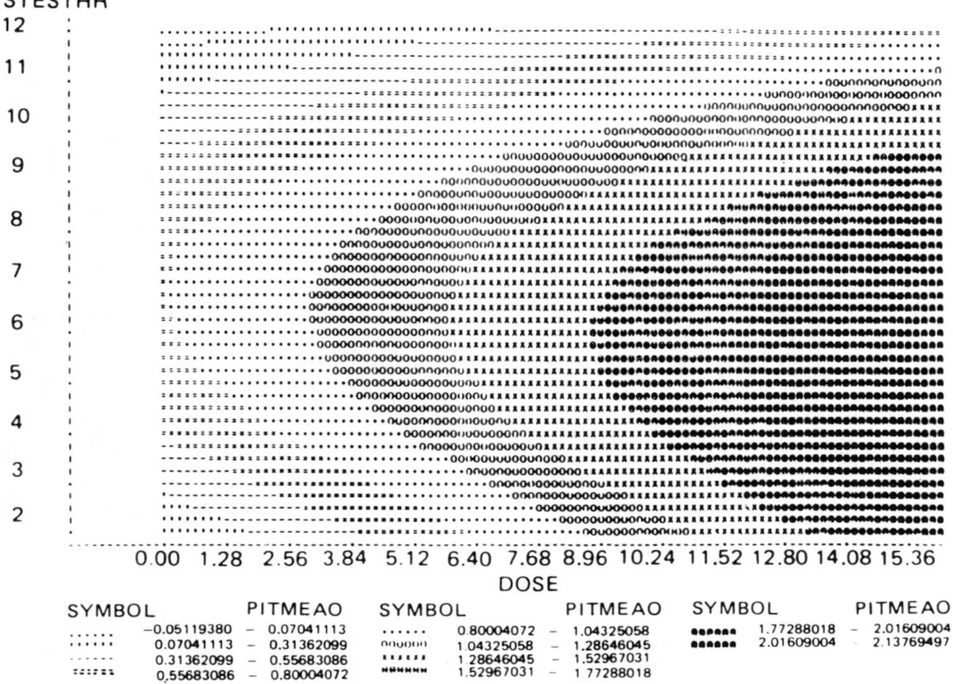

FIGURE 5.4

test at 2 h is predicted. To achieve a clinically significant predicted delay of 1.60 min (30% above baseline) a total daily dose of at least 7.6 mg must be given. However, this effect at a total daily dose of 7.6 mg would be predicted to be maintained for only 2–5 h. To maintain this effect out to 7–8 h maximally requires 16 mg.

It was felt clinically that an antianginal drug would have to prolong the onset of exercise-induced angina by at least 30% above baseline in order to warrant continued clinical development. Each RSM analysis predicted a dose that would achieve this, with two predicting that such an effect would last from 7 to 9 h after dosing. Therefore, it was recommended that Phase III trials be conducted with a t.i.d. regimen using divided daily doses of 4, 6, and 6 mg.

TABLE 5.12 ANOVA summary for RSM analysis 3: 0, 2, 4, 6 mg b.i.d., 6 mg t.i.d.

Response mean	1.1708				
Root MSE	0.71460575				
R-square	0.47636196				
Coef. of variation	0.61033943				
Regression	DF	Type I SS	R-square	F-ratio	Prob.
Linear	2	15.7222	0.3839	15.39	0.0001
Quadratic	2	1.225	0.0274	1.10	0.3426
Crossproduct	1	2.6667	0.0651	5.22	0.0274
Total regress	5	19.5114	0.4764	7.64	0.0001
Residual	DF	SS	Mean square	F-ratio	Prob.
Lack of fit	1	1.6044	1.6044	3.315	0.0760
Pure error	41	19.8433	0.48398374		
Total error	42	21.4478	0.51066138		
Parameter	DF	Estimate	SD	T-ratio	Prob.
Intercept	1	1.4333	0.20628891	6.95	0.0001
χ_1	1	0.69444444	0.16843419	4.12	0.0002
χ_2	1	−0.62546279	0.16843419	−3.71	0.006
$\chi_1 * \chi_1$	1	−0.31666667	0.29173658	−1.09	0.2839
$\chi_1 * \chi_2$	1	−0.76980036	0.33686838	−2.29	0.0274
$\chi_2 * \chi_2$	1	−0.38333333	0.29173658	−1.31	0.1960
Factor	DF	SS	Mean square	F-ratio	Prob.
χ_1	3	11.9489	3.9830	7.80	0.0003
χ_2	3	10.5900	3.5300	6.91	0.0007

TABLE 5.13 Comparison at baseline of patients in RSM analysis 1 but not in RSM analysis 2 and vice versa

Group	Mean	SD	*n*
122[a]	5.37	0.54	6
124[b]	5.60	0.44	6

[a] 16 mg Total daily dose; receive 6 mg b.i.d.
[b] 16 mg Total daily dose; receive 4 mg t.i.d.

TABLE 5.14 Comparison at baseline of patients in RSM analysis 1 but not in RSM analysis 3 and vice versa

Group	Mean	SD	*n*
162[a]	5.33	0.69	6
163[b]	5.27	0.12	6

[a] 16 mg total daily dose; receive 6 mg b.i.d.
[b] 16 mg total daily dose; receive 4 mg t.i.d.

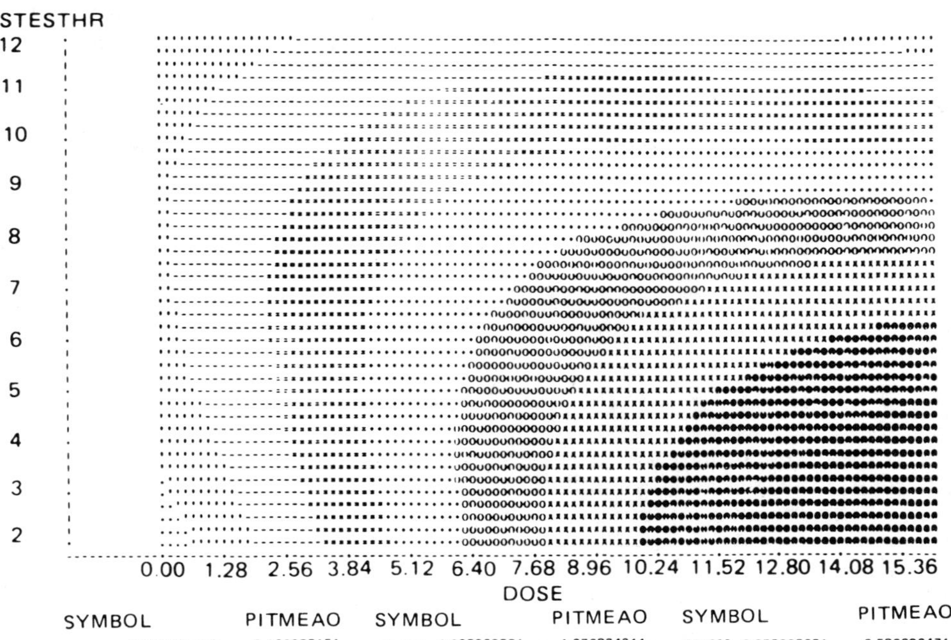

FIGURE 5.5

TABLE 5.15 RSM analysis summary

Desired effect	Predicted dose	Predicted time
	RSM Analysis 1	
Maximal	Increase	Decrease
(2.98 min; 3.16 min) (55%; 59%)	16 mg	2 h
(1.60 min;) (30%;)	8 mg	2–5 h
(1.60 min;) (30%;)	16 mg	8.5–9.5 h
	RSM Analysis 2	
Maximal	Increase	Decrease
(2.02 min; 2.14 min) (38%; 40%)	16 mg	3–7 h
(1.60 min;) (30%;)	9–14 mg	2–9 h
	RSM Analysis 3	
Maximal	Increase	Decrease
(2.58 min; 2.73 min) (48%; 51%)	16 mg	2 h
(1.60 min;) (30%;)	7.6 mg	2–5 h
(1.60 min;) (30%;)	16 mg	7–8 h

REFERENCES

Addelman, S., Gaylor, D. W., and Bohrer, Q. E. (1966). Sequence of combination chemotherapy experiments. *Biometrics*, *22:* 730–746.

Berger, R. L. (1989). Uniformly more powerful tests for hypotheses concerning linear inequality and normal means. *Journal of the American Statistical Association*, *84:* 192–199.

Bonnadonna, G.., et al. (1961). Dose-response effect of adjuvant chemotherapy in breast cancer. *New England Journal of Medicine*, *304:* 10–5.

Box, G. E. P. (1958). Discussion of experimental design in combination chemotherapy by N. Mantel. *Annals of NY Academy*,

Burdette, W. U., and Gehan, E. A. (1970). *Planning and Analysis of Clinical Studies*. Springfield, IL, Charles C. Thomas.

Carter, W. A., Wampler, G. L., Crews, S. L., and Howells, R. (1977). On determining the levels of treatment to optimize the probability of a favorable response. *Cancer Treatment, 61:* 849–853.

Carter, W. H., Stablein, D. M., and Wampler, G. L. (1979). An improved method for analyzing survival data from combination chemotherapy experiments. *Cancer Research, 39:* 3446–3453.

Carter, W. H., Wampler, G. L., and Stablein, D. M. (1983). *Regression Analysis of Survival Data in Cancer Chemotherapy*. New York: Marcel Dekker.

Cohen, A., Gatsonis, C., and Marden, J. (1983). Hypothesis tests and optimality in discrete multivariate analysis. In *Studies in Econometrics, Time Series and Multivariate Statistics*, S. Karlin (Ed.). New York: Academic Press.

Frei, and Cannellos (1980).

Goldin, A., Vendetti, J., Mantel, N., Kline, I., and Gang, M. (1958). Evaluation of combination chemotherapy with three drugs. *Cancer Research, 28:* 950–1.

Guttman, S. (1987). Tests uniformly more powerful than uniformly most powerful monotone tests. *Journal of Statistical Planning and Inference, 17:* 279–292.

Hollander, D., and Harlan, J. (1973). Antacids vs. placebo in peptic ulcer therapy: A controlled double blind investigation. *Journal of the American Medical Association, 226:* 1181–1185.

Inada, K. (1978). Some bivariate tests of composite hypotheses with restricted alternatives. *Rep. Fac. Sci., Kagoshima University (Math. Phys. Chem.), 11:* 25–31.

Laska, E. M., and Meisner, M. (1986). Testing whether an identified treatment is best: The combination problem. *Proceedings of the Biopharmaceutical Section of the American Statistical Association*, pp. 163–170.

Laska, E. M. and Meisner, M. (1989). Testing whether an identified treatment is best. *Biometrics*, in press.

Lehman, E. L. (1952). Testing multiparameter hypotheses. *Annals of Mathematical Statistics, 23:* 541–552.

Lehman, E. L. (1975). *Nonparametrics: Statistical Methods Based on Ranks*. San Francisco, Holden-Day.

Mantel, N. (1959). Experimental design in combination chemotherapy. *Annals of the New York Academy of Science, 76:* 909–9.

Miller, R. G., Jr. (1981). *Simultaneous Statistical Inference*, 2nd ed. New York: Springer-Verlag.

Myers, R. (1971). *Response Surface Methodology*. Boston, Allyn and Bacon.

Peterson, W., Sturdevant, R., Frankl, H., Richardson, C., Isenberg, J., Elashoff, J., Sones, J., Gross, R., MacCallum, R., and Fordtran, J. (1977). Healing of duodenal ulcer with an antacid regimen. *New England Journal of Medicine, 297:* 341–345.

Sasabuchi, S. (1981). A test of a multivariate normal mean with composite hypotheses determined by linear inequalities. *Biometrika, 67:* 429–439.

Sasabuchi, S. (1988). A multivariate one sided test with composite hypotheses when the covariance matrix is completely unknown. *Memoirs of Faculty of Science, Kyushu University, Japan, Ser. A 42:* 37–46.

Stablein, D. M., Carter, W. H., and Wampler, G. L. (1980). Survival analysis of drug combinations using a hazards model with time-dependent covariates. *Biometrics*, *36:* 537–546.

Stablein, D. M., Carter, W. H., and Wampler, G. L. (1983). Confidence regions for constrained optima in response surface experiments. *Biometrics*, *39:* 759–763.

Wampler, G. L., Carter, W. H., and Williams, V. R. (1978). Combination chemotherapy arriving at optimal treatment levels by incorporating size effect constraints. *Cancer Treatment Reports 62:* 33–40.

6
Dosing in the Elderly

Arthur F. Johnson* *Smith, Kline and French Laboratories, Philadelphia, Pennsylvania*

Rukmini Rajagopalan *Boehringer Ingelheim Pharmaceuticals, Inc., Ridgefield, Connecticut*

David S. Salsburg *Pfizer Laboratories, Inc., Groton, Connecticut*

I. THE ELDERLY IN CLINICAL TRIALS: WHO AND HOW MANY?

Arthur F. Johnson

A. Introduction

Considerable attention is currently being focused on the elderly portion of the population. Part of this attention is directed at the use of pharmaceutical drugs in treating the elderly. The stereotyped health care situation for an elderly person involves a patient who will not follow directions, forgets medication, can not open the bottle, self medicates or over medicates, does not recognize side effects, suffers from physiological deficits and multiple chronic disease, and is dismissed with a diagnosis of senility, which may well be drug interaction or side effects, by a health

**Present affiliation:* Hahnemann University, Philadelphia, Pennsylvania

care provider who does not have the time or the concern to establish a caring relationship.

Discounting the stereotype, there is still concern as to how age-associated decrement in physiological function affects the use of the pharmacopeia in the elderly. Indeed it is fair to ask whether there even exists a group—elderly—to which general recommendation on the use of a drug can be made or whether the elderly are sufficiently diverse in terms of age-associated deficits that they must be considered on an individual basis. In the following discussion it will be assumed that there is a substantial fraction of the elderly population that can provide subjects for drug evaluation studies, that is, are otherwise healthy apart from the disease process under investigation and to which the results of such studies will be broadly applicable. I emphasize that I am not at all sure how reasonable this assumption is. Our concern, then, is with the relationship between the elderly part of our population and the process of new drug evaluation. What portion of the elderly can be involved in the drug evaluation process, and what problems may arise if the elderly are included in efficacy trials either as a part of the subject pool or in separate trials?

B. Study Date/Birth Date/Age

In reading the original literature to understand the characteristics of "the elderly" one has to continually remind oneself that "the elderly" are a constantly changing group as far as study results and study implications are concerned. In a recent review article most of the studies cited were published in the late 1970s. Subjects in their seventh decade (61–70) at the time when they were studied were thus born in the years around 1910. If one were now to attempt to replicate such a study or to take direction from it for further work, the available seventh-decade cohort would be subjects born around 1920. People who lived from 1910 to 1970 and were accessible at the first study location are going to be different from people who lived from 1920 to 1980 and are now accessible at a different study location. Ethnic background, socioeconomic history, exposure to medical care, and losses to wars and other disasters are some of the factors responsible for difference. People who live from 1930 to 1990, born and raised in the depression era, are the likely beneficiaries of the results of today's studies. How will the study results apply to them? The chronological part of the problem is as shown:

Age at time of study

Study year	Birth year 1890	1900	1910	1920	1930
1950	60	—	—	—	—
1960	70	60	—	—	—
1970	80	70	60	—	—
1980	90	80	70	60	—
1990	—	90	80	70	60

All of which is not to suggest abandoning study of the elderly. After all, most clinical trials include a fairly wide age range of subjects, and any lack of homogeneity from life history is assumed to be negligible or at least acceptable as part of the variability from subject to subject. However, for concerns focused on "the elderly," a relatively narrow age grouping, one must consider the history that has produced the subjects available for study and that is producing the subjects to whom the study results will be applied.

C. Will the Elderly Be All That Different?

Unfortunately, much of the thinking in regard to the elderly is greatly influenced by the stereotype of the elderly person as deteriorating if not deteriorated. The observations in the preceding section are greatly relevant here. In the interpretation of literature on "the elderly" with respect to the "nonelderly" the effect of aging is almost always confounded with birth date. Today's 60-year-olds are compared with today's 30-year-olds and any difference is marked up to age's account. C. Everett Koop (Moore and Teal, 1985) has pointed out that each new generation of elderly has a better health history with more emphasis on responsibility for personal health than the one before. Koop attributes much of the remarked "deterioration" of our present aged population to health history. If we tie our programs and proposals too closely to present difficulties we will develop measures that will be obsolescent when the next cohort comes along. A second area of difficulty is that the medical profession inevitably sees more frequently the more severely compromised elderly subjects. For every elderly subject seen that misuses or abuses prescription and nonprescription drugs and thus supports the generalization that this is what the elderly do, there is an indefinitely larger number whose habits have not been observed. Again, recommendations and programs based on the disease-based sample may not be relevant to the rest of the elderly population.

D. Effect of Age-Compromised Physiology

While it is not always clear in an individual patient whether a physiological deficiency is age-related or disease-related, there is general agreement that bodily changes do occur as subjects age. One may remark in passing that with increased attention to such changes there is mounting evidence that a greater number can be attributed to subclinical or previously unrecognized systemic problems other than age itself. Among the changes one may list (McGlone, 1982) the immune response, hepatic function, renal function, cardiac output, body mass composition, tissue metabolism, protein-binding capacity, and membrane composition. Without going into detail, it is apparent that all of these changes may have an effect on the way on the body handles a drug.

Accept that there is a segment of the elderly population that is eligible for a clinical trial with respect to general health status and the existence of the target disease. In a clinical trial for evaluating a new drug, what consideration needs to be given to the known decrements in physiological function between the older subjects and younger subjects considered as groups? Should one expect a wider variation in function among the eligible elderly than with the young, and will this be associated with a wider variation in response? Should one expect a different level of response with the elderly? Whether or not information on these issues is available in a particular situation will have to be determined. The assistance of our clinical colleagues in accessing and interpreting the available literature is essential. The wise statistician will not hesitate to explore *Index Medicus* independently.

In a trial of a given drug the particular physiological function most likely to influence the response may be specifiable. If there is a marker variable that can conveniently be measured to provide the level of functioning, then the marker variable can be included as a covariate in the analysis of the response. Of course, the analysis and its interpretation will have to proceed cautiously since the relation of the response to the marker variable is not necessarily linear. Note that age per se is not an adequate marker variable. Though age might adjust for changes in level of response, it would not adjust for changes in variability.

The question of age-compromised function means, at the very least, that if the elderly are included in a clinical trial the analysis will have to consider both the possibility of inhomogeneity of variance with age and the possible interaction of treatments by age. For the variance question one would require an examination of residuals versus age of variance estimates by age group. For the elderly to remain as part of the principle analysis both these possibilities must be excluded and the usual problems regarding power in such decisions pertain.

E. How Many of the Elderly Are Needed?

The otherwise healthy elderly should not, it is recommended, be excluded from participation in clinical trials. Otherwise healthy, that is, in that they have the condition or disease under investigation and only the condition or disease under investigation. However, we have just discussed some of the potential problems that age may engender that may set even the otherwise healthy elderly in a separate category. There is nothing to be gained by including the elderly in a clinical trial and then taking them out again at the analysis stage because they are not homogeneous with the rest of the subjects. In the previous section mention was made of the possibility of employing marker variables to define the degree of physiological deficit in subjects and the incorporation of the marker variables as covariates in the analysis. In most cases the success of such a maneuver will only be determinable after the trial and there is thus still the problem that the elderly will be separate.

Stratification will of course attempt to assure than an overall estimate of efficacy will not be biased by an uneven distribution of subject ages between regimens. Stratification does not take care of inhomogeneity of variance nor of interaction between treatments and strata. In reality even if everything is satisfactory as regards the elderly being part of a homogeneous group, the response of the elderly group is going to be looked at separately and conclusions drawn for the elderly on this basis.

All of which is simply to say that one must confront directly the fact that there are not going to be very many elderly in a clinical trial involving a wide age range of subjects. One does not have enough elderly subjects—enough power—to distinguish clinically meaningful differences between regimens in the elderly group, nor to detect clinically meaningful interactions between treatment and age group, nor to provide comfortable confidence intervals on treatment differences in the elderly group.

Consider an example (Table 6.1) in which the subjects are arranged in four age groups of equal size and the risks are 5% for both Type I and Type II errors with regard to a difference of concern between treatments. Then, setting the variance of treatment difference across age groups to 1.0, the relative variance of treatment difference for the oldest group will

TABLE 6.1 Analysis of an age-stratified trial with equal numbers in each stratum

	Contrasts		
	A	B	C
Plac. young	−1/4	0	+1/3
Plac. middle-lo	−1/4	0	+1/3
Plac. middle-hi	−1/4	0	+1/3
Plac. elderly	−1/4	−1	−1
Test young	+1/4	0	−1/3
Test middle-lo	+1/4	0	−1/3
Test middle-hi	+1/4	0	−1/3
Test elderly	+1/4	+1	+1
Sum of squares	1/2	2	8/3
Rel-variance	1	4	5.3

		Characteristics of analysis			
Contrast	Rel-variance		Sensitivity	Risk I	Risk II
A	1.0		D	5%	5%
Overall					
B	4.0		2.0D	5%	5%
Elderly		OR	D	5%	50%
C	5.3		2.3D	5%	5%
Interact		OR	D	5%	>50%

be 4.0 and the relative variance of the interaction between treatments and oldest versus the other three age groups will be 5.3. Focusing on the oldest group we can say either that we are satisfied with half the sensitivity for which the trial was designed or that we are satisfied with a risk of false negatives of 50%. It would be specious to pretend that either of these options is acceptable.

If one is interested in the elderly population then one must be prepared to carry out an adequately sensitive trial with appropriate risks on the elderly. One cannot expect to derive useful information from the few elderly subjects that are picked up in a clinical trial with a wide age specification for entry.

F. Power and Responsibility

On occasion when I have presented arguments on sample size as in the previous section I have encountered the comment "Oh, he's just talking about power," with the implication that we all know all there is to know about that. Of course I am talking about power, but I am also talking about the responsibility of the statistician in the design of clinical trials. It is our responsibility to inform the client of the information content of the experimental program options being considered and to guide the client to the selection of an option that is scientifically and ethically sound. In a particular case with a particular client we may or may not be successful but the effort must be made. Professional responsibility does not permit the statistician simply to crank out a risk of Type II error for a fortuitous sample size and go on to other business. This is despite the fact that most of us have been exposed to the dictum that "setting risks is the responsibility of the client."

Particularly in clinical trials work where the ethical content is so apparent, the responsibility of the statistician is critical. The ethical imperative is that the clinical trial must address an important question and must be able to resolve the issue. Now the statistician may defer to the clinician as to what constitutes "an important question," although I would expect the statistician to be sufficiently knowledgeable in the substantive area to recognize the importance of the question. The statistician will assist in formulating the question so that it can be adequately addressed by a clinical trial.

With regard to "resolving the issue," the statistician has a critical role. There are some medical issues—the equivalence of antibiotics, for instance—where professional peer assessment of a modest trial is accepted as adequate for resolution of an issue. In most situations a statistical test and power considerations come to the fore, particularly if the regulatory agency is involved. Either a statistically significant result or a statistically not significant result must resolve the question. The question of significance is de facto resolved at the 5% risk level. There must also be an acceptable level for risk of Type II error. Parenthetically, in drug development economic considerations alone would seem to indicate a low risk for Type II error. In the absence of an accepted norm for Type II error risk each organization (or statistician) will have to set a standard. My own practice over the last 30 years has been to set the risk of Type II error at 5%. This is, not entirely coincidentally, the choice of SK&F Labs. While one would not cavil at another choice, unacceptable practice would be no choice at all. Textbooks aside, there is never sufficient information available to establish a specific set of risks for each occasion.

G. Conclusions

In conclusion, in dealing with questions involving the elderly it is essential to avoid stereotyping and to consider carefully the relevance of literature to present populations. Three points about the elderly and clinical trials for evaluating drugs were discussed.

1. Otherwise healthy elderly subjects can participate in clinical trials for evaluation of new drugs for their presenting condition. Age alone should not be an exclusion.
2. Otherwise healthy elderly subjects may to varying extent manifest age-associated physiological deficits that may interfere with drug evaluation and that usually mandiate separate consideration for the response of elderly subjects.
3. If there is an issue, or a suspicion of an issue, as regards the elderly in a drug evaluation, then sufficient elderly subjects must be involved in a trial to ensure resolution of the issue. This entails a full-scale clinical trial on the elderly. A subgroup of elderly in a trial of all ages is not ethically acceptable.

II. STEADY-STATE BLOOD LEVELS

Rukmini Rajagopalan

A. Introduction

Steady-state is said to be achieved when the amount of drug administered is equal to the amount of drug eliminated from the body. The time to achieve steady state is estimated as follows:

To achieve 50% steady state it takes 1 half-life.
To achieve 75% steady state it takes 2 half-lives.
To achieve 82.5% steady state it takes 3 half-lives.
To achieve 93.75% steady state it takes 4 half-lives.
To achieve 100% steady state it would take approximately 4–5 half-lives.

Steady-state blood level ($C_{B,ss}$) is an important factor in calculating the maintenance dose:

$$\text{Maintenance dose} = (C_{B,ss})\text{CL} \times \tau$$

where Cl is the clearance and τ is the time interval between doses.

Properties of steady-state blood level that are pertinent for use in statistical analysis are:

1. By first-order kinetics, drug level in plasma diminishes logarithmically over time.
2. Depending on how the medication is administered, the blood level can be fixed or fluctuating within limits. Figures 6.1–6.3 demonstrate some examples of such variations (Winter, 1980).

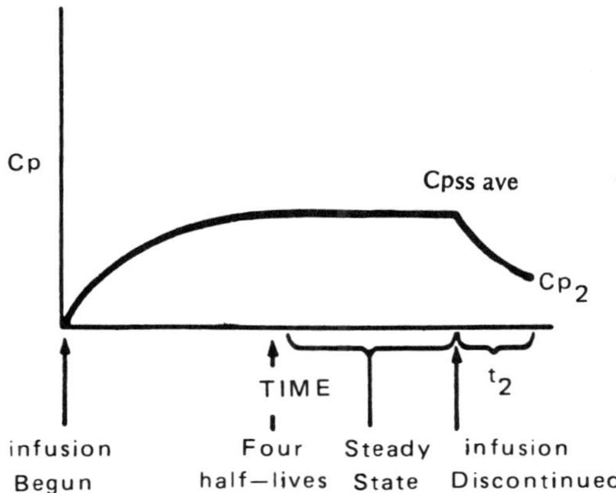

FIGURE 6.1 Graphical representation of the plasma concentration versus time curve which results when an infusion is continued until steady state is reached and then discontinued. $C_{PSS\,ave} = (S)(F)(\text{Dose}/\tau)/CL$ and $CP_2 = (S)(F)(\text{Dose}/\tau)/CL \times (e^{-Kdt_2})$.

3. When a patient was given medication three times a day compared to the same total daily dose once a day, steady-state blood level was found to be higher (Cooper et al., 1975).
4. There is some evidence to suggest that drug effects are a function of free drug concentration rather than total drug con-

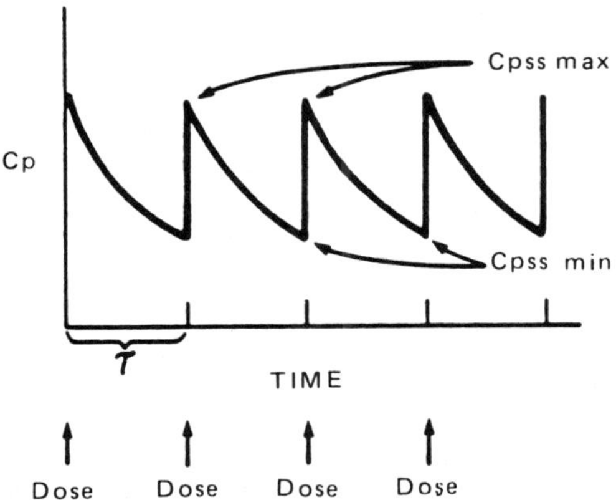

FIGURE 6.2 Graphical representation of the steady state plasma concentration versus time curve which occurs when drugs are given intermittently at regular dosing intervals. $C_{PSS\,ave} = (S)(F)(\text{Dose}/\tau)/CL$, $C_{PSS\,max} = (S)(F)(\text{Dose}/Vd)/(1 - e^{-Kdt})$ and $C_{PSS\,min} = [(S)(F)(\text{Dose})/Vd]/(1 - e^{-Kd\tau})(e^{-Kd\tau})$.

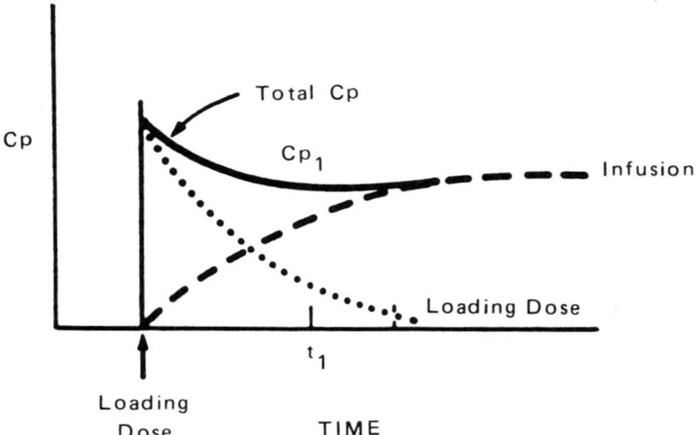

FIGURE 6.3 Graphical representation of the plasma level time curve which results from a loading dose followed by a maintenance infusion. $CP_1 = [(S)(F)(\text{Loading dose})/Vd \times (e^{-Kdt_1})] + [(S)(F)(\text{Dose}/\tau)/cl \times (1 - e^{-Kdt_1})]$.

centration (Gibald and Koup, 1981). Free drug concentration in blood at steady state ($C'_{\mathrm{B,ss}}$) is defined by equations of the form

$$C'_{\mathrm{B,ss}} = f_{\mathrm{B}} C_{\mathrm{B,ss}}$$

where f_{B} is the fraction of free drug concentration in blood, whereas total drug concentration in any given organ or tissue (compartment) relative to total drug concentration in the blood is defined by equations of the form

$$C_{\mathrm{T,ss}} = R_{\mathrm{T}} C_{\mathrm{B,ss}}$$

where R_{T} is a partition coefficient calculated as $f_{\mathrm{B}}/f_{\mathrm{T}}$, that is, the ratio of free drug concentration in blood to the free drug concentration in the tissue.

B. Factors That Affect Steady-State Blood Levels

1. Absorption

When drug is administered intravenously, it is absorbed straight into the circulation and is 100% bioavailable. When it is administered through other routes, the bioavailability of the drug depends on the efficiency of the organ (e.g., skin, digestive system) to absorb, which in turn affects the drug concentration of the blood.

Many drugs have been known to be absorbed better with increased gastric acidity. Sommers et al. (1984) examined the effect of reduced gastric pH on the bioavailability of two prodrug β-lactam antibiotics, bacampicillin and cefuroxime axetil. They found that reduced pH enhanced the absorption of both these prodrugs, even though the presence of food had contrasting effects on them. When gastric pH was sufficiently low, presumably cefuroxime axetil was better dissolved in the gastric juices. Now, pH levels has been shown to sharply increase after the age of 50 (Levin et al., 1951). Such increase may alter the absorbability of certain drugs.

However, in spite of many physiological changes that occur within the alimentary tract with aging, only a few major changes occur in absorption. In most cases, these changes are also balanced by alterations in binding, metabolism, clearance, and distribution such that the net effect on the plasma drug concentration is well controlled (Massoud, 1984).

2. Distribution

Ritschel (1976) suggested the following correction factor for the volume of distribution (V_d) for the aged; it is slightly different for males and females.

$$V_d(\text{elderly males}) = \frac{V_{25}[54.25 - 0.199(\text{age} - 25)]}{54.25}$$

$$V_d(\text{elderly females}) = \frac{V_{25}[49.25 - 0.130(\text{age} - 25)]}{49.25}$$

where V_{25} is the volume of distribution determined in healthy young individuals (i.e., 25 years old).

3. Drug Binding

When considering binding changes in the elderly, the albumin, red blood cell (RBC) binding, alpha-acid glycoprotein concentration, numbers/types of binding sites, sex, underlying disease processes, and renal function should be considered. A change in blood binding will affect drug clearance from the blood as well as average steady-state blood level.

A change in tissue or liver binding will affect partition coefficient and volume of distribution but will have no effect on the steady-state blood level of either total or free drug.

4. Plasma Protein Binding

For highly protein-bound drugs, diminished plasma protein binding does not necessarily mean an increase in free drug concentration because the drug finds binding sites in other nonspecific tissues. Therefore diminished plasma protein binding with no corresponding increase in free drug concentration is associated with a decreased plasma drug concentration (total bound plus free drug). Thus steady-state blood level also decreases with decreased plasma protein binding.

Carbamazepine is a highly protein-bound drug and it has been shown (Wichlinski et al., 1983) that elevated total cholesterol and lipid levels diminish its protein binding and thereby diminish the steady-state blood levels of carbamazepine. The relationship between pharmacokinetic parameters of the drug carbamazepine and total cholesterol levels is biphasic in character (Fig. 6.4) and has been described by Wichlinski et al. using biexponential equations.

In this study, even though the association of elevated total cholesterol levels and diminished steady-state blood levels is demonstrated, it is not established a priori that subjects with normal total cholesterol and lipid levels had comparable steady-state blood levels. Also, it is not shown that in the same patient as total cholesterol level goes high the steady-state blood level proportionately decreases.

Some other researchers seem to think that the receptor availability for the drug and receptor response are more crucial factors than unbound plasma drug levels. In a recent study to predict the pharmacodynamics of diazepam (Ellinwood et al., 1984), it was illustrated that the wheel-tracking and digit-symbol substitution performance by young healthy adults was more significantly correlated with relative receptor occupancy (RRO) than with unbound plasma drug levels; for

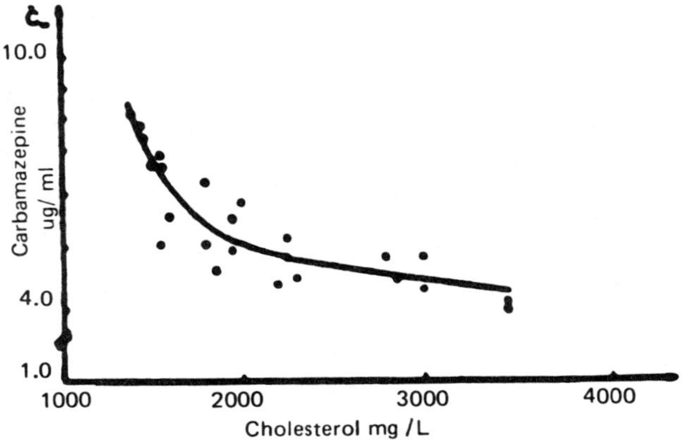

FIGURE 6.4 Relationship between Css of carbamazepine and serum cholesterol values in individual patients.

both tasks, greater similarity was found between performance and RRO than between performance and blood concentration. This result supports the theory that to predict the drug performance, both receptor-binding kinetics and the plasma drug concentration should be used as criterion variables.

5. Cardiac Output

The variations in rate and/or extent of blood flow to different organs can alter the distribution of drugs. With age, the amount of body water decreases and the body fat increases, precipitating localized deposits of drugs after intramuscular, subcutaneous, or intradermal injections in the elderly. These factors, along with changes in permeability of various tissues and barriers and conditions such as atherosclerosis and congestive heart failure, result in an abnormal distribution profile and mask the real picture of plasma drug concentration.

6. Clearance

In terms of liver function, the effect of a decreased function in an eliminating organ (in drug clearance) with or without an accompanying decrease in apparent volume of distribution due to a decrease in tissue binding is an elevation in steady-state blood level (Winter, 1980) (Fig. 6.5).

In terms of renal function, in a clinical trial (Mylan Laboratories, 1984) comparing Dyazide (triamterene 50 mg and hydrochlorothiazide 25 mg) and Maxzide (triamterene 75 mg and hydrochlorothiazide 50 mg), it was found from the plasma and urine data (Table 6.2) that the elderly had lower renal clearances for hydrochlorothiazide and triamterene sulfate and showed larger areas under curves (AUCs) and C_{max} following administration of both Dyazide and Maxzide.

In a study on amobarbital blood levels comparing subjects aged 20–40 years with those aged over 65 years with use of data on absorption, distribution, and metabolism (Ritschel et al., 1978), no change was found in volume of distribution with age; however, biologic half-life was increased from 20.8 h in young subjects to 86.62 h in the elderly subjects as a result of decreased metabolism. This means that to maintain the same steady-state blood level as in the young subjects, the nightly dose in the elderly has to be reduced to 25%.

Besides these physiological factors, the wide variations in pharmacokinetic parameters found among subjects caution the researcher to pay attention to any subtle details he finds extraordinary in his subjects, especially the elderly. In a 1983 review of literature on tricyclic antidepressants (TCAs) (Van Brunt, 1983) the following facts were compiled:

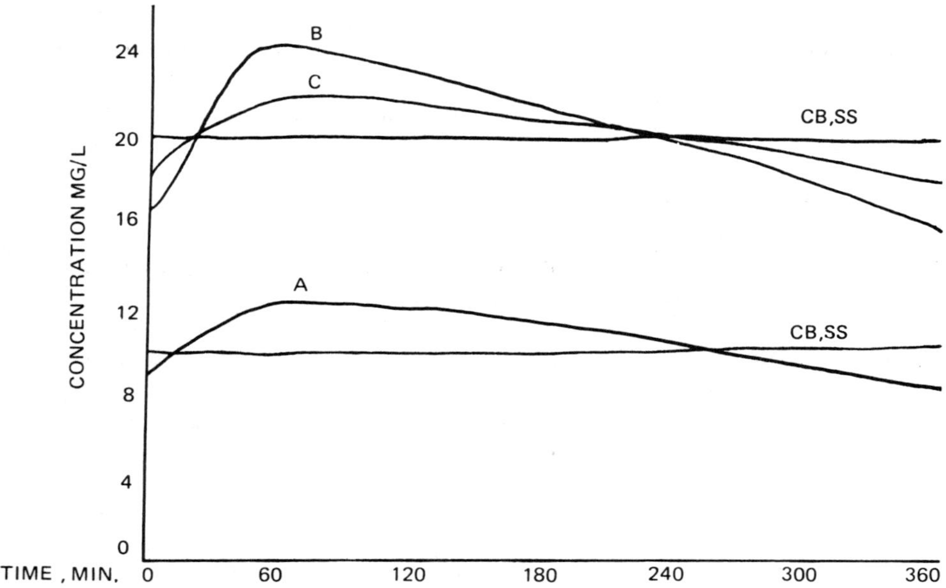

FIGURE 6.5 Effect of a change in intrinsic clearance on steady state blood level of a low clearance drug

Curve	CL_{int} (l/min)	$C_{B,ss}$	Fraction of free drug in tissue
A	0.286	10 mg/l	0.8
B	0.143	20 mg/l	0.8
C	0.143	20 mg/l	0.2

Bioavailability of TCAs ranged from 30 to 70%.

Forty-two percent of subjects who received the same daily dose of Amitryptyline had a serum concentration outside the therapeutic range of 80–200 ng/ml.

Elimination half-lives ranged from 8 to 198 h.

Volumes of distribution ranged from 6.4 to 60 l/kg.

Interpatient variation of free drug levels ranged from a 9.3-fold difference for imipramine to a 1.7-fold difference for protriptyline.

Furthermore, concomitant medications may also affect the steady-state blood levels of drugs requiring adjustment of maintenance dose.

Even though evidence exists as to how physiological factors change

TABLE 6.2 Dyazide versus maxzide study[a]

	Plasma AUC (ng h/ml) (CV%)		Plasma C_{max} (ng/ml) (CV%)		Renal clearance	
	2 × Dyazide	Maxzide	2 × Dyazide	Maxzide	2 × Dyazide	Maxizide
Elderly:						
HCT	3008.7 (43%)	4764.9 (35%)	296.1 (36%)	599.2 (29.7%)	8.5 (47%)	8.2 (49%)
TMT	272.5 (143%)	599.9 (108%)	41.8 (90%)	208.2 (84%)	13.7 (53%)	8.0 (55%)
TMT–SO_4	6991.9 (38%)	10791.7 (40%)	629.8 (46%)	2278.5 (43%)	5.0 (36%)	5.5 (36%)
Nonelderly:						
HCT	1768.1 (41%)	2718.5 (33%)	224.9 (36%)	461.8 (41%)	15.0 (67%)	13.9 (37%)
TMT	224.0 (80%)	592.5 (51%)	49.1 (76%)	192.3 (54%)	18.7 (68%)	11.2 (61%)
TMT–SO_4	3553.7 (46%)	6302.5 (49%)	443.8 (61%)	1678.2 (39%)	7.7 (62%)	8.0 (40%)

[c]Composition of active ingredient, mg/tablet: Maxizide (triamterene, USP, 75 and hydrochlorothiazide, USP, 50); Dyazide (triameterene 50, hydrochlorothiazide 25).

with age, extrapolation of pharmacokinetic parameters for the elderly is not recommended since competing factors influence steady-state blood levels. For example, Rubin et al. (1982) found that Atenelol disposition as an effective hypotensive agent was not significantly changed by age.

An important thing to remember is that although the average steady-state plasma concentration remains the same as in the young, the fluctuations between the maximum and the minimum will be blunted in the elderly. With plasma drug concentrations similar to those in the younger populations, the amount of drug at the receptor site could be varied in the elderly. The pharmacokinetic parameters in the elderly are also affected by their mobility, sex, numbers or types of diseases, and/or number of medications, rather than mere age alone.

C. Conclusions

Given the wide variations in the pharmacokinetic parameters regardless of age and the variations due to age, the question is how important and useful a variable steady-state blood level is in evaluating the efficacy or determining the maintenance dose in the clinical trials for the elderly. The appropriate thing to do is to evaluate the predictive value of the steady-state blood level for the drug in question in terms of drug efficacy and/or its correlation to adverse experiences, (e.g., lidocaine digoxin). Blood levels below and above the therapeutic range are signalled promptly by EKG and adverse experiences. Close association of blood levels with efficacy or safety parameters is a necessary condition to include steady-state blood level as a variable in designing studies on the dosing of the elderly for the drugs exclusively used for them.

When steady-state blood level is used as a variable in statistical analyses, its wide interpatient variation should be dealt with using an appropriate transformation.

III. THE DISTRIBUTION OF PATIENT-SPECIFIC ELIMINATION RATES IN SINGLE-DOSE PHARMACOKINETIC STUDIES

David Salsburg

A. Introduction

One of the considerations in current proposals for the examination of the effects of drugs in the elderly is the fear that patients with impaired renal or hepatic function may have modified pharmacokinetics. This could lead to a build-up of potentially toxic levels of drug in tissue or, on the other extreme, to a lack of efficacy due to more rapid elimination of drug from the system. Thus, a first step in evaluating possible differences between younger and older patients would involve determining if there is, in fact, a difference in pharmacokinetics.

The usual working pharmacokinetic model for drugs is the two-compartment model (see Fig. 6.6), where the ingested drug is assumed to be absorbed at a constant rate into the bloodstream from the site of application and eliminated from the blood at a constant rate. The elimination of drug from the blood is assumed to represent elimination of active drug from the entire body and is the total of several modes of action such as metabolism, excretion, or irreversible binding. A simple two-compartment linear pharmacokinetic model seldom describes the true situation, but it allows us to compute a single measure of residual activity, the elimination rate constant(or its reciprocal, the half-life of the drug.) It has been proposed that we can estimate this single measure of residual activity in each patient, following a fixed dosing pattern, and use these patient-specific estimates to determine if one group has a different pharmacokinetic profile from another.

If patient-specific estimates of elimination rates or half-lives are going to be used to test for differences between groups, then we need to know something about the statistical properties of these estimates, in order to plan studies and to derive reasonably powerful tests of hypotheses. The presentation that follows is an attempt to derive the statistical properties of these estimates from data in the files of Pfizer Central Research. The data are drawn from five drug programs, where the compounds tested have different patterns of pharmacokinetics. The compounds examined are:

1. Lithium carbonate. This is a simple salt that apparently comes closest to the classical two-compartment model in its pharmacokinetics. It is eliminated at a steady rate via the kidney and is neither bound to tissue nor metabolized.

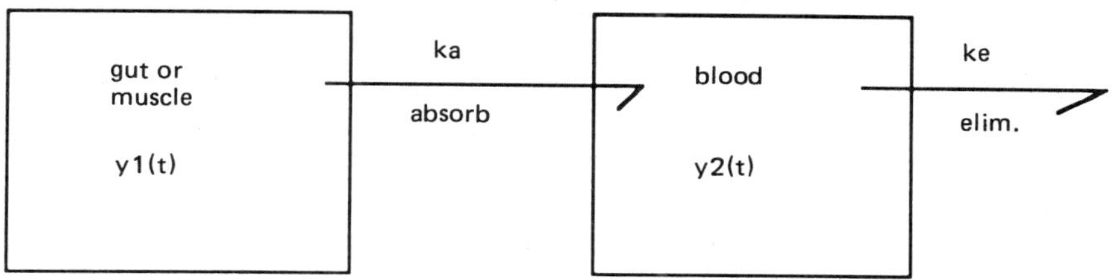

FIGURE 6.6 Simple two-compartment pharmacokinetic model where $dy1(t)/dt = -ka^*y1(t)$ and $dy2(t)/dt = ka^*y1(t) - ke^*y2(t)$.

2. Ampicillin. This is a drug that is also eliminated almost entirely through the kidney at what appears to be a constant rate. It is not metabolized but there may be some reversible tissue binding.
3. Compound A. This is an antibiotic with a long half-life. The compound is stored in the fatty tissues of the body and tends to be eliminated via the kidney. However, there is a secondary route of elimination via the bile, which comes into play as the first route becomes saturated.
4. Compound B. This compound is highly metabolized before being eliminated via several routes. There is a measurable amount of protein binding. It has a relatively short half-life in the blood but the pharmacological effect is still measurable 4–5 half-lives after absorption.
5. Compound C. This compound circulates in the blood without much tissue binding and is eliminated almost entirely by being metabolized into inactive moieties that are then eliminated by the kidney. Its extremely long half-life is probably due to saturation of the metabolic enzymes.

Thus, of the five compounds, only one (lithium carbonate) fits the simple two-compartment model in its pharmacokinetics. Ampicillin comes close to following the model. The pharmacokinetics of compound A must be modeled in terms of at least four compartments. With compound B, we violate the assumption that drug measurable in the blood is equivalent to drug active in the system. And with compound C, the assumption of first-order kinetics is violated. These drugs, however, are representative of the spectrum of different patterns of pharmacokinetics we can expect to see. From each of them, we hope to derive a single patient-specific measure of residual activity (the "elimination rate") in order to determine differences between younger and older patients.

B. Estimating the Elimination Rate

This section deals entirely with data from a single dose-comparative study of two formulations of lithium carbonate. Because this is the compound that most closely follows the assumptions of the two-compartment model, it is the appropriate one with which to compare the statistical behavior of competing methods of estimation.

Two methods of estimation are examined here. One requires that we fit the predicted blood levels from a two-compartment model to the observed blood levels in a given patient, using nonlinear least squares, thereby estimating the three parameters of the model, the initial "dose," the absorption rate (into the blood), and the elimination rate (out of the blood). The least-squares estimates were derived with a Nelder–Mead minimization for each subject and for each formulation.

The second method fits the final portion of the blood level curve to a simple exponential with linearized least squares. That is, we plot the logarithm of the blood level, starting at some point past the peak, against the time post dose and take the negative of the slope of the ordinary least-squares line as an estimate of elimination rate. There are a number of variants of this method. The "infinite" version attributes additional values beyond those observed by extrapolating an exponential decay from the last point. The choice of the first point in time at which to start plotting can vary. Some methods allow the individual patient values to dictate that point. Others require that the same point in time be picked for all patients. The method used here was to pick the first point in time past the peak of the average values across all patients as the common starting point for all patients. The last observed point was the last one used in the estimate. When values were indicated as below the level of the assay, the following procedure was used: If this was the first below-

TABLE 6.3 Estimates of elimination rate constant for lithium carbonate

	Nonlinear LS, full model		OSL slopes on tailing values	
Subject	Form. 1	Form. 2	Form. 1	Form. 2
1	0.672	0.552	0.490	0.489
2	0.497	0.738	0.475	0.449
3	0.549	0.494	0.620	0.559
4	0.566	0.621	0.470	0.559
5	0.398	0.659	0.565	0.580
6	0.652	0.528	0.518	0.502
7	0.549	0.299	0.562	0.450
8	0.412	0.559	0.454	0.506
9	0.229	0.246	0.338	0.333
10	0.542	0.676	0.662	0.692
11	0.504	0.910	0.569	0.541
12	0.086	0.460	0.439	0.420
13	0.542	0.858	0.621	0.710
14	0.611	0.079	0.690	0.511
15	0.525	0.525	0.539	0.623
16	0.738	0.559	0.457	0.535
17	0.549	0.528	0.488	0.492

assay value in time, it was replaced by one-half the minimum detectable level of the assay. If it was a second or third value below the assay, it was treated as a missing value.

Table 6.3 displays the results of the two methods of estimation for the 17 subjects in this study. It can be seen that there is a slight but nonsignificant shift in the mean. Morgan's test (as described in Salsburg, 1975) was used to compare the variances of the methods. The full-model nonlinear least-squares estimates had significantly higher variances, whether we consider the between-patient variance ($p < 0.05$) or the within-patient variance ($p < 0.001$). This is reflected in the sample correlations between estimates for the two different formulations, $r = 0.121$ for the full model estimates and $r = 0.692$ for the simple slope estimates.

Thus, these data display a result that has been a "folk theorem" in the industry for some time: we do better with a simple estimate based on the tailing-off portion of the curve than with an elaborate model-derived estimate that uses all the data. This is shown here to hold for a situation where the two-compartment model is the correct one. It can be expected to be true, *a fortiori*, where the two-compartment model is not the correct one.

C. Elimination Rates, Half-Lives, or some Transformation Thereof

Table 6.4 displays the numbers of patients, the observed averages, and the between- and within-patient variances for the simple slope estimates of elimination rate for the five compounds. It can be seen that the variance is a function of the mean for both the within- and the between-patient variances. In fact, if we model the variance (Y) as a function of the mean (X), we can account for 97.7% of the overall variance of Y by

TABLE 6.4 Between and within subject variances, individual elimination rates derived from slopes

Compound	n	Pooled avg.	Sample variance: Between	Sample variance: Within	Within subject corr.
Li CO_2	17	0.527	0.00809	0.00520	0.692
Ampicillin	16	0.648	0.00203	0.01033	0.261
Compound A	26	0.0242	6.74×10^{-5}	5.76×10^{-5}	0.264
Compound B	12	0.269	0.00360	0.00878	−0.578
Compound C	19	0.0222	8.09×10^{-5}	12.57×10^{-5}	0.123

the simple formula

$$Y = kX^2$$

where $k = 0.031$. The transformation that stabilizes the variance of a random variable whose variance is proportional to the square of the mean is the logarithm.

Table 6.5 displays the results of examining the original estimates of the elimination rates, their logarithms, and the half-lives:

Half-life = log(2)/elimination rate

There is a general assumption that variance-stabilizing transformations are also normalizing transformations. To check on this, I tested the goodness of fit for each of the transformations for each of the compounds, with a chi-square test based on 10 equiprobable intervals. Thus, for each transformation and for each compound, I computed a statistic that should behave approximately like a chi square with eight degrees of freedom. The sum of these chi squares across all five compounds should behave like a chi square with 40 degrees of freedom. It can be seen from Table 6.5 that elimination rate itself is closest to being normally distributed, and that the chi squares for the two others lie within the 25% tails of the distribution.

It can also be seen from Table 6.5 that the logarithm succeeds in stabilizing the variance.

Thus, we can conclude that the most powerful statistical tests will probably result from running normal theory tests on the patient specific elimination rates themselves. However, the log values are sufficiently close to normal that we can use a single estimate of the stabilized variance to compute sample size and power—as if the final analysis were on the logs.

D. The Power of a Comparison of Two Groups

Table 6.5 displays a pooled variance estimate of the log (elimination rate). This is sometimes called the "rel-variance" of the distribution. If we use normal theory to compute confidence bounds on the true underlying rel-variance, we get the 80% bounds displayed in the last line of Table 6.5. We now have three rel-variance estimates on which to base power calculations.

The rel-variance has the advantage in computing power and sample size that we can examine power in terms of the difference between treatments as a percent of the mean of one of them. Thus the ap-

TABLE 6.5 Tests for normality of elimination rates and transformations

Compound	n	Elimination rate			Half-life			$\log_e$(Elim. rate)[a]		
		Avg.	SD	χ^2	Avg.	SD	χ^2	Avg.	SD	χ^2
Li CO_2	17	0.527	0.900	7.118	1.355	0.2511	4.765	−1.996	0.5081	18.882
Ampicillin	16	0.648	0.0450	2.750	1.750	0.0731	1.500	−0.437	0.0687	1.500
Compound A	26	0.02417	0.00821	5.538	31.991	8.508	12.462	−3.801	0.2508	5.538
Compound B	12	0.269	0.06002	6.333	2.717	0.6804	18.000	−1.339	0.2387	11.333
Compound C	19	0.02221	0.00899	7.842	37.665	21.187	9.947	−3.884	0.4534	9.778
Total chi square				29.581			46.674			47.031
Sig. level				>0.50			0.217			0.207

[a] Pooled variance estimate for $\log_e$(elimination rate) = 0.119; 80% upper and lower bounds (based on normal theory) = [0.098, 0.148].

TABLE 6.6 Numbers of patients needed per group to detect differences in mean elimination rates between two groups, $\alpha = 0.05$ Two-Sided Testing

Differences between group I and group II as a percent of mean rate for group I	Lower bound = 0.098 power			Median = 0.119 power			Upper bound = 0.148 power		
	50%	80%	95%	50%	80%	95%	50%	80%	95%
1%	7,605	>10,000	>10,000	9,235	>10,000	>10,000	>10,000	>10,000	>10,000
5%	317	647	1,070	385	786	1,300	478	977	1,617
10%	83	170	281	101	206	341	126	256	424
25%	16	31	52	19	38	63	23	47	78
50%	5	10	16	6	12	19	7	15	24
100%	3	4	4	3	4	4	3	5	9

proximate power equation (for n patients per group in a two-group comparison) is

$$d^2 = [\log(1 + D)^2]/(2 \times \text{rel-variance}/n)$$

where

$$D = (\text{group II mean} - \text{group I mean})/(\text{group I mean})$$

and d is the sum of the $N(0, 1)$ cut-off values for Type I and Type II error.

Table 6.6 displays the values of n (rounded up to the nearest integer) for three levels of power (50%, 80%, and 95%), for the three estimates of rel-variance and for several choices of D. If we consider a feasible clinical trial to be one with 50 or fewer patients in a group, then it can be seen that we can be reasonably sure of detecting a difference in elimination rates between two groups only if the difference is greater than 25%. Since the half-life is the reciprocal of the elimination rate, the same figure holds for half-life. Thus, if we have a drug with a half-life in healthy volunteers of 12 h, we will need about 50 patients per group to detect an increase to 15 h, and a study using only 20 patients per group has reasonable power to detect an increase to 18 h.

REFERENCES

Cooper, T. B. et al. Butaperazine pharmacokinetics, *Archives of General Psychiatry*, *32:* 906, 1975.

Ellinwood, E. H., et al. Prediction of pharmacodynamics from pharmacokinetics, *Psychopharmacology (Berlin)*, *83*(3): 297, 1984.

Gibaldi, M., and Koup, J. R. Pharmacokinetic concepts—Drug binding, apparent volume of distribution and clearance, *European Journal of Clinical Pharmacology*, *20:* 299, 1981.

Levin, E., et al. 'A simple measure of gastric secretion in man. *Gastroenterology*, *19*(1): 88, 1951.

Massoud, N. Pharmacokinetic considerations in geriatric patients, in *Pharmacokinetic Basis for Drug Treatment* L. Z. Benet et al., eds.). New York, Raven Press, 1984.

McGlone, F. B. *Journal of the American Geriatric Society*, *30* (November), 1982.

Moore, E., Sr., and Teal, T. W. *Geriatric Drug Use—Clinical and Social Perspectives*. New York, Pergamon Press, 1985.

Mylan Laboratories. Summary basis for approval—Clinical trials by Mylan Laboratories, 1984.

Ritschel, W. A. Pharmacokinetic approach to drug dosing in the aged. *Journal of the American Geriatric Society*, *24:* 344, 1976.

Ritschel et al. 'Age-dependent disposition of amobarbital: Analog computer evaluation, *Journal of the American Geriatric Society*, *XXVI*(12): 540–1978.

Rubin, P. C., et al. Atenolol disposition in young and elderly subjects. *Journal of Clinical Pharmacology*, *13:* 234, 1982.

Salsburg, D., Estimating differences in variance when comparing two methods of assay. *Technometrics*, *17:* 381–382, 1975.

Sommers, D. K., et al. Influence of food and reduced gastric acidity on the bioavailability of bacampicillin and cefuroxime axetil. *British Journal of Clinical Pharmacology*, *18:* 535, 1984.

Van Brunt, N. The clinical utility of tricyclic antidepressant blood levels: A review of the literature, *Therapeutic Drug Monitoring*, *5*(1): 1, 1983.

Wichlinski, L. M., et al. Correlation between the total cholesterol serum concentration data and carbamazepine steady-state blood levels in humans. *Drug Intelligence and Clinical Pharmacy*, *17:* 812, 1983.

Winter, M. E., et al., *Basic Clinical Pharmacokinetics*. San Francisco, Applied Therapeutics, 1980.

7
Intention to Treat in Clinical Trials

Lloyd D. Fisher *University of Washington and Fred Hutchinson Cancer Research Center, Seattle, Washington*

Dennis O. Dixon *M. D. Anderson Cancer Center, University of Texas, Houston, Texas*

Jay Herson *Applied Logic Associates, Inc., Houston, Texas*

Ralph K. Frankowski *University of Texas, Houston, Texas*

Martha S. Hearron *The Upjohn Company, Kalamazoo, Michigan*

Karl E. Peace* *Biopharmaceutical Research Consultants, Inc., Ann Arbor, Michigan*

I. ANALYSIS OF RANDOMIZED CLINICAL TRIALS: INTENTION TO TREAT

Lloyd D. Fisher, Dennis O. Dixon, Jay Herson, and Ralph F. Frankowski

A. Introduction

This chapter reviews the background for, rationale behind, and need for the randomized clinical trial (RCT). It is argued that to preserve the benefits of randomization one type of analysis, the intent-to-treat analysis, is preferable; this approach may not be the preferred analysis from other points of view. The reasons for this tension are discussed and it is

**Previous affiliation:* Warner-Lambert Company, Ann Arbor, Michigan.

argued that for well-designed and well-executed experiments the intention-to-treat analysis is appropriate and congruent with the other desired analyses.

1. Background

The historical background of medical clinical trials is presented in an excellent article by Bull (1959). In the context of more recent events and clinical trials some of this material appears in Meinert (1986) and Frye et al. (1987). A few highlights are given here, but the more interested reader should consult the Bull article.

Even in biblical times, Daniel resolved "not to defile himself" with the royal food and wine and requested "Please test your servants for ten days: give us nothing but vegetables to eat and water to drink. Then compare our appearance with that of the young men who eat the royal food, and treat your servants in accord with what you see." The experiment turned out well (*The Holy Bible*, 1978). Avicenna, who lived between 980 and 1037, noted that remedies must be tried on man "for testing a drug on a lion or a horse might not prove anything." He also noted that a comparative trial was needed—"two opposed cases be observed." Other investigators noted that similar groups must be used for comparing therapies. For example, the American physician Elisha Bartlett (1804–1855) noted that "In therapeutic investigations cases which are to be compared must have equal disturbing factors of location, social class, and the like . . . ." The advocation of a clinical trial on comparable groups has a long and distinguished tradition within medicine. The problem of assuring "equal disturbing factors" was to prove difficult in practice. This may be especially because (as argued in Frye et al., 1987) the human mind apparently cannot act randomly—and indeed much important information that might influence the trial could be available in a form not amenable to conscious and objective recording.

The need for a fair unbiased experiment and to have a known probability distribution to examine the difference in outcome in separate treatment groups was bothering R. A. Fisher, later to become Sir R. A. Fisher, in the 1920s. It is not known precisely when he developed the concept of the randomized experiment, but it was between 1918 and 1923 (Box, 1978). The idea led to the first reported randomization of patients in 1931 [as given in Meinert (1986) referring to Amberson et al. (1931)].

2. The Randomized Clinical Trial (RCT)

The method of randomization conveyed three important benefits in clinical research (Meier, 1983; Ederer, 1975; Green, 1982).

1. The method guards against bias (in a statistical sense) when the randomization process is correctly carried out. The potential investigator biases controlled include unconscious biases with unmeasured variables as well as the conscious concerns. We view this as an exceedingly important property of randomization.
2. Closely related to this is the fact that the groups are balanced statistically, or on the average, because of the method of randomization; again, *a most important point is that this balance occurs not only for known factors but even for unknown and/or unrecorded variables*. Thus the method of the randomized clinical trial assures statistical balance between therapeutic groups in all regards.
3. The validity of appropriate statistical tests is assured by the process of randomization. Observational data analyses of necessity depend on assumptions; the known distribution of the randomization process and the subsequent statistical tests depend only on the fact that the randomization was a true randomization.

These benefits apply also to the randomized clinical trial in humans; the RCT is widely considered to give the highest level of proof and cogency to the development of new therapies.

3. Design and Analysis of RCTs

To reiterate, the benefits described above apply to clinical trials in humans and are sufficiently compelling that the RCT is considered the most cogent and highest level of scientific proof of the usefulness of a new therapy. Note that to preserve the benefits of the randomization process, the groups to be compared are the groups of individuals as they were randomized. Analyses that analyze patients, or subjects, in the groups to which they were randomized are called *intent-to-treat analyses*. We do not have time to argue at length the following proposition: the well-designed and well-executed randomized clinical trial would be analyzed by the intent-to-treat method; in this case the intent-to-treat method of analysis would be the most satisfactory analysis from a biological and statistical point of view.

One crucial problem in clinical trials in humans is that they rarely, if ever, can be performed without flaw. Suppose that some of the patients randomized to receive a new drug never received any of the drug (possibly because they refused, because of administrative error, or even an earthquake). Is it not biologically absurd to require such a person to be analyzed in the drug treatment group? Suppose individuals in a drug group comply very poorly with their assigned therapy: how can the drug work when taken only occasionally? Is it rational to try to find drug efficacy using such cases? In any event, what does intent-to-treat analysis mean when crucial needed follow-up data are missing? As one individual replied to a questionnaire about intent-to-treat analyses, *is the purpose of the experiment to study the drug or is the purpose of the experiment to study the randomization process*?

This is the crux of the debate about intent-to-treat analyses: to the extent that the experimental design is inappropriate or executed less than perfectly there may be tension between the statistical and biological claims about the best analysis. More biologically oriented individuals who worry less about biased comparisons and the validity of statistical methods may argue against intent-to-treat analyses (i.e., for other "efficacy" analyses); those more concerned about statistical issues may argue for intent-to-treat analysis and great effort to perform RCTs as designed in order that the intent-to-treat analysis also be biologically compelling.

Stated more operationally, the intent-to-treat debate concerns methodologic principles governing the qualification and disqualification of randomized subjects and outcome events for the purpose of assessing treatment benefits (Gent and Sackett, 1979).

The issue arises because of special and, at times, unique problems posed by the exclusion and attribution of subjects in a randomized clinical trial. In addition to the points discussed above, subjects may be misdiagnosed and treated for a disease that they do not have. Subjects may withdraw from the study unexpectedly. Subjects may deviate from their assigned course of treatment under medical advice. These and other similar problems resulting from the execution of a randomized clinical trial raise serious questions concerning how to properly assign subjects and outcomes to treatment groups and how to best combine the resulting complete and incomplete information. These two divergent viewpoints focusing on the identification of which endpoints should be assigned to a treatment group and the disqualification of randomized subjects can be found in the literature. Two opposing positions on the postrandomization deletion of subjects and outcome events have been clearly stated. One position holds that regardless of the kind of randomized trial performed or the kind of events measured, all subjects meeting admission criteria and subsequently randomized should be counted in their originally assigned treatment groups without regard to deviations from assigned treatment. Within the statistical community this policy of "analyze as randomized" is identified with the intention-to-treat principle; as discussed above, it is based primarily on the danger of observational bias connected with disqualification of subjects or events (Peto et al., 1976; Friedman, Furberg, and DeMets, 1985, Chapter 16; Gail, 1985).

The opposing and more lenient position holds that "There are no hard and fast rules concerning the qualification and disqualification of patients and events in clinical trials" (Gent and Sackett, 1979). These and other authors note their exceptions to the intention to treat principle on the argument that the objectives and type of clinical trial conducted, as well as collateral evidence, should rule the cases and events used to determine the outcomes of treatment (Sackett, 1983; Detre and Peduzzi, 1982).

Armitage (1983), in a careful review of the opposing positions, recommended that the primary analysis of a randomized clinical trial should generally follow the intention-to-treat principle and that liberal exclusion of subjects from treatment group be considered as the object of secondary analysis of the data. He noted, however, that there is room for further discussion.

We proceed to examine the strengths and weaknesses of the opposing positions on the qualification and disqualification of subjects in randomized clinical trials in order to provide direction for the development of standards for use in statistical practice.

Before proceeding to consider further the intent-to-treat principle, we discuss briefly the meaning of the term. The first and most obvious meaning is that the randomized assignment was indeed the treatment that was intended to be given to the subject. But it is also important to note that physicians de facto act under the intent-to-treat principle. They can prescribe drugs or physical therapy, say, but they cannot assure that we contrary human beings will follow the plan. Thus the intent-to-treat analysis often most closely models the possible clinical scenario. On the other hand, one could argue that the biology is best investigated by restricting attention (for active drugs) to those who comply with their therapeutic assignment. This leads to distinctions among clinical trials according to their purpose.

B. Classification of Clinical Trials

Trials can be classified by their general objectives. Previous writers have classified them into one of two broad categories: (1) trials designed to test a specific biological or therapeutic hypothesis, and (2) trials designed to evaluate specific relative benefits of competing treatment regimens in practice. These two categories have been variously named as "explanatory" versus "pragmatic" trials (Schwartz and Lellouch, 1967), "efficacy" versus "effectiveness" trials (Cochrane, 1972), and "explanatory" versus "management" trials (Sackett, 1983).

The purpose of a pragmatic or management trial is to ascertain a rank ordering of treatment regimens for use in general medical practice. The pragmatic clinical trial logically implies the statistical policy of intention-to-treat, namely, the total groups formed by randomization are compared without deletion of subjects or events to evaluate treatments. As stated above, the intention-to-treat recommendation represents a realistic clinical option where the treatment question reduces to a choice of the best treatment regimen to initiate with the medical (or surgical, etc.) intention to continue the regimen, if possible (Armitage, 1983). Thus, the pragmatic or management randomized clinical trial is a comparison of treatment strategies or policies (Peto et al., 1976).

In contrast, the explanatory randomized clinical trial represents an earlier stage of inquiry designed to unravel the chain of events and medical interventions that might lead to the prevention or delay of a specified outcome. The distinction between pragmatic and explanatory clinical trials is closely analogous to the biometric problem of finding improved strains of a new crop. In crop improvement at an explanatory stage, the best of many new strains are selected for specific merits and then the explanatory trial is followed by a large-scale field trial to evaluate the general merits of improved strains. In medical trials, this is illustrated by comparing the early VA trials (Veterans Administration, 1967) on the evaluation of antihypertensive drugs with the large-scale management trial (HDFP, 1979) evaluating treatment strategies in the general hypertensive population. In this section we will be primarily concerned with pragmatic randomized clinical trials. In any event in practice the distinction blurs and the long-term, and usually short-term, goal is to find a therapy that gives an overall benefit when intended to be given in some group of patients.

C. Exclusions, Withdrawals, and Losses

Following Peto et al. (1976) we will distinguish among three distinct categories of subjects in a RCT: (1) exclusions, subjects never randomized; (2) withdrawals, subjects randomized but not analyzed, as though never entered; and (3) losses, subjects inadvertently lost during follow-up and whose treatment experience is known only up to the date of loss.

1. Exclusions

The design of a RCT requires that explicit criteria for the inclusion and exclusion of subjects be stated as a formal part of the trial design. Furthermore, it is incumbent that the design assures that case entry criteria be carefully and systematically applied to all potential subjects in advance of randomization.

Since exclusions never enter the clinical trial and hence are never randomized, exclusions cannot directly affect or bias treatment comparisons. The influence of exclusions, if present to any considerable number, will be to limit the generalizability of the results of the trial. Those randomized may not fully represent the target population of interest. This limitation of inference will also obtain when patients who meet diagnostic criteria of the trial decline participation under medical advice or for other reasons, some of which may be related to the course of the disease. This limitation can be partially addressed by use of a registry that characterizes eligible but excluded cases (Frommer et al., 1983; CASS et al., 1984), but if certain types of eligible cases are never or rarely randomized, the objectives of a management trial will not be met; the inference will be more restricted than planned.

2. Withdrawals

The diagnosis of disease is rarely unequivocal and thus, despite careful attention to inclusion and exclusion of subjects, randomization errors may result, and cases without the disease may be randomized to treatment. Since it is often unethical to delay treatment for a disease, if sufficient evidence suggests its presence, a preliminary diagnosis is often used to randomize and thus promptly initiate a treatment regimen. Results from confirmatory testing such as lab testing of a prerandomization biopsy or computer-assisted interpretation of physiological parameters may be delayed until after randomization. It is clearly uninformative to analyze treatment outcomes for subjects without the disease of interest yet they have been randomized. Worst yet noise is added by including such individuals when searching for a treatment effect. How will such subjects and their outcomes influence final treatment comparisons?

If the original clinical trial design did not take into account rates of prerandomization errors, then in fixed sample size designs the statistical power of the design will be compromised. This is the case whether or not these subjects are withdrawn, so that the final comparison of treatments is diluted by the inclusion of subsets in each group for whom no benefit is expected. As emphasized by Ingelfinger et al. (1983), "Inaccurate diagnosis followed by randomization can result in finding no benefit when in fact there are benefits in properly diagnosed patients. It cannot often explain away observations suggesting benefit."

Although the effects of misdiagnosis could be minimized by delaying randomization until a confirmed diagnosis can be obtained, such an expedient option may not always be possible. In potentially life-threatening conditions treatment must be started promptly but confirmation of the specific condition will be unavoidably delayed beyond the time of randomization and thus a fraction of randomized cases will be misdiagnosed.

It may therefore be argued that randomized cases disqualified based on information obtained during the prerandomization time period may, at the option of the analyst, be withdrawn from final treatment comparisons without risk of misleading results. The important point is the loss of statistical power in the design that will result from misdiagnosed cases and the possibility that important treatment differences will not be detected. Administrative procedures to withdraw misdiagnosed cases and a discussion of the delicate balance between liberal and conservative entry criteria can be found in Peto et al. (1976) and Armitage (1983).

Among the various types of withdrawals that have been discussed in the literature, one that seems easy to decide is the patient found to be ineligible after randomization, on the basis of objective data *knowable* prior to randomization. As Gail states (1985, p. 1110), "Removing [such a patient] will not bias the the treatment comparison provided the detection of this eligibility violation was unrelated to the treatment assignment." The main example is clerical error, such as the simple misreporting of the patient's age. Naturally, there is potential for trouble if those conducting the study check eligibility more carefully in selected subgroups. Since it would be difficult or impossible to be certain on this point, it may be best to follow the advice of Friedman et al. (1982, pp. 245–246): "Every effort should be made to establish the eligibility of subjects for entry into the study within the constraints of the design. No withdrawals should be allowed . . . ."

Gent and Sackett (1979, p. 128) take the opposing view, that clinical trials are blunt instruments, and that one cannot afford to sacrifice any power by including subjects for whom the null hypothesis is almost certainly true: ". . . *strict* adherence to protocol is essential. This class of patient should be discarded for the very simple reason that they are outside the defined population in which the potential benefit of the drug is being assessed."

Gent and Sackett's concern applies in a practical way only if there are more than a few patients involved. If that is true, the trial probably has other major problems as well. On balance, therefore, we recommend that patients not be withdrawn from analysis, even if found to be ineligible after randomization. In any event it is best that a prestated policy exist, and that any exclusion be done blindly to treatment assignment and outcome (see Friedman, Furberg, and DeMets, 1982).

A different problem arises when investigators enter patients before all eligibility checks can be completed. In emergency situations, for example, treatment must begin promptly, even if there is insufficient time to obtain the results of all the laboratory tests. Another example common in multicenter trials is centralized review of material, such as pathology review of slides in cancer and other diseases. These procedures sometimes create a sizable group of patients declared ineligible retrospectively.

Several authors have issued warnings about the dangers in such circumstances. Gail (1985, p. 1110) is typical: "Eligibility violations [due to errors on subjective data] are problematic, and the potential for biased removals is great enough that such analyses should be avoided and must be viewed skeptically. The potential for abuse is great if subjective data . . . are re-evaluated at the time of analysis."

There is a further difficulty that we view as more important, having to do with the interpretability of trial results. It seems basic that a clinical trial addresses a specific question in a defined population, and that *the definition of the population must be applicable at the time a treatment choice is made*. Thus, if one excludes patients from an analysis on the basis of information available only after the start of treatment, then to what identifiable population do the results apply?

Preplanned stratified analyses based on later evaluation of data collected at baseline (i.e., before randomization) may help to preserve statistical power and suggest important predefined subgroup analyses.

Our suggestion is to restrict the eligibility criteria to those that are knowable at the time of entry. Data derived from centralized expert review might be useful in ancillary analyses and quality control reports, but should not lead to withdrawal of patients meeting all preentry eligibility criteria.

3. Losses

During the course of a clinical trial patients may become lost to follow-up. Many investigators prefer to analyze the results of the trial ignoring their existence. The intention-to-treat policy dictates that these patients be included in all analyses.

For a survival end point a policy of censoring all patients at the time of loss is usually followed, regardless of intention-to-treat persuasion. Note that biases may enter here: sicker patients may be less likely to take off; adverse events may trigger drop-out in one group but not another. But this policy is acceptable providing that investigators do not intentionally alter their follow-up operations based on patient survival and that the percent lost to follow-up is small.

When outcome is dichotomous, such as objective response to treatment, patients lost to follow-up are often classified as failures. This approach is considered conservative and motivates intensive follow-up.

Again biases can occur. Patients may be lost to follow-up in separate groups for different reasons. To ignore the existence of lost-to-follow-up patients can cause biased results when loss is related to treatment and presents outcomes that are not representative of medical practice. For graded response, the corresponding policy is to classify lost patients in the most unfavorable category. Every effort must be made to minimize lost data; bias can potentially enter in.

Often end points are continuous, such as a lipid determination. Here a baseline and 6-month follow-up may be required by the protocol and lost patients will not have, for example, a 6-month measurement. In these cases loss may be related to outcome because patients can have their lipids, blood pressure, or weights determined independently of the trial and drop out if they feel that they are not benefiting from the program. Investigators may wish to impute 6-month values for patients lost to follow-up. Imputed values may be estimated using regression methods based on data for patients with complete data; either average or conservative values could in principle be used.

In fact, imputation of values for missing continuous-endpoint data seems extremely uncommon. One reason may be the feeling that there is no completely objective approach to the problem.

In general, if there is much missing data one should do some sensitivity analyses to see how sensitive the results are to the missing data. For example, if survival is being compared in two groups and one group appears to have superior survival and if those in the group with the best survival lost to follow-up are coded as dead at the last contact while those in the other group are assumed to survive until the last scheduled follow-up, and the result still holds, no would dispute the difference. This is an extreme case, but intermediate scenarios could be evaluated (Fisher and Kanarek, 1974). For other types of end points, similar sensitivity analyses could be envisioned.

D. Issues That Are Not Intent-to-Treat Issues

Sometimes the intent-to-treat debate gets sidetracked about important and sometimes controversial decisions that are not logically related to the reasons for doing an intent-to-treat analysis. A few of these issues are discussed here.

1. Cause-Specific End Points

Selection of the end points of a trial is an important decision. There is the opportunity for bias to enter here. For example, if cause-specific mortality is to be used, (1) the classification could be inappropriate and (2) this end point could ignore important unexpected mortality due to other causes. But as long as the cause-specific end point is applied to all subjects, the intent-to-treat principle is intact. This is not to say that cause-specific end points are not appropriate in certain cases; for example, in bone marrow transplantation there is agreement that some causes of death, such as relapse and severe graft versus host disease, are fairly reliably assessed.

2. Length of Follow-Up Used

The length of a patient's follow-up used for analysis may be decided to be less than full. For example, in studying an antihypertensive therapy certain findings may be predetermined to be a treatment failure. Assuming the trial is for the change in blood pressure, the last measurement when the therapy failed might reasonably be used for analysis. In studying congestive heart failure some individuals who have an unsatisfactory therapeutic response might receive a heart transplant; one might arguably predefine this to be a death for purposes of data analysis.

3. Method of Dealing with Missing Data

The method of dealing with missing data is not part of the intent-to-treat principle. Whether one imputes, declares failures, or does a sensitivity analysis, as long as the decision includes all patients in their original group the analysis is an intent-to-treat analysis. Note that all methods of handling missing data are unsatisfactory to various degrees and may be the subject of debate. Also note that the reason data are unavailable is important in the interpretation. For example, if the missing data are at the site of one inept investigator at a multicenter trial and fall across treatment groups generally, this would be perceived as less likely to introduce bias than the same amount of missing data spread across clinics and primarily in one treatment group.

E. Design Considerations

It is worth emphasizing that study design can influence the extent to which exclusions from analysis is an issue. For example, as mentioned above, Friedman, Furberg, and DeMets (1985) advise adding to the protocol a statement of policy on withdrawal of enrolled but ineligible patients. Assuming a defensible policy, then at least one avoids "the concern that the withdrawal policy was dependent on the outcome of the trial." [They specifically warn of the dangers of this policy-statement approach in the case of exclusions due to postentry events, such as noncompliance or loss to follow-up. See the Coronary Drug Project (1980) in this regard.] Though the ideal would be to eliminate the possibility of enrolling ineligible cases, the policy would allow exclusions when the errors were demonstrably made on information available at the time of randomization.

Another aspect of the issue was considered by Gent and Sackett (1979). They argue that treatment comparisons are diluted by the inclusion of ineligible and noncompliant patients. Ineligible patients are by definition ones thought unlikely to exhibit large differences in response to experimental and control treatments. Noncompliant patients often receive treatment appropriate to a study group different from the one assigned, so that final groups receive a mixture of treatments. Gent and Sackett recommend "increasing our efforts to (a) maximize patient drug compliance, (b) minimize co-interventions, (c) increase our effectiveness in keeping study clinicians and patients on the protocol," and "make an explicit declaration of criteria for disqualification of patients and events a mandatory section of both the original protocol and the subsequent publications of such studies.

Note that most concerns can be addressed by innovative study design. For example, if one feels that there is a class of responders to a drug along with many nonresponders, a different design might be used. A preliminary trial with a drug response could be used to qualify patients for the randomized study. This restriction to apparent early responders would need to be taken into account in interpreting the trial but could be used to show a beneficial drug effect if the underlying ideas were correct. Similarly, an initial screen could be used for those who could not tolerate a drug in some situations. Where appropriate a placebo run-in period would use patient compliance as one possible entry criterion. There is still room for considerable ingenuity and advancement in the design of trials.

F. Is the Intent-to-Treat Analysis Always the Best Analysis?

To establish the position that an intent-to-treat analysis is not always the best position, consider the following hypothetical situation. A trial is to be run to compare the antihypertensive effects of placebo versus drug X. The data center prepares the randomization schedule and sends it with the code for placebo and active drug to the pharmacy by electronic transmission. Against all experience the trial is perfectly run with 100% compliance, every visit on time and with complete data. Contrary to the animal data and Phase I and II studies drug X has statistically significant *less of an* effect. This triggers investigation where it is discovered that there was a documentable error in data transmission that led the pharmacy to reverse the packaging—patients intended for placebo received drug X and visa versa. Clearly the intent-to-treat analysis would be wrong. As "a foolish consistency is the hobgoblin of small minds," the drug should be labeled a success.

Now, however, consider another situation. Overall there is no statistically significant difference between a placebo group and an active therapy group. However, when attention is restricted to the 24% who complied, the active drug looks better. Briefly, no or little intent-to-treat efficacy but a result comparing placebo and the minority of those with good compliance gives a result. Does the drug work? Do we go with biology at the great risk of bias (Coronary Drug Project, 1980), or do we play it safe? We would argue that the experiment was poorly conducted; although the results may be encouraging, another experiment is needed if one is to establish efficacy.

When the intent-to-treat principle is dropped in analysis one loses some, or sometimes even most, of the protection of the randomization process. Thus the data analysis is to some unknown degree an observational data analysis. Even though data from a randomized trial will tend to have more balance by treatment than most observational databases, the protection of randomization is diminished or gone. The scientific cogency is less. The randomized trial is not a cureall execution, and appropriate analyses are needed to accrue the benefits of randomization.

We feel the intent-to-treat analysis may not always be the best analysis but when it is not this usually indicates that (1) the experiment was designed or run suboptimally and (2) the results are more debatable.

G. Conclusions

In summary, the authors of this section feel that:

Randomization was one of the great intellectual advances of the twentieth century. It is especially important for avoiding bias and assuring statistical balance even on unmeasured variables.

The most scientifically sound and cogent method of demonstrating a treatment effect is the randomized clinical trial.

Because the protection of randomization depends on an intent-to-treat analysis, such an analysis should always be done—usually as the first primary analysis. (A notable exception is the allowable removal of patients not meeting eligibility criteria on the basis of information available at the time of randomization. Such exclusions should be written into the protocol.)

The debate about the intent-to-treat principle and other methods of analyzing clinical trials occurs because of a conflict between statistical and biological cogency.

If the interpretation of a trial needs an "efficacy" analysis eliminating patients based on postrandomization information, then the protection of randomization is diminished and the analysis is to some extent observational. One should expect much more debate and criticism about the meaning of the RCT. Often an additional experiment(s) would be needed to have firm proof of the finding.

Usually one can design a trial so that if it is well executed the intent-to-treat and most biologically compelling analyses are one and the same.

DISCLAIMER

This section resulted from the establishment of the ASA working group on who to include in analyses. The group was not able to reach a consensus position; thus these views while authored by and congruent with many members of the working group do not represent the group as a whole.

II. INTENTION TO TREAT—A SUMMARY VIEW

Lloyd D. Fisher

Sir Ronald Alymer Fisher made one of the great intellectual advances of the twentieth century with the concept of randomization, introduced in the 1920s. In the late 1940s the British, under the leadership of Sir Austin Bradford Hill, applied the randomized experiment to clinical medicine, giving us the randomized clinical trial.

The randomized clinical trial is important in medicine because it is so difficult to get known comparable groups to evaluate different therapies. It seems impossible for the human to allocate individuals into two balanced groups. There is suggestive evidence to indicate that the gifted diagnostician or physician may have at his or her disposal more information than can be conveniently quantitated on forms and by objective tests. Note that the process of randomization assures statistically comparable groups for comparing therapeutic options, not only with respect to known recorded variables but also with respect to unknown and/or unrecorded variables. This point cannot be emphasized enough.

If, however, individuals are omitted from the analysis of a randomized study by using variables that occur after the randomization, (for example, individuals who do not comply in taking their drugs, individuals who have an adverse response to therapy, and individuals who are lost to follow-up), there is no way of showing that the individuals removed from the different treatment groups are comparable; thus groups left for comparison may not be comparable. One can look at important known recorded factors to see if the individuals left for analysis are comparable, but this does not and cannot assure that the patients are comparable with respect to unknown factors. Further, if a large number of individuals "need" to be removed from analysis, this would indicate an experiment that in point of fact did not adhere closely to the desired experimental design; some suspicion should be evident.

For these reasons it is felt that for all randomized clinical trials an intent-to-treat analysis should be the first analysis done and presented. It is agreed that there are very important difficult issues about how to do this when there are individuals lost to follow-up or without recorded data. Nevertheless, the intent-to-treat analysis is the desirable analysis from which other analyses would proceed and need to be justified. The intent-to-treat analysis assures the statistical balance due to the process of randomization. It forces the disclosure of what happens to all patients, and it gives a benchmark from which to consider differences resulting from other analyses. The intent-to-treat analysis also emphasizes the importance of good science and comparability of treatment groups.

This is not to say that other analyses are never appropriate. There are many circumstances where other analyses are not only desirable but should be done. However, by virtue of the fact that another analysis is done, one acknowledges some departure from the original experimental design.

Most of the commonly raised objections to intent-to-treat analyses (such as the feeling that it is nonsensical to include patients with noncompliance to drug therapy) have solutions. One can have a pretrial period to see if patients reasonably comply with their medication. Randomization after the pretrial period would help to eliminate poor compliance. If side effects are a big issue, one can have early studies and even dose ranging on an active drug to try to make sure that individuals tolerate the drug before randomization and respond to the therapy. A protocol can reasonably define as a treatment failure a person with (what would appear to be) an intolerable side effect, or so little therapeutic response that other drugs must be used. In this case these failures would be included in the analysis.

III. INTENTION TO TREAT—ANOTHER VIEW

Martha S. Hearron

Whom one includes in an analysis depends on the hypothesis to be tested. Consider the following:

Response = medication group + evaluability + treatment + error

Intent-to-treat analysis looks for differences in effects of group membership. If one wishes to compare the effects of "treatment + error" some other approach may be more appropriate.

With respect to treatment, where two major divisions emerge, the first case is when a patient is randomized but receives no treatment at all. In the second case, inadequate treatment is received. Here, there are several scenarios. The patient may receive inadequate treatment but achieve the end point. The patient may receive inadequate medication for therapeutic efficacy because of an adverse reaction that leads to discontinuation of therapy. In yet another case, a patient may refuse to continue treatment or may simply be lost to follow-up.

Study protocols all include evaluability criteria. The motivation for this is twofold. The first purpose is to provide a homogeneous population for study. The second is for reasons of patient safety. In either case, what might be called "errors in randomization" may occur, that is, patients who are not truly eligible for randomization still receive treatment. An example of the first case is when a patient on reexamination clearly does not have the disease which was to be studied. The second case, where for instance a patient may be too old, not taking reliable birth control measures, etc., is further complicated by the time frame at which the error is discovered. If the violation is discovered during the treatment period, the decision to continue the patient on therapy is a medical one based on risk to the patient in continuing. This may then revert back to the problem of adequate versus inadequate treatment. If the patient has completed the full treatment period, a different decision may be made.

The third part of evaluability is described by the term "protocol violation." The simplest example of this is taking concomitant therapy specifically excluded in the protocol usually because it interferes with evaluation of the effect of the study treatment on the end point.

In general, if one finds approximately equal deletions in each of the treatment groups for the various reasons, the trial is as "random" as one considered in the intent-to-treat analysis. If unequal dropouts are found, this may be informative in terms of the conclusions to be drawn, and analyses with and without the questionable patients are probably appropriate.

The entire discussion above refers to questions of efficacy. All patients receiving any medication should, of course, be used in any analysis of safety data.

In summary, which analyses are selected depends on the hypothesis one wishes to test.

IV. INTENTION TO TREAT—WHAT IS THE QUESTION?

Karl E. Peace

I first began statistically analyzing data from clinical trials as a graduate student in biostatistics at the Medical College of Virginia in 1973 (–1976). Whether to include or exclude some patients from the analysis never arose, as clinical researchers presented their data on hand-written sheets to the statistical laboratory for analysis. Whether some patients were excluded from the sheets, in retrospect, is unknown. At any rate, all data presented were analyzed. Following completion of the Ph.D. in biostatistics in 1976, I entered the pharmaceutical industry as a senior statistician in 1977.

During the years 1977–1980, I analyzed many clinical trials of drugs being developed for a variety of uses: as antiinfectives or antibiotics, as anticancer agents, antiviral agents, antihypertensive agents, and cough-cold and CNS compounds. One of the most important exercises that had to be completed before proceeding with analysis, was to determine what patients should be included in efficacy analyses. This exercise was a joint one between the responsible clinical trial clinician and the statistician. Efficacy evaluatable criteria were developed and included in the study protocol. These criteria were applied in a proactive, ongoing, and blinded manner as the data came in house on case reporting forms. Only after completing the efficacy evaluatibility assessment was the blind broken and the trial statistically analyzed. The efficacy evaluatable analysis was the only analysis of efficacy data performed. This analysis almost always excluded some patients, whereas analysis of safety data excluded none.

Defining which patients were to be included in the efficacy evaluatable analysis seemed to me to be a most scientifically compelling exercise to do. The idea was that any patient who violated the conditions of the protocol sufficient to confound, cloud, or mask the efficacy of the drug being developed and evaluated should not be included in analysis of efficacy of the drug. It was not until 1980, following the Sackett and Gent publication in December 1979, that clients with whom I interacted began to question whether we should be performing efficacy analysis of all patients who entered the trial. Surely such interest has been the focus of much attention over the last nine to ten years. Analysis of all patients has evolved in the pharmaceutical industry to the point where most regulatory agencies specifically request the analysis, and it seems to have been named the intent-to-treat analysis.

Based upon a recent (December 30, 1988) literature search using MEDLINE (1966–1988), EMBASE (1974–1983), RINGDOC (1963–1982), University of Michigan Graduate and Medical Libraries, various medical and legal dictionaries, HISTLINE, MATHSCI (1959–1988), JOUR, IRCS, and the Parke-Davis biometrics department and library journals, it appears that Sherry (1980) was the first to use the phrase "intent-to-treat" for the analysis of all randomized patients. Schwartz and Lellouch (1967) previously referred to this type of analysis as reflecting a "pragmatic attitude" versus the efficacy evaluatable only analysis as reflecting an "explanatory attitude." However, Bjerkeland (1957) may have been the first to propose that the interpretation of clinical trials results should be based on all patients entering the trial. In addition, other publications prior to those of Sackett and Gent and Sherry that reflected the "pragmatic attitude" are those by Lovell et al. (1967), Ebert et al. (1969), the International Collaborative Group (1970), and Lovell (1977), whereas those by Harvald et al. (1962) and the Medical Research Council (1970) appear to reflect the "explanatory attitude."

I prefer to use the phrase "efficacy evaluatable only" analysis rather than "explanatory attitude" or "explanatory analysis" or "explanatory approach," as I believe that all analyses should be explanatory. After about ten years of dealing with whether one or both of the analyses "efficacy evaluatable only" or "intent-to-treat" should be performed, I recognize that in most situations, both should. As Lovell (1977) and Hearron (Section III) have pointed out, what analysis one embraces depends on the trial objective or question. In my opinion, the intent-to-treat analysis addresses the question of randomization group differences—not treatment or drug differences. The full benefits of the randomization itself not withstanding, it seems to me that proponents of the intent-to-treat analysis as the only or primary analysis are saying that patients who were randomized were intended to be successfully treated according to the treatment regimen delineated in the protocol and anything, such as premature withdrawal or failure, that censors therapeutic success from being observed is considered a failure of the treatment regimen. Such information is informative and may represent the clinician's goal. However, the intent-to-treat analysis does not address the most relevant question or objective of clinical trials on (new) drugs in clinical development prior to regulatory market approval. The question is, "Is the drug efficacious?" I consider such trials to be bioassays in humans of efficacy as a characteristic of the drug. Therefore, the efficacy evaluatable only analysis should be the primary analysis. Any patient who sufficiently violates the conditions of the protocol so as to make it unclear as to whether the drug or the violations caused (or did not cause) the effect should be excluded from analyses. The intent-to-treat analysis should be presented, but only as a check of possible bias inherent in the exclusion of patients from the evaluatable only analysis. I agree with Fisher et al. (Section I), although I say it a bit differently, that a goal of clinical research in the development of new drugs is to design protocols and conduct the clinical trials so that the evaluatable only analysis is also the intent-to-treat analysis.

REFERENCES

Amberson, J. B., Jr., McMahon, B. T., and Pinner, M. A clinical trial of sanocrysin in pulmonary tuberculosis. *Am. Rev. Tuberc. 24:* 401–435, 1931.

Armitage, P. Exclusions, losses to follow-up, and withdrawals in clinical trials. In *Clinical Trials* (eds. S. H. Shapiro and T. A. Louis). New York, Marcel Dekker, 1983.

Bjerkelund, C. J. The effect of long term treatment with dicoumarol in myocardial infarction: A controlled clinical study. *Acta Med. School Suppl.* 330, 1957.

Box, J. F. *R. A. Fisher, The Life of a Scientist.* New York, John Wiley and Sons, 1978.

Bull, J. P., The historical development of clinical therapeutic trials. *J. Chronic Dis. 10:* 218–248, 1959.

CASS Principal Investigators and their Associates. Coronary Artery Surgery Study (CASS): A randomized trial of coronary artery bypass surgery. Comparability of entry characteristics and survival in randomized patients and nonrandomized patients meeting randomization criteria. *J. Am. Coll. Cardiol. 3:* 114–128, 1984.

Cochrane, A. L. *Effectiveness and Efficiency.* London, Nuffield Provincial Hospitals Trust, 1972.

Coronary Drug Project: Influence of adherence to treatment and response of cholesterol on mortality in CDP. *N. Engl. J. Med. 303:* 1038–1041, 1980.

Detre, K., and Peduzzi, P. The problem of attributing deaths of nonadherers: The VA coronary bypass experience. *Controlled Clinical Trials 3:* 355–364, 1982.

Ebert, R. V., Borden, C. W., and Hipp, H. R. Long-term anti-coagulant therapy after myocardial infarction: Final report of the Veterans Administration Cooperative Study. *J. Am. Med. Assoc., 27:* 22–63, 1969.

Ederer, F. Why do we need controls? Why do we need to randomize? *Am. J. Opthalmol. 76:* 758–762, 1975.

Fisher, L., and Kanarek, P. Presenting censored survival data when censoring and survival times may not be independent. *Proceedings of the SIAM Conference on Biometry and Reliability*, Tallahasse, Florida, pp. 303–326, 1974.

Friedman, L. M., Furberg, C. D., and DeMets, D. L. *Fundamentals of Clinical Trials*. John Wright PSG, 1982.

Frommer, P. L., Fisher, L. D., Mock, M. B., et al. The Coronary Artery Surgery Study: A randomized trial in the context of a registry, in *Coronary Bypass Surgery, the Late Results* (K. E. Hammermeister, ed.). New York, Prager, 1983, pp. 83–97.

Frye, R. L., Fisher, L. D., Schaff, H. V., et al. Randomized trials in coronary artery bypass surgery. *Prog. Cardiovasc. Dis. 30:* 1–22, 1987.

Gail, M. H. Eligibility exclusions, losses to follow-up, removal of randomized patients and uncounted events in cancer clinical trials. *Cancer Treat. Rep. 69:* 1107–1113, 1985.

Gent, M., and Sackett, D. L. The qualification and disqualification of patients and events in long-term cardiovascular clinical trials. *Thrombos. Haemostas. 41:* 123–134, 1979.

Green, S. B. Patient heterogeneity and the need for randomized clinical trials. *Controlled Clin. Trials 3:* 189–198, 1982.

Harvald, B., Hilden, T., and Lung, E. Long-term anti-coagulant therapy after myocardial infarction. *Lancet, 2:* 626, 1962.

International Collaborative Group. Collaborative analysis of long-term anti-coagulant administration after acute myocardial infarction. *Lancet I:* 203, 1970.

Lovell, R. R. H., Denborough, M. A., Nestel, P. J., and Goble, A. J. A controlled trial of long-term treatment with anti-coagulant after myocardial infarction in 412 male patients. *Med. J. Aust., 2:* 97, 1967.

Lovell, R. R. H. Problems of interpretation in secondary prevention trials in coronary heart disease. *Med. J. Austr. 1:* 224–226, Feb. 12, 1977.

Medical Research Council. An assessment of long-term anti-coagulant administration after cardiac infarction. *BR. Med. J. I:*, 803, 1970.

Meier, P. Statistical analysis of clinical trials, in *Clinical Trials* (S. H. Shapiro and T. A. Louis, eds.). New York, Marcel Dekker, 1983.

Meinert, C. L. *Clinical Trials, Design, Conduct, and Analysis*. New York, Oxford University Press, 1986.

Peto, R., Pike, M. C., Armitage, P., et al. Design and analysis of randomized clinical trials requiring prolonged observation of each patient, I. Introduction and design. *Br. J. Cancer 34:* 585–612, 1976.

Sackett, D. L. On some prerequisites for a successful clinical trial. In *Clinical Trials* (S. H. Shapiro and T. A. Louis, eds.). New York: Marcel-Dekker, 1983.

Schwartz, D., Lellouch, J. Explanatory and pragmatic attitudes in therapeutic trials. *J. Chron. Dis. 20:* 637–648, 1967.

Sherry, S. The Anthrome Reinfarction Trial. *Circulation 62:* 73–78, 1980.

The Holy Bible, New International Version, Daniel 1: 12–16. Grand Rapids, MI, Zondervan Bible Publishers, 1978.

8
Dual Control Groups in Rodent Carcinogenicity Studies

Joseph K. Haseman *National Institute of Environmental Health Sciences, Research Triangle Park, North Carolina*

Gerald Hajian *Burroughs Wellcome Corporation, Research Triangle Park, North Carolina*

Kenneth S. Crump *Clement Associates, Inc., Ruston, Louisiana*

Murray R. Selwyn *Statistics Unlimited, Inc., Auburndale, Massachusetts*

Karl E. Peace* *Biopharmaceutical Research Consultants, Inc., Ann Arbor, Michigan*

I. INTRODUCTION

Joseph K. Haseman, Gerald Hajian, Kenneth S. Crump,
Murray R. Selwyn, Karl E. Peace

There are a number of important statistical issues associated with the design of laboratory animal carcinogenicity studies. One of the most important of these is the selection of a proper control group on which to base statistical comparisons. There is general agreement that concurrent rather than historical controls should be given primary emphasis in the overall evaluation (Gart, Chu, and Tarone, 1979; Haseman et al., 1984; Gart et al., 1986). However, it is not always clear how best to formulate

---

**Previous affiliation:* Warner-Lambert Company, Ann Arbor, Michigan.

and utilize the concurrent controls, as evidenced by an increased interest in using two (or more) such control groups (e.g., Society of Toxicology, 1982).

Whether or not to use multiple concurrent control groups in carcinogenicity testing is an important experimental design issue. One increasingly common practice is to use "dual controls," that is, to add a second concurrent control group to the study. Survival and tumor incidence in the two control groups are compared, and the results of these analyses determine how the control data are utilized for evaluating tumor incidences in the various dosed groups. Decisions regarding how to use dual control information (e.g., whether or not to pool the two control groups) are critical in the overall evaluation of the study.

In its laboratory animal carcinogenicity studies, the National Toxicology Program (NTP) frequently uses three dosed groups and a concurrent control with 50 animals per group. The total cost of such a study is between 1 and 2 million dollars, and modifying the experimental design to add a second concurrent control group of 50 animals for each sex–species group would increase this cost by approximately 10–20%. Thus, the decision of whether or not to use dual controls has important practical implications. However, financial considerations should not be paramount if dual controls are necessary for the study to be scientifically defensible.

II. EVALUATING THE ARGUMENTS THAT SUPPORT DUAL CONTROL GROUPS

Joseph K. Haseman, Gerald Hajian, Kenneth S. Crump, Murray R. Selwyn, Karl E. Peace

A number of arguments have been advanced to support dual controls, most involving the general concept of better assessing biological variability by providing additional information on spontaneous tumor incidence. For example, it has been suggested that use of dual control groups will increase the power of the experiment for detecting carcinogenic effects.

If the two control groups are simply pooled, thus increasing the control group sample size, then this will certainly increase the power of the study for detecting carcinogenicity. Moreover, since each dosed group is compared with the same control, it makes some sense to argue that the control tumor incidence is more important than the dosed group rates and should be known with greater accuracy (see, e.g., Dunnett (1955) or Finney (1964) for a discussion of this issue and a proposed allocation of animals in the context of continuous variables.]

However, it is not difficult to show that if power is the primary consideration, there are other ways to allocate additional animals that would increase the study's power beyond that associated with dual control groups (Hsu, 1987). Indeed, the most powerful design would be to eliminate the lower dosed group(s) altogether and allocate the animals to high-dose and control groups in approximately equal proportions. However, such a design is not used in practice because of the need to better characterize the dose-response curve. Moreover, the use of several dosed groups also provides a measure of protection against the possibility that the high dose will produce overt toxicity, causing animals to die before they are at risk for developing tumors, and thereby reducing study sensitivity for detecting carcinogenic effects.

Furthermore, historical control data are often available to provide additional information on spontaneous tumor incidences. Although there is currently no consensus regarding whether or not historical control data should be used in a formal testing framework, such information is certainly utilized informally in many studies to help interpret the biological significance of observed carcinogenic responses. The availability of historical control data reduces to some extent the need to double the concurrent control group sample size. Thus, while the use of additional animals may increase the power of the study, this should not be the primary justification for utilizing dual control groups.

A second, frequently, cited, argument to support the use of dual controls is that use of two control groups will reduce the false positive rate of laboratory animal carcinogenicity studies. Those who hold this view feel that the assay currently yields too many carcinogenic results, and that the use of dual controls will reduce the false positive rate (as well as study sensitivity). At first it seems contradictory that additional animals could actually reduce study sensitivity, but advocates of this argument generally do not intend to pool the two control groups. Rather, they would compare the dosed groups to each control group separately and regard an effect as meaningful only if it were significant relative to both groups.

This conservative approach is perhaps understandable, particularly if the primary study objective is to protect against false positive results. A typical carcinogenicity study involves four sex–species groups, several dose levels, and approximately 30 different organ sites. Under these conditions it would not be unusual to find a statistically significant difference in tumor incidence occurring by chance alone.

However, while concerns about multiple comparisons and overall false positive rates are important scientific issues in the design, analysis, and interpretation of laboratory animal carcinogenicity studies, these problems are well recognized and generally taken into account in the overall evaluation of carcinogenicity results. In addition to the statistical significance of an observed tumor increase, biological factors must also be considered. These include whether or not a dose-response relationship was observed, historical control tumor incidences, and whether or not supporting nonneoplastic effects were observed. Thus, for example, the International Agency for Research on Cancer (IARC) cites a number of studies that have demonstrated that "rules which attempt to model the actual decision process indicate that the false-positive rates are close to the nominal level" (Gart et al., 1986).

If an investigator is concerned that his study may have an unacceptably high false positive rate, he should consider use of one of several statistical procedures that have been proposed to deal with this particular problem (e.g., Fears et al., 1977; Gart et al., 1979; Brown and Fears, 1981; Haseman, 1983; Heyse and Rom, 1988; Farrar and Crump, 1988). Methods specifically designed to address the multiple comparisons issue seem preferable to ultraconservative data analyses with dual controls.

A third argument to support use of two control groups is that dual controls provide a measure of replication. A common criticism of laboratory animal carcinogenicity studies is that results are seldom replicated, due to the high cost involved in repeated testing. A replicate experiment would help determine whether an observed carcinogenic response is reproducible (and thus likely to be a "real" effect) or limited to a single study (and thus likely to be a false positive result).

However, merely replicating a control group within a study does little to alleviate the concerns of these critics, since this is not the type of replication they have in mind. If replication is the true objective, the whole study should be replicated, not merely the control group.

In summary, none of these particular arguments (increased power, reduction of the false positive rate, replication) is a strong reason to employ an experimental design that uses dual control groups.

The strongest argument in support of dual controls is the following: There may be unknown factors operating during the in-life, necropsy, or pathology evaluation phases of the study that could introduce group-to-group differences in tumor incidence (or other key variables) in excess of what would be expected by chance alone. Dual controls is one method of assessing the extent of these differences.

Some control animals develop tumors and others do not, due to normal biological variation. If animals are randomly assigned to two control groups, subsequent differences in tumor responses between these groups must be due either to binomial variability associated with the chance assignment of the animals or to the additional influence of some (perhaps unknown) factor in the experimental design. In the first instance, use of dual controls does not provide any information on the inherent biological variability of the animals beyond that obtained by combining the animals into a single control group.

The second case is somewhat more difficult. When a dosed group is compared with a control, it is possible that factors unrelated to chemical treatment are selectively influencing the responses in certain groups, resulting in an increased tumor incidence in a dosed group that does not reflect a true chemically related effect. Use of dual controls might possibly provide a means of estimating the extent of this unknown "extrabinomial" variability and its effect on the interpretation of study results. Gart et al. (1986) note that "while two control groups serve no useful purpose in a properly randomized experiment (other than to increase the number of control animals), this practice could act as a quality control mechanism in terms of identifying unsuspected biases in design."

There are studies in the literature that have suggested that certain environmental factors such as cage shelf level may be related to increased tumor incidence. However, such associations have generally been somewhat inconsistent (Lagakos and Mosteller, 1981) or quite subtle, requiring large sample sizes to attain statistical significance (Greenman et al., 1984). Young (1987) reported a single instance in which liver tumors in the NTP eugenol study (NTP, 1983) appeared to show "local room effects," but Haseman (1988), utilizing the broader database of all NTP studies, demonstrated that the frequency with which such differences occur is virtually identical to chance expectation. Similarly, Haseman et al. (1986) examined a large database of 18 studies with dual control groups housed at different locations in the animal room and found that the frequency of significant differences between the two controls agreed closely with chance expectation.

It is important to distinguish between inherent biological (binomial) variability and "excessive" (extrabinomial) variability that may be induced by unknown factors. A proper randomization of animals should reduce or eliminate the extrabinomial variability, but cannot eliminate the inherent binomial variability.

III. ISSUES RELATED TO THE USE OF DUAL CONTROL GROUPS

Joseph K. Haseman, Gerald Hajian, Kenneth S. Crump,
Murray R. Selwyn, Karl E. Peace

If an investigator has decided that dual controls are appropriate for his particular study, he is immediately faced with a number of important experimental design and data analysis questions. The first problem is how to form the two control groups. This basic experimental design issue is not as simple a matter as it might first appear. If dual controls are to be used in a meaningful way, there must be a sound basis for determining how the two distinct control groups should be formed.

Past studies that have utilized dual control groups have often taken the following approach: Animals are divided at random into two control groups. The first is housed at one location in the animal room, while the second is housed at a different location for the entire study period. Thus, differences between the two control groups could reflect any potential systematic effects associated with the animal room environment.

However, this is not the best way to design a carcinogenicity study. Because of concerns regarding systematic room effects, most investigators now employ some type of randomized (or stratified randomized) design. Some investigators (e.g., Freedman and Zeisel, 1988) go so far as to recommend a completely randomized housing protocol for the animals. Others regard this as somewhat impractical, because of difficulties in dosing, possible cross-contamination of cages, and other associated problems. In addition to randomly assigning animals to cages, current NTP toxicology and carcinogenicity studies also employ random assignment of columns of cages in a rack to dosed or control groups and periodic rotation of cage location (NTP, 1984).

The point is that if some type of randomization scheme is employed in the housing of the animals, then it may not always be clear how to divide the controls into two meaningful groups. Clearly, the two groups can not be merely formed at random. As noted by Gart et al. (1986), "With a completely randomized design, any difference between the two groups would be due solely to chance, so that, in effect, the two groups form one large control group."

That is, if two control groups are formed at random, then the number of significant differences between them will simply reflect chance expectation. Thus, there would be no valid scientific reason not to pool the two control groups for purposes of statistical evaluation. While comparing random dichotomizations of the control animals may provide some information on the overall false positive rate of the experiment, the false positive issue is well recognized, and, as indicated above, there are a number of statistical procedures that have been proposed to deal specifically with this problem.

Thus, there must be a scientifically meaningful way to form two control groups. How this is done will not always be obvious, particularly if the study is designed in such a manner as to minimize potential extraneous sources of variability that might be associated with potentially confounding factors.

A second problem is how dual control groups should be used in the data analysis. Most investigators would agree that if a comparison of the two control groups reveals no significant differences in tumor incidence, then they can be combined into a single control group and the subsequent data analysis becomes relatively straightforward.

What if significant differences are seen? If such differences are relatively minor, they may not preclude combining the two control groups. Because of the large number of tissue sites being evaluated, it is not unusual to find instances of significant differences between the two control groups occurring by chance alone. For example, in one series of 18 carcinogenicity studies that used dual controls, Haseman et al. (1986) concluded that, "even without extra-binomial variability, the overall false positive rate associated with a $p < 0.05$ pairwise comparison is quite high (47–50%)."

What if major differences in tumor incidence are observed between the two control groups? The proper course of action in this situation is unclear. Some would argue that if the target organ shows little or no evidence of differences in tumor incidence between controls, then combining the groups for that particular tumor type may be appropriate, since the unknown factors that produced variability in tumor incidence had no apparent effect on the target organ. Others would argue that in this situation the two control groups should not be combined for any tumors. In this case, the only alternatives would seem to be (1) comparing the dosed group to each control group separately (as indicated in Table 8.1, such an approach may be quite conservative and relatively insensitive for detecting carcinogenic effects) or (2) declaring the study to be inadequate for evaluating the presence or absence of a carcinogenic effect because of this problem.

Finally, there is the question of how one should interpret the results of a study with dual controls. This will generally become an issue only if the two control groups show strong evidence of variability in tumor incidence; otherwise the two groups can simply be combined and the usual evaluation carried out.

If separate comparisons are made with each control group, then it may be possible for a study to be considered positive if, despite the variability in control tumor incidence, the dosed group(s) show obvious carcinogenic effects. Similarly, certain studies may show no evidence of carcinogenic effects in dosed groups irrespective of the control variability. However, even in these situations (which should be evaluated on a case-by-case basis), the overall confidence one places in the study results will be reduced.

Perhaps the most difficult experimental outcome to interpret is one in which both (1) the dual control groups differ significantly in tumor incidence, thus requiring that the dosed groups be compared to each separate control, and (2) the carcinogenic response observed in the dosed animals is significant relative to one control group, but not relative to the other. Such situations should be evaluated on a case-by-case basis, since many additional factors could influence the final interpretation of the data in these experiments. In the absence of such information, the most prudent course of action in these cases may be either (1) to regard the study as providing only equivocal evidence of carcinogenicity or (2) to consider the study to be inadequate for a meaningful evaluation because of this problem.

TABLE 8.1 False positive rate and power associated with possible pairwise comparison procedures that utilize dual controls[a]

	Underlying tumor rates		Probability of $p < 0.05$ difference		
	Controls	Dosed	Single control group (50 vs. 50)	Combined control group (100 vs. 50)	Comparison with each separate control group (50 vs. 50; 50 vs. 50)
Significance level for nominal $p < 0.05$ test	0.05	0.05	0.011	0.027	0.002
	0.10	0.10	0.024	0.029	0.004
	0.20	0.20	0.029	0.033	0.005
	0.30	0.30	0.032	0.034	0.007
Power	0.05	0.20	0.663	0.810	0.526
	0.10	0.30	0.748	0.869	0.623
	0.20	0.50	0.917	0.972	0.861
	0.30	0.60	0.880	0.959	0.801

[a]Comparisons made by Fisher's exact test (similar results would hold for other procedures, such as a Cochran–Armitage trend test). In the first instance a single control group of size 50 is compared with a dosed group of 50 animals; in the second, two control groups of size 50 are pooled and compared with the dosed group; in the third, each control group is compared separately with the dosed group and it is required that both be significant ($p < 0.05$). For this exercise it is assumed that the underlying probability of tumor response is the same in the two control groups. Significance level and power are determined by complete enumeration.

IV. FACTORS THAT INFLUENCE THE NEED FOR DUAL CONTROL GROUPS

Joseph K. Haseman, Gerald Hajian, Kenneth S. Crump, Murray R. Selwyn, Karl E. Peace

Because of the potential difficulties associated with the use of dual controls, it is important that an investigator consider possible ways to reduce or eliminate the need for such a design. Since the primary scientific basis for dual control groups is to assess the magnitude of extrabinomial variability, it follows logically that attempts should be made to identify these sources of variation and if possible control for them by an appropriate experimental design.

To date, certain potential sources of variation that have been identified (e.g., location in the animal room) do not appear to have a major impact on tumor incidence; others, such as litter membership, have not been as well studied. If extrabinomial variability is suspected, the experiment should be designed to control for any potentially confounding factors that have been identified.

For example, dosed and control animals should be housed in the same room, and some type of randomization scheme should be employed to control potential systematic environmental differences that may be associated with the housing of the animals. Similarly, at necropsy the same prosector should prepare slides for dosed and control groups and a single pathologist should examine the slides in each group to ensure that slide preparation and diagnostic differences are minimal. The amount of tissue examined for each target organ should be comparable in all groups. Also, the order of histopathological examination should be random to control for time-related variability in diagnosis (pathologists frequently prefer evaluating the control group first to better assess the spontaneous rate of various neoplastic and nonneoplastic lesions).

Although blind pathology is traditionally a source of debate between pathologists and statisticians (e.g., Fears and Schneiderman, 1973; Weinberger, 1980; American College of Veterinary Pathologists, 1986; Freedman and Zeisel, 1988), it seems appropriate to employ this technique at least during the quality assurance and pathology review phases of the study to ensure objectivity of diagnoses. There is at least one instance that can be cited in which two different groups of pathologists, examining the same slides, reached remarkably different conclusions concerning the pathology diagnoses (Huff et al., 1985; Reuber, 1985). The one notable difference in approach that may have produced this striking variability was that one group employed blind pathology while the other did not.

It is important to reemphasize that the identification and control of potentially confounding factors reduce the need for dual controls by eliminating the basis by which two distinct control groups can be formed. That is, as indicated above, animals cannot be merely assigned at random to one of two control groups; there must be some meaningful biological basis for forming two distinct groups. However, if a meaningful dichotomization of the two groups can be formulated (e.g., by different locations in the animal room), then prior to the start of the study, the experimental design could be modified to minimize or eliminate this potential source of variability. That is, rather than using dual control groups to assess the impact of a particular source of variability, a better approach would be to modify the experimental design to eliminate this source of variability.

V. CONCLUSION

In the final analysis the decision regarding whether or not to utilize dual controls may depend on the investigator's ability to identify and deal with the major factors likely to produce extrabinomial variation among groups. While dual controls may be useful in some instances, in a properly randomized carcinogenicity study that controls for potential biases, dual controls should be unnecessary.

REFERENCES

American College of Veterinary Pathologists (1986). Letter to the Editor. *Toxicol. Appl. Pharmacol. 83:* 184–185.

Brown, C. C., and Fears, T. R. (1981). Exact significance levels for multiple binomial testing with application to carcinogenenicity screens. *Biometrics 37:* 763–774.

Dunnett, C. W. (1955). A multiple comparisons procedure for comparing several treatments with a control. *J. Am. Stat. Assoc. 50:* 1096–1121.

Farrar, D., and Crump, K. (1988). Exact statistical tests for any carcinogenic effect in animal bioassays. *Fundam. Appl. Toxicol. 11:* 652–663.

Fears, T. R., and Schneiderman, M. A. (1973). Pathologic evaluation and the blind technique (Letter to the Editor). *Science 183:* 1144.

Fears, T. R., Tarone, R. E., and Chu, K. C. (1977). False-positive and false-negative rates for carcinogenicity screens. *Cancer Res., 37:* 1941–1945.

Finney, D. J. (1964). *Statistical Method in Biological Assay*. New York, Hafner Publishing, 318–322.

Freedman, D. A., and Zeisel, H. (1988). From mouse to man; The quantitative assessment of cancer risk. *Stat. Sci. 3:* 3–56.

Gart, J. J., Chu, K. C., and Tarone, R. E. (1979). Statistical issues in interpretation of chronic bioassay tests for carcinogenicity. *J. Natl. Cancer Inst. 62:* 957–974.

Gart, J. J., Krewski, D., Lee, P. N., Tarone, R. E., and Wahrendorf, J. (1986). *Statistical Methods in Cancer Research*, Vol. 3. *The Design and Analysis of Long-Term Animal Experiments*. IARC Scientific Publication No. 79. New York, Oxford University Press, 34–35.

Greenman, D. L., Kodell, R. L., and Sheldon, W. B. (1984). Association between cage shelf level and spontaneous and induced neoplasms in mice. *J. Natl. Cancer Inst. 73:* 107–113.

Haseman, J. K. (1983). A reexamination of false-positive rates for carcinogenicity studies. *Fundam. Appl. Toxicol. 3:* 334–339.

Haseman, J. K., Huff, J., and Boorman, G. A. (1984). The use of historical control data in carcinogenicity studies in rodents. *Toxicol. Pathol. 12:* 126–135.

Haseman, J. K., Winbush, J. S., and O'Donnell, M. W., Jr. (1986). Use of dual control groups to estimate false positive rates in laboratory animal carcinogenicity studies. *Fundam. Appl. Toxicol. 7:* 573–584.

Haseman, J. K. (1988). Lack of cage effects on liver tumor incidence in B6C3F1 mice. *Fundam. Appl. Toxicol. 10:* 179–187.

Heyse, J. F., and Rom, D. (1988). Adjusting for multiplicity of statistical tests in the analysis of carcinogenicity studies. *Biom. J. 8:* 883–896.

Hsu, J. P. (1987). Allocation of animals in a long-term carcinogenicity study. Paper presented at the 147th Annual Meeting of the American Statistical Association, San Francisco, August 17, 1987.

Huff, J. E., Bates, R., Eustis, S. L., Haseman, J. K., and McConnell, E. E. (1985). Malathion and malaoxon: Histopathological reexamination of the National Cancer Institute's carcinogenesis studies. *Environ. Res. 37:* 154–173.

Lagakos, S., and Mosteller, F. (1981). A case study of statistics in the regulatory process: The FD & C Red 40 experiments. *J. Natl. Cancer Inst. 66:* 197–212.

National Toxicology Program (1983). Carcinogenesis Studies of Eugenol in F344/N Rats and B6C3F1 Mice (Feed Studies). NTP Technical Report 223, U.S. Department of Health and Human Services, National Toxicology Program, Research Triangle Park, NC.

National Toxicology Program (1984). General Statement of Work for the Conduct of Acute, Fourteen-Day Repeated Dose, 90-Day Subchronic, and 2-Year Chronic Studies in Laboratory Animals. National Toxicology Program, Research Triangle Park, NC.

Reuber, M. B. (1985). Carcinogenicity and toxicity of malathion and malaoxon. *Environ. Res. 37:* 119–153.

Society of Toxicology (1982). Animal data in hazard evaluation: Paths and pitfalls. *Fundam. Appl. Toxicol. 2:* 101–107.

Weinberger, M. A. (1980). How valuable is blind pathology in histopathologic examinations in conjunction with animal toxicity studies? *Toxicol. Pathol. 7:* 14–17.

Young, S. S. (1987). Are there room effects on hepatic tumors in male mice? An examination of the NTP eugenol study. *Fundam. Appl. Toxicol. 8:* 1–4.

Index